PROGRESS IN UNDERSTANDING CYSTIC FIBROSIS

Edited by **Dinesh Sriramulu**

Progress in Understanding Cystic Fibrosis
http://dx.doi.org/10.5772/63263
Edited by Dinesh Sriramulu

Contributors

Jorge Leitão, Joana Feliciano, Sílvia Sousa, Tiago Pita, Soraia Guerreiro, Theerthankar Das, Jim Manos, John Widger, Bernadette Prentice, Shihab Hameed, Keith C. Y. Ooi, Charles F. Verge, Teiji Sawa, Yoshifumi Naito, Kiyoshi Moriyama, Ibrahim Janahi, Abdul Rehman, Scott O'Grady, Milena Rikalovic, Nataša Avramović, Ivanka Karadzic

Published by InTech
Janeza Trdine 9, 51000 Rijeka, Croatia

Publishing Process Manager Romina Skomersic
Technical Editor SPi Global
Cover InTech Design team

First published July, 2017
Printed in Croatia
Legal deposit, Croatia: National and University Library in Zagreb

Additional hard copies can be obtained from orders@intechopen.com

Progress in Understanding Cystic Fibrosis, Edited by Dinesh Sriramulu
p. cm.
Print ISBN 978-953-51-3291-2
Online ISBN 978-953-51-3292-9

For EU product safety concerns:
IN TECH d.o.o., Prolaz Marije Krucifikse Kozulić 3, 51000 Rijeka, Croatia,
info@intechopen.com or visit our website at intechopen.com.

Meet the editor

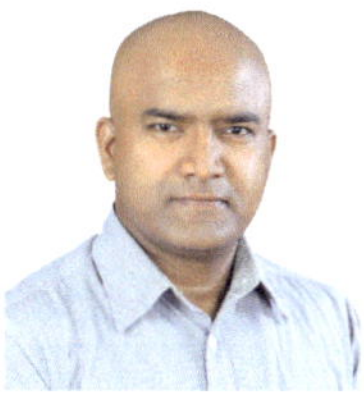

Dinesh Sriramulu graduated from the Technical University of Braunschweig, Germany, with his doctorate degree in Medical Microbiology. He started his research career at the Helmholtz Centre for Infection Research, Braunschweig, Germany, in collaboration with the Karolinska Institutet, Stockholm, Sweden. His area of expertise is on the adaptation of bacteria toward diverse niches, ranging from the human lung to the cattle rumen. He also worked on tumor microenvironment in the case of esophageal and breast cancers. He continued his research work at various reputed institutions worldwide: University College Cork, Ireland; University of Medicine and Dentistry of New Jersey, USA; Food and Drug Administration, Rockville, USA; University of Southern California, Los Angeles, USA; University of Trento, Italy; and University of Cape Town, South Africa. He has published his research findings in various international peer-reviewed journals and presented his works at international conferences. He has been serving as an editorial board member, a peer reviewer, and an expert referee for scientific journals and research funding agencies.

Contents

Preface

The Open Access Initiative has been making its stride toward liberal dissemination of scientific knowledge to the world community through unrestricted access to full-text articles, chapters, and other contents. Since the inception of virtual media science publishing has been adopting a constant fast-track update of information as and when it occurs. In this line, InTech has been making its footprint all along by identifying and openly involving eminent scientists worldwide. The book, *Progress in Understanding Cystic Fibrosis,* is the successor of *Cystic Fibrosis – Renewed Hopes Through Research.*

Cystic fibrosis (CF), also known as mucoviscidosis, is an autosomal recessive multisystem genetic disorder that occurs predominantly among Caucasians. Though found highest among Irish population, the incidence of CF is on the rise among other populations including the least-affected ones. The interdisciplinary approach toward better understanding the CF condition and the development of sensitive early diagnostic methods have contributed toward efficient diagnosis, treatment, and management of the disease. The CF condition is characterized by abnormal transport of chloride and sodium across the epithelium that leads to thickening of secretions especially in the lungs, pancreas, liver, and intestine. The complex nature of this disease involving multiple organs and subsequent secondary infections by microbes is the basis for mortality in CF population. Decades of research by scientists worldwide has narrowed down the cause of CF to a single target gene. But the complexity of the disease is the most challenging impediment to finding a single-shot cure. This book is a simple collection of chapters on CF-related cellular biochemistry, diabetes, microbiome, and immunotherapy that highlight the progress in CF research. From the information contained in the chapters of this book, it is obvious that only with the help of interdisciplinary research, better understanding and management of the CF disease condition would be possible and this approach has certainly increased the level of life expectancy among CF patients. In addition, a cohort- or patient-specific treatment strategy supported by intense bench-to-bedside research flow seems to be a feasible option to reduce morbidity and mortality in CF population.

I thank InTech for appointing me as the editor of this book and for providing me the opportunity to contribute to the scientific community. I thank the authors of the chapters for their valuable contributions. I thank Helmholtz Centre for Infection Research, Braunschweig, Germany, which served as the knowledge center for me to gain expertise in this field.

Dinesh Sriramulu
Division of Cell and Immune Biology
Helmholtz Centre for Infection Research
Braunschweig, Germany

Chapter 1

CFTR Involvement in Cell Migration and Epithelial Restitution

Scott M. O'Grady

Additional information is available at the end of the chapter

http://dx.doi.org/10.5772/66309

Abstract

Over the past decade, research has shown that *c*ystic *f*ibrosis *t*ransmembrane conductance *r*egulator (CFTR) plays an important role in epithelial cell migration and wound healing. Experiments with airway epithelium, ovarian epithelial cells, placental epithelium and epidermal keratinocytes demonstrated that CFTR function is necessary to achieve maximum migration rates during restitution and in certain cancer cells, CFTR activity contributes to tumor cell invasion. Multiple mechanisms appear to underlie the motility-promoting actions of CFTR, and although many details remain to be established, our present understanding indicates that processes such as electrotaxis (galvanotaxis), integrin-mediated cell adhesion and lamellipodia protrusion are dependent on normal CFTR function. In this chapter, the role of CFTR in epithelial cell migration and its implications in cystic fibrosis (CF) will be reviewed with emphasis on the underlying mechanisms that may explain observations made in various epithelial tissues, particularly in airways. Ultimately, a better understanding of CFTR involvement in epithelial repair may lead to new therapeutic approaches to improve barrier function and reduce airway infection and inflammation associated with CF.

Keywords: cystic fibrosis, CFTR, wound healing, collective migration, barrier function, inflammation

1. Introduction

1.1. Ion channels and cell motility

The role of ion channels and membrane transporters in cell migration has been the subject of several recent reviews [1–4], so only a few examples will be highlighted in this section to provide the reader with an appreciation of their importance in cell motility. Ion channels and other membrane transport pathways participate in multiple housekeeping functions within cells that include regulation of membrane potential, intracellular [Ca^{2+}], cytoskeletal assembly, integrin-mediated signaling, cell volume regulation, as well as the maintenance of intracellular and extracellular pH. Each of these housekeeping functions can influence cell migration. For instance, changes in ion channel activity produces changes in membrane potential that can facilitate uptake of Ca^{2+} from the extracellular media. A recent example involves the slow calcium wave that develops approximately 1 h after wounding of corneal endothelial cells [5]. The rise in intracellular [Ca^{2+}] is associated with plasma membrane depolarization of cells along the margin of the wound and serves to increase the rate of cell migration. This depolarization has been attributed to increased expression and activity of epithelial Na^+ channels (ENaC) within cells that boarder the wound, resulting in elevated intracellular [Na^+]. The combined effect of depolarization and increased Na^+ load drives Na^+/Ca^{2+} exchange (NCX) activity in reverse mode to produce Ca^{2+} uptake, which propagates from the border of the wound into the epithelium. There may also be an additional role for transient receptor potential (TRP) channels in this process since inhibition of NCX activity does not completely block Ca^{2+} uptake, whereas inhibition of both NCX and TRP activity abolishes the increase in intracellular [Ca^{2+}].

Membrane hyperpolarization can also stimulate Ca^{2+} uptake and enhance the rate of cell migration. Differentiated intestinal epithelial cells with increased expression of voltage-gated K^+ channels (Kv1.1/Kv1.5) exhibit membrane hyperpolarization and increased intracellular [Ca^{2+}] as a result of a greater driving force for electrogenic Ca^{2+} uptake across the plasma membrane [6]. The elevation in intracellular [Ca^{2+}] was shown to augment formation of myosin II containing stress fibers necessary for efficient cell migration. Similarly, ionotropic $P2X_7$ receptors have also been shown to contribute to changes in intracellular [Ca^{2+}] and cell migration. During injury of corneal epithelial cells, $P2X_7$ receptors redistribute to the leading edge of cells that border the wound [7]. Adenosine triphosphate (ATP) is released from the damaged cells leading to activation of these receptors and subsequent uptake of Ca^{2+} from the extracellular solution. The increase in intracellular [Ca^{2+}] induces actin cytoskeletal rearrangements that facilitate the formation of branched dendritic networks of actin within lamellipodia, promoting the dynamic regulation of focal adhesions within cells at the wound margin.

ATP release and $P2X_7$ receptor activation have also been shown to be initiated in response to ligand-activated $\alpha_V\beta_3$ integrin and syndecan-4 engagement leading to increased formation of focal adhesions and an enhanced rate of migration in astrocytes [8]. The mechanism of ATP release involved activation of PI3K, PLCγ and IP_3 receptors following integrin activation. This resulted in opening of Cx43/Panx-1 hemichannels in the plasma membrane, facilitating ATP release, transactivation of $P2X_7$ receptors and ultimately, an increase in intracellular [Ca^{2+}]. Furthermore, enhanced expression of both $\alpha_6\beta_4$ integrin and TRPV1 receptors at the leading edge of keratinocytes after wounding has also been linked to increases in intracellular [Ca^{2+}]. Evidence appears to support a model where TRPV1-mediated increases in intracellular [Ca^{2+}] trigger the activation of transcription factors such as nuclear factor of activated T cells (NFAT) and cAMP response element binding protein (CREB) to stimulate expression of β_4 integrins in cells at the margin of the wound leading to an increase in directional migration [9]. Direct coupling between the β_1 integrin and $K_{Ca}3.1$ channel expression has been demonstrated in alveolar type II cells grown on a fibronectin matrix and inhibition of channel activity was shown to decrease the rate of migration [10]. This inhibitory effect may be due in part to reducing Ca^{2+} uptake through TRPC4 channels which were also shown to participate in migration during wound repair. TRP channel-associated Ca^{2+} uptake has also been shown to be stimulated by mechanical stretch of the plasma membrane associated with tension and cell shape changes occurring during migration. A specific example involves activation of TRPM7 which mediates transient and highly localized increases in intracellular [Ca^{2+}] known as Ca^{2+} flickers that take place within lamellipodia in response to mechanical forces linked to contraction [11]. This initial Ca^{2+} response is amplified by localized Ca^{2+}-induced Ca^{2+} release from internal stores leading to transactivation of protein kinase A (PKA) through stimulation of Ca^{2+}-sensitive adenylyl cyclases. PKA is known to have multiple cell migration-associated targets including components of the cytoskeleton and the focal adhesion proteome that can have both positive and negative effects on migration depending on intracellular localization.

An interesting example of enhanced cell migration linked to K^+ channel regulation has been reported in glioblastoma cells [12]. In astrocytes and oligodendrocytes from normal brain tissue, the $\alpha_9\beta_1$ integrin is not expressed; however, expression has been shown to increase with glioma grade and appears to be critical for sustaining increased migration rates following exposure to urokinase receptor (uPAR), agonists. A unique feature of the α_9 subunit is that its cytoplasmic domain specifically interacts with spermidine/spermine-N-acetyl transferase (SSAT), which catalyzes the breakdown of higher-order polyamines (spermidine and spermine) to putrescine. Spermidine and spermine are known to regulate the rectification properties of Kir channels by binding to negatively charged residues within the channel pore, significantly reducing K^+ efflux from the cell. In contrast, putrescine is a much less effective blocker of outward K^+ current in Kir channels. In glioma cells, the α_9 subunit colocalizes with Kir4.2 and silencing of the channel inhibits uPAR-enhanced cell migration. A proposed mechanism to explain the increase in migration rate involves activation of SSAT in response to uPAR-dependent $\alpha_9\beta_1$ integrin activation, which produces a localized decrease in the [spermidine/spermine] ratio ultimately leading to reduced rectification, increased K^+ efflux and membrane hyperpolarization.

1.2. Airway inflammation and epithelial damage

Loss of CFTR function in the airways of CF patients leads to reduced anion secretion, enhanced Na^+ absorption and a decrease in the depth of airway surface liquid that ultimately impairs mucociliary clearance and the removal of pathogens from the lungs [13–15]. Reduced pathogen clearance facilitates infection that induces neutrophilic inflammation, leading to progressive epithelial damage within the conducting airways [16–19]. Over time, a recurrent cycle of intense inflammation, epithelial injury and airway remodeling produce irrevocable damage that dramatically compromises lung function [20–22]. Mounting evidence from in vitro studies and animal models of CF indicate that CFTR malfunction appears to alter the innate immune response of the airways leading to increased release of proinflammatory mediators evoking an amplified, yet less effective inflammatory reaction that is unable to eliminate airway pathogens [17, 18]. In some cases, elevated cytokine levels, neutrophil infiltration and neutrophil elastase (NE) concentrations within the bronchial alveolar lavage (BAL) fluid have been reported in infants without signs of infection, although other studies support the concept that infection is necessary to initiate inflammation [17, 23–25]. Neutrophils represent the major inflammatory leukocyte recruited into CF airways where they release a variety of mediators including oxidants and proteases such as neutrophil elastase (NE), which possess bacteriocidal properties [26, 27]. Moreover, NE catalytic activity is also known to damage the epithelium and reduce structural integrity of the airways leading to bronchiectasis and deteriorating lung function [28–31]. Furthermore, the airways of CF patients encounter various reactive oxygen species (ROS) derived from bacterial pathogens or from the environment [32]. ROS production can exceed the endogenous oxidative defense capacity of the airways leading to oxidative stress and additional injury. In adults, the concentration of reduced glutathione (GSH), a major ROS scavenger present in the airway surface liquid, is significantly reduced in CF patients [33, 34]. This condition may be directly related to the loss of CFTR function since the channel is known to transport GSH in addition to anions in normal airways [35].

Decreases in CFTR channel activity also result in acidification of airway surface liquid coupled to an increase in intracellular pH, which reduces antimicrobial function of the airway surface liquid, promoting bacterial infection [36–41]. Intracellular alkalinization also appears to enhance the accumulation of ceramide, a metabolite of sphingomyelin, within lysosomes [42–44]. Ceramide is thought to amplify the inflammatory response by triggering tumor necrosis factor (TNF)α signaling pathways involving mitogen-activated protein kinases (MAPK), IκB-kinase degradation [an inhibitory regulator of necrosis factor (NF)-κB] and NF-kB nuclear localization [45–47]. Additionally, for class II CFTR mutations, the accumulation of misfolded CFTR protein within the endoplasmic reticulum (ER) induces stress and stimulates what is known as an unfolded protein response, which involves activation of signaling pathways that mitigate ER stress [48–51]. For the most common class II mutation, retention of misfolded ΔF508 CFTR within the ER causes an unfolded protein response that stimulates inflammation by activating NF-κB and inducing cytokine secretion that can result in apoptosis.

1.3. Evidence for defective epithelial regeneration in CF

In an earlier investigation, a humanized airway xenograph model was created by inoculation of CF and non-CF airway epithelial cells onto epithelium-deleted rat trachea that was then subcutaneously implanted into nude mice over a period from 4 to 35 days [52]. This model was then used to investigate the process of reepithelialization following injury and to determine if remodeling of CF epithelium is a consequence of defective epithelial regeneration independent of infection. The results showed that CF epithelial cells exhibited enhanced proliferation along with continuous expression of IL-8, matrix metalloproteinases (MMP7, MMP9) and tissue inhibitor of metalloproteinase (TIMP)-1. Moreover, regeneration was delayed and final restitution resulted in a remodeled epithelium that appeared to be a product of aberrant regeneration unrelated to bacterial contamination. A relationship between abnormal regeneration and loss of CFTR function was not identified in this study, although it was concluded that it might be a consequence of altered MMP/TIMP/IL-8 expression observed in CF epithelium. In a subsequent study, wound healing experiments using immortalized normal (NuLi-1 cells) and CF (CuFi-1 cells) human airway epithelial cells revealed that CuFi-1 cell migration was significantly delayed relative to NuLi-1 cells [53, 54]. This difference in migration activity was attributed to defective epidermal growth factor (EGF)/epidermal growth factor receptors (EGFR) signaling and reduced K^+ channel expression. Interestingly, no significant effect on migration was reported in the presence of the CFTR inhibitor, $CFTR_{inh}$-172 [53]. In subsequent investigations described below, loss of CFTR function was shown to directly contribute to delayed epithelial repair in CF airways and that expression of normal CFTR augments epithelial restitution.

2. Anion channels, cell migration and epithelial restitution

2.1. Volume-sensitive anion channels in cell migration and invasion

Earlier electrophysiological studies of human glioma cells showed that they express voltage-sensitive Cl^- channels that were blocked by chlorotoxin (Ctx), a peptide isolated from scorpion venom as well as tamoxifen, an estrogen receptor modulator [55–57]. Furthermore, hypotonic solutions were also shown to activate tamoxifen and 5-nitro-2-(3-phenylpropylamino)-benzoate (NPPB)-sensitive, outwardly rectifying Cl^- currents carried by channels that were shown to contribute to the resting Cl^- conductance under isotonic conditions [55]. Treatment with either Ctx or NPPB inhibited glioma cell migration and invasiveness in transwell migration assays. Similarly, osmotically activated cell swelling and regulatory volume decrease (RVD) were also blocked by Ctx and tamoxifin indicating a role in the regulation of cell volume that contributes to migration and tumor cell invasion [56]. Simultaneous time lapse imaging and patch clamp recording of glioma cells demonstrated detectable changes in cell shape and movement that was associated with activation of volume-sensitive Cl^- currents. Changes in cell shape and motility were attributed to Cl^- efflux coupled to K^+ and water movement across the plasma membrane resulting in cell shrinkage, which appeared to be localized at the leading edge of the cell. Consequently, cell flattening at the leading edge was proposed to facilitate protrusion through restricted extracellular spaces required for tumor cell invasion [58].

Experiments with murine primary microglial cells or a microglial (BV-2) cell line demonstrated that exposure to hypotonic saline or an elevated extracellular [K^+] produced localized swelling and protrusion of lamellipodia at the leading edge of these cells [59]. Blockade of volume-activated Cl^- channels or inhibition of K-Cl co-transporters (KCC) effectively inhibited lamellipodia formation. The migratory response induced by localized increases in extracellular [K^+] may likely result from cell death caused by injury. Ischemia for example, has been shown to increase extracellular [K^+] by more than 20 fold [60]. Such increases in [K^+] would provide a favorable driving force for KCl uptake by KCC leading to cell swelling and produce membrane depolarization. This would establish conditions for electrogenic Cl^- influx through volume-activated anion channels which also contributes to localized swelling. Furthermore, signaling proteins such as the chemokine ligand CCL21 is released by damaged neurons and is known to induce a chemotaxis response in microglia which is inhibited by Cl^- channel blockers [61]. This response was not dependent on activation of the canonical CCL21 receptor CCR7, but instead was shown to stimulate CXCR3 receptors. Short-duration exposure (30 s) to CCL21 or the selective CXCR3 ligand CXCL10 in either brain slice preparations or microglial cells in culture produced a sustained increase in Cl^- channel activation that appears to represent an initial trigger for stimulating directed cell migration in response to neuronal injury.

2.2. CFTR and epithelial wound repair

The first direct evidence of a role for CFTR in cell migration was obtained from studies of airway epithelial cells [62]. Experiments using Calu-3 cells, a human airway adenocarcinoma cell line and normal human bronchial epithelial cells revealed that inhibition of CFTR channel activity with the selective CFTR blocker, $CFTR_{inh}$-172 or silencing CFTR expression by RNAi significantly slowed cell migration and epithelial restitution (see **Figure 1**). Moreover, CFTR channel inhibition or silencing also reduced the extent of lamellipodia protrusion during migration. These results demonstrated that the ion transport activity of CFTR was necessary for airway epithelial cells to achieve a maximum rate of migration during wound closure and that lamellipodia protrusion was at least one aspect of the migration process that was affected by the loss of CFTR function. Following publication of this initial investigation, Sun et al. (2011) showed that epithelial wound repair in a tracheal preparation from rhesus monkeys was delayed following treatment with $CFTR_{inh}$-172 [63]. Experiments employing the use of a noninvasive vibrating probe demonstrated that inhibition of CFTR activity inhibited the spontaneous outward current induced by wounding and that treatment with aminophylline, a phosphodiesterase inhibitor and CFTR activator, stimulated this outward current. These results suggested that CFTR activity contributes to the wound current that serves as a guidance cue for directed migration and that inhibition of CFTR activity disrupts the process of electrotaxis, thus delaying wound closure. Further support for the importance of CFTR in airway cell migration and epithelial restitution was provided by a set of rescue experiments involving (i) expression of wild-type CFTR into CF airway epithelial cell lines to restore the normal rate of wound closure and (ii) treatment with VRT-325, a CFTR corrector molecule that facilitates apical membrane localization of CFTR with the ΔF508 mutation in CFBE-ΔF508 cells and in primary bronchial epithelial cells obtained from CF patients [64].

Involvement of CFTR in cell migration has also been observed in other epithelial cell types besides airways. For example, in human trophoblast (BeWo) cells, CFTR activation with forskolin increased cell migration into the wound and subsequent addition of $CFTR_{inh}$-172 significantly inhibited the response to forskolin [65]. Poor trophoblast migration/invasiveness and associated spiral artery remodeling represent early recognizable pathologies that underlie preeclampsia and previous studies demonstrated that CFTR expression is reduced in preeclamptic placentas [66]. Thus, changes in CFTR function not only appear to have consequences on placental ion and fluid transport but may also contribute to altered trophoblast invasion in preeclampsia. Another example based on experiments with human ovarian carcinoma cells showed that CFTR silencing by RNAi significantly reduced cell migration and invasion under in vitro conditions and that the tumorigenic potential of these cells in vivo was suppressed compared to controls [67]. This result was consistent with the observation that CFTR expression in ovarian cancer was higher relative to normal ovarian epithelial cells or benign ovarian tumors and that enhanced CFTR expression was associated with advanced International Federation of Gynecology and Obstetrics (FIGO) staging and poor histopathology grade. Lastly, CFTR was also shown to play a role in cutaneous wound healing, where ΔF508*cftr*$^{-/-}$ mice that lack plasma membrane localization and normal CFTR channel function exhibited delayed wound closure compared to wild-type mice [68].

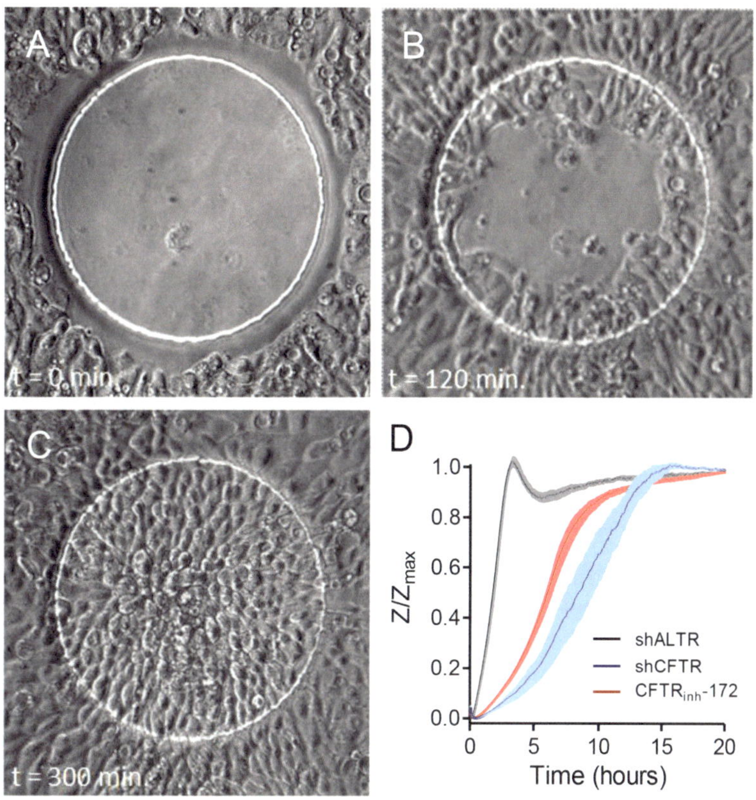

Figure 1. Inhibition of CFTR channel activity or silencing expression by RNAi delay airway epithelial restitution. (**A**)–(**C**) Impedance-sensing arrays were used to track the process of Calu-3 cell migration over the surface of a 250 μm diameter electrode following wounding by electroporation. Images show the extent of Calu-3 cell confluence at three time points (0, 120 and 300 min). (**D**) Normalized impedance (Z/Z_{max}) measurements as a function of time for Calu-3 cells expressing shRNAs designed to selectively target CFTR (shCFTR cells) or have an altered sequence that no longer recognizes CFTR mRNA (shALTR cells). Note that as cells reach confluence on the electrode surface, the normalized impedance value approaches 1, which indicates complete epithelial restitution. For these experiments, shALTR cells were used as controls where the black line represents the mean Z/Z_{max} values and the shaded grey area corresponds to the SEM ($n = 8$). The blue line (mean) and light-blue-shaded area (SEM) shows the effects of silencing CFTR on wound closure, where the slope provides a measure of the average rate of cell migration into the wound ($n = 8$). Finally, the red line (mean) and pink-shaded area (SEM) are the results from shALTR cells treated with 20 μM $CFTR_{inh}$-172, a selective inhibitor of CFTR channel activity, throughout the process of restitution ($n = 8$). Images were adapted from Ref. [114].

Exceptions to the migration-promoting actions of CFTR can be found in studies of non-small cell lung cancer (NSCLC) cells and human keratinocytes [69]. Experiments with NSCLC cells showed reduced CFTR expression which correlated with an advanced stage of the cancer, lymph node metastasis and enhanced malignant behavior which manifested as an increase in epithelial-mesenchymal transition, invasion and migration. In contrast, overexpression of CFTR reduced cancer progression and metastasis, supporting the observation that in some types of cancer, CFTR appears to function as a tumor suppressor. Similarly, CFTR silencing by RNAi in human keratinocytes was shown to promote cell migration and inhibit differentiation, whereas overexpression inhibited migration and stimulated differentiation [68]. The effects of manipulating CFTR expression on migration appeared to be related to its role in the formation of epithelial junctions since silencing the channel downregulated adhesion molecule (E-cadherin, ZO-1 and β-catenin) expression and intercellular junction formation while overexpression promoted junction formation.

2.3. ANO1, cell migration and cystic fibrosis

TMEM16A/ANO1 is one of the 10 known members of the anoctamin family (TMEM16A-K) of proteins, some of which function as anion channels. Certain members of this family, such as ANO1, ANO2 and ANO6, can be activated by increases in intracellular [Ca^{2+}] and are classified as Ca^{2+}-activated chloride channels (CaCCs) [70–72]. CaCCs exhibit voltage dependence, outward rectification and are perhaps best known for their role in Ca^{2+}-dependent Cl^- secretion in various epithelial tissues. Compounds including T16Ainh-A01, CaCCinh-A01 and NS3728 block channel activity to varying degrees depending on cell type [73]. Prior to the discovery of its anion channel activity, ANO1 was regarded as either a tumor cell marker or as an oncogene in human cancers with poor prognosis [74, 75].

In prostate cancer (LNCaP and PC-3) cells, ANO1 is highly expressed and these cells exhibit large CaCC currents in response to increases in cytosolic [Ca^+] [76]. Silencing ANO1 by RNAi in PC-3 cells significantly inhibited cell proliferation and migration/invasion. Studies using Ehrlich Lettre ascites (ELA) cells revealed that they express both ANO1 and ANO6 [71]. Interestingly, silencing ANO1 expression was shown to alter directionality of ELA migration while knockdown of ANO6 was shown to cause a ~40% decrease in the overall rate of migration. Although the mechanism responsible for ANO1-dependent control of directionality is not understood, it is likely that some contribution to outward current associated with wounding may be important in electrotaxis. Various pancreatic ductal adenocarcinoma cells have also been shown to have increased expression of ANO1 and enhanced CaCC activity. Knockdown of ANO1 or inhibition by CaCC blockers including CaCCinh-A01, and NS3728 delay migration in BxPC-2 cells, however, T16Ainh-A01 exhibited no effect [77]. The authors speculated that activation of ANO1 was important for cell volume changes necessary to control cell shape and that the channel may serve as a potential target for reducing the metastatic potential of pancreatic tumor cells.

Investigations of bronchial epithelial cell repair in cystic fibrosis (CF) demonstrated that the expression of ANO1 and CaCC channel activity were significantly reduced in CF cells compared to bronchial epithelial cells from normal subjects [78]. Consequently, epithelial restitution in wound healing assays was delayed in CF cells relative to non-CF cells. Moreover silencing ANO1 expression in non-CF cells reduced the rate of migration, whereas overexpression of ANO1 in CF cells partially restored cell motility, although complete recovery was not achieved. To establish whether ANO1 channel function was necessary for supporting cell migration, primary non-CF cells were treated with T16Ainh-A01 which produced a significant delay in wound closure. These findings indicate that reduced rates of cell migration in bronchial epithelial cells from CF patients may be attributed to an overall decrease in apical membrane Cl^- conductance resulting from loss of both CFTR and ANO1 anion channel activity.

3. Mechanisms of CFTR-dependent cell migration and epithelial repair

Although the molecular mechanisms underlying the contribution of CFTR to the processes of cell migration and epithelial restitution remain to be fully characterized, the data collected so far have identified three important aspects of migration that merit further investigation. These include the process of lamelliopdia protrusion, electrotaxis and the dynamics of integrin-mediated adhesion, each of which are discussed in more detail below.

3.1. Lamellipodia protrusion

Lamellipodia are actin-containing, sheet-like structures that protrude from the leading edge of migrating cells [79]. They are capable of sensing environmental cues and are necessary for sustained directional migration. A key force contributing to the protrusion of lamellipodia is provided by the extension of actin filaments at the leading edge of the cell. Within lamellipodia, actin forms networks of branched filaments with highest density near the membrane at the leading edge, where the barbed (positive) ends of the filaments are directed toward the plasma membrane to form brush-like assemblies [80, 81]. Elongation occurs primarily at junctions formed by a multiprotein structure known as the Arp2/3 complex, which functions as a nucleation site for new actin monomers to attach to the sides of existing actin polymers to create a branched arrangement of fibers [82]. As these monomers add to the growing meshwork at the barbed end, cleavage and dissociation of monomers takes place at the pointed (minus) end of filaments located in the more proximal regions of the lamellipodium. ATPase activity associated with actin filaments facilitates accumulation of ADP-actin at the pointed ends as filament disassembly takes place. This dynamic process of simultaneous actin monomer addition to the barbed end and dissociation at the pointed end of the filament is known as treadmilling and is controlled by several actin-regulatory proteins [82, 83] as well as intracellular pH [84, 85]. Previous studies have shown that during polarization along the axis of movement, a redistribution of the Na^+-H^+ exchanger (NHE1) occurs, which localizes toward the leading edge of the cell. Redistribution of NHE1 results in the development of a steady-state pH gradient extending from the front of the cell, which becomes more alkaline, to the rear, developing a more acidic pH relative to the leading edge [86–88]. A key regulator of polarization is Cdc42, a small guanosine-5'-triphosphatase (GTP)ase that accumulates at the leading edge where it stimulates actin polymerization. Cdc42 activation is pH sensitive, requiring NHE1 activation and proton efflux to produce localized alkalinization of the cytoplasm to enhance its activity [86]. Moreover, alkalinization also promotes F-actin cleavage by cofilin, an actin binding protein that facilitates treadmilling by causing depolymerization at the pointed ends of actin filaments [87]. Other acid extruding or base loading transport mechanisms could potentially contribute to this alkalinization process, including CFTR and its ability to conduct bicarbonate ions, provided that a favorable electrochemical driving force exists.

As previously mentioned localized osmotic swelling can also contribute to the force that powers lamellipodia protrusion [59]. Solute uptake serves as a driving force for fluid uptake into the cell, often involving electroneutral transporters that couple cation uptake with Cl^- transport (e.g. KCC or NKCC cotransporters). It is also possible that if the plasma membrane is depolarized to a voltage that is more positive than the reversal potential of anion channels such as CFTR or ANO1, then the inwardly directed Cl^- concentration gradient would facilitate influx, setting up a favorable osmotic gradient for fluid uptake and lamellipodia protrusion. Whether Cl^- influx or efflux is occurring at the leading edge may not be predicable, since this would depend on the activity of multiple electrogenic transport pathways or conditions associated with injury. It is worth emphasizing that depending on the electrochemical gradient for Cl^-, CFTR could contribute instead to retraction taking place at the rear of the cell. In this case, efflux of Cl^-, perhaps coordinated with K^+ channel activity, would enable localized solute and fluid exit at the trailing edge of the cell, promoting forward movement [3].

3.2. Electrotaxis

Epithelia engaged in active electrolyte transport typically generate spontaneous transepithelial potentials (TEP) that provide an electrical driving force for paracellular ion movement across the epithelium [89]. Following wounding, the TEP at the site of the wound collapses as laterally oriented electric fields develop with the cathode (negative pole) located at the center of the wound. In dermal, corneal and airway epithelia, for example, outward current can be detected using a noninvasive technique that employs a self-referencing vibrating probe [90]. Many epithelial cell types respond to wound-induced electric fields by migrating toward the cathode although some cell types exhibit anodal migration in response to electric field stimulation [91, 92]. In fact, changing the polarity of the field will reverse the direction of migration. In experiments with primate tracheobronchial epithelial cells, an applied electric field with a threshold intensity of 23 mV/mm was effective at stimulating migration with a displacement speed that increased with field strength [63]. The displacement speed reflected greater migration efficiency and in the case of tracheobronchial epithelial cells, the increase in speed primarily resulted from improved directionality, which was quantitatively expressed using a directedness parameter for the migrating cells. Directedness was expressed as the angle (θ) that individual cells moved relative to the electric field vector, where cosine θ was defined as the directedness value. Cells moving randomly in the absence of an electric field have an average directedness value near zero, whereas those that move entirely along the electric field lines toward the cathode have a value approaching 1. Experiments with tracheobronchial epithelial cells showed that directedness increased with increasing field strength such that when the voltage achieved 90 mV/mm, a number of the cells migrated directly toward the cathode. The finding that inhibition of CFTR reduces the electric field evoked by wounding and that CFTR inhibition or silencing decreases lamellipodia protrusion [62], strongly suggests that CFTR activity plays an important role in sustaining directed migration in airway epithelial cells.

The cellular mechanisms underlying the increase in directed migration induced by wound-evoked electric fields are complex and cell type dependent. Studies of corneal epithelial cells and keratinocytes, for instance, revealed changes in the localization of epidermal growth factor receptors (EGFR) toward the cathode-facing borders of migrating cells, and in at least one study, EGFRs appeared to be activated by the electric field independently of ligand binding to the receptor [93–97]. Moreover, inhibition of EGFR-MAPK signaling was shown to alter the actin cytoskeleton at the leading edge and diminish directed migration of epithelial cells, demonstrating an important role for EGFR in detecting and initiating the epithelial response to electric field stimulation [96]. Additionally, electric fields can redistribute and activate PI3K/Akt signaling in a polarized manner at the cathode-oriented leading edge of the cell [98]. When PI3K is activated, membrane protrusion and lamellipodia formation is initiated at that site, facilitating directed migration toward the cathode. Pharmacological inhibition of PI3K activity or selective disruption of the PI3K-γ isoform has been shown to block electrotaxis in wound healing assays and organ cultures [98, 99]. Furthermore, in keratinocytes, deletion of phosphatase and tensin homolog (PTEN), a phosphatase that functions as a negative regulator of PI3K, resulted in increased Akt phosphorylation and enhanced electrotaxis. Other kinases linked to the control of cell motility such as extracellular signal-regulated kinase (ERK) have also been shown to be involved in electric field-evoked migration [97, 100, 101]. In experiments with glioma and fibrosarcoma cells, electric field stimulation induced NADPH oxidase activation, resulting in the production of reactive oxygen species (ROS) [100]. Intracellular accumulation of ROS stimulates ERK phosphorylation/activation which leads to reorganization of the cytoskeleton and an increase in directed migration [101]. Based on these observations, it appears likely that further studies will uncover additional molecular targets and signaling pathways involved in the detection and regulation of directionality by injury-induced electric fields.

3.3. Dynamics of integrin-mediated adhesion

A recent study examining the consequences of CFTR silencing on cell migration and epithelial repair in human airway (Calu-3) epithelial cells demonstrated a ~60% reduction in GM1 ganglioside content within the plasma membrane of CFTR deficient cells compared to controls [102, 103], which was restored following expression of wild-type CFTR. Similarly, treatment of cells with the selective CFTR blocker, $CFTR_{inh}$-172, also produced comparable reductions in GM1 content in cells expressing wild-type CFTR. These observations were consistent with earlier studies showing reduced levels of sialylated gangliosides in cells expressing CFTR with the ΔF508 mutation [104, 105]. Furthermore, previous investigations have also shown that gangliosides are capable of regulating integrin signaling and cell migration [106, 107]. Experiments with Calu-3 cells revealed that CFTR knockdown did not directly affect β_1 integrin surface expression; however, the level of activated β_1 integrin was significantly lower than observed in CFTR expressing control cells [102]. β_1-integrin activation could be completely recovered by incubating CFTR deficient cells with exogenous GM1, but not with GM3 gangliosides, confirming that integrin activation was dependent on GM1 and CFTR expression. Reduced β_1 integrin phosphorylation was associated with lower levels of focal adhesion kinase (FAK) and Crk-associated substrate (CAS) phosphorylation which was

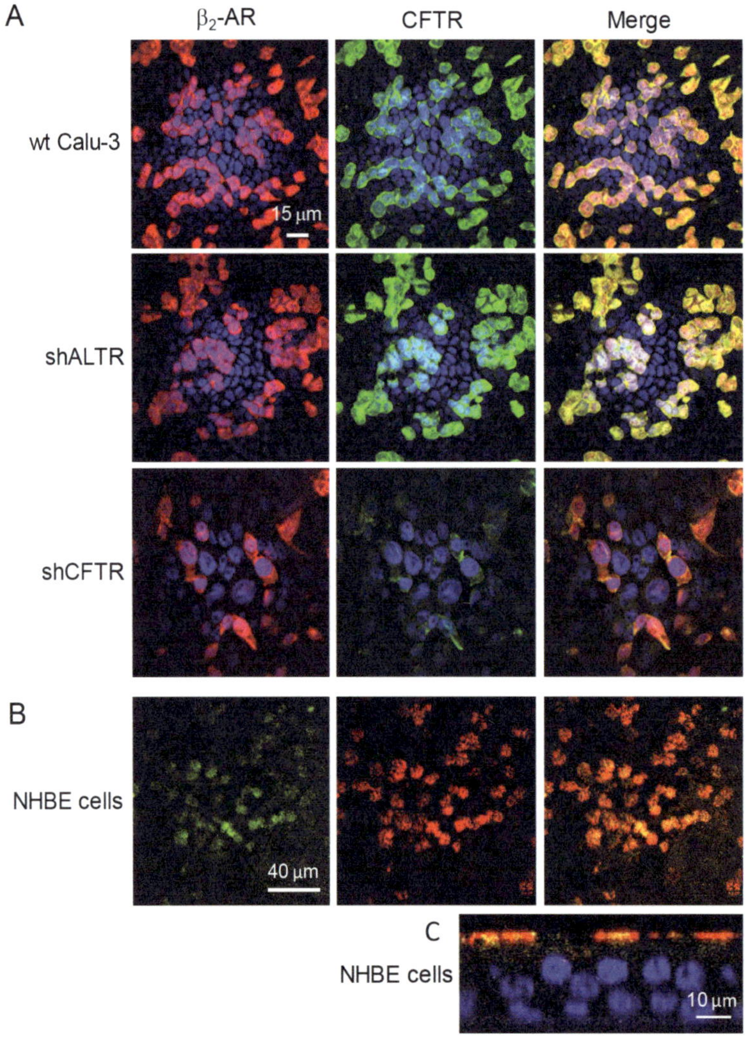

Figure 2. Colocalization of CFTR and the β_2-adrenergic receptor (β_2-AR) in the apical membrane of Calu-3 cells and in cilia of differentiated primary normal human bronchial epithelial (NHBE) cells grown under air-liquid interface conditions. (**A**) Antibody labeling of the β_2-AR, CFTR and merged images (where yellow represents colocalization) collected from wild-type Calu-3 cells (wt Calu-3), Calu-3 cells expressing shRNA that does not recognize CFTR (shALTR) and CFTR-deficient cells were CFTR expression was silenced by RNAi (shCFTR). (**B**) Labeling of the β_2-AR and CFTR within the cilia of differentiated primary NHBE cells. Yellow-orange represents colocalization of the receptor and channel. (**C**) Cross section of differentiated, pseudostratified primary NHBE cells showing colocalization of the β_2-AR and CFTR within the cilia. Note the layering of nuclei reflecting pseudostratification. Images were adapted from Refs. [114] and [115].

also restored by incubation with exogenous GM1 ganglioside. A possible explanation for the reduction in β_1 activation may be related to loss of localization to specific membrane microdomains that function as integrin signaling platforms. This would be consistent with GM1 localization within lipid raft domains where it is known to associate with CFTR [108, 109]. Moreover, recovery of FAK and CAS phosphorylation along with β_1 integrin activation with GM1 repletion also produced partial restoration of cell migration, suggesting that reduced integrin engagement with the extracellular matrix, presumably at the leading edge of the cell, accounts for at least part of the effect that loss of CFTR expression or inhibition of channel activity has on epithelial restitution.

More recently, stimulation of β_2-adrenergic receptors (β_2-AR) expressed on the apical membrane of normal human bronchial epithelial cells and Calu-3 cells caused a significant delay in cell migration and wound closure. This effect could be reproduced using carvedilol, a β_2-AR agonist that functions as a bias ligand to activate cAMP-independent, β-arrestin-dependent signaling cascades [110]. The inhibitory effects of β_2-AR agonists could be blocked if cells were pretreated with an inhibitor of PP2A phosphatase, indicating that PP2A activation was a critical step in regulating cell migration [111, 112]. Interestingly, in airway epithelial cells, β_2-ARs form a tightly coupled signaling complex with CFTR in the apical membrane (see **Figure 2**) such that receptor activation by endogenous ligands, such as epinephrine, or by selective β_2-AR agonists, like salbutamol, stimulate CFTR channel activity [113]. The reduced rate of migration following β_2-AR activation was associated with a reduction in lamellipodia protrusion, similar in magnitude to the effect produced by CFTR channel inhibition with $CFTR_{inh}$-172 or silencing by RNAi. Furthermore, β_2-AR agonists, including carvedilol, decreased β_1-integrin activation, and in CFTR-deficient Calu-3 cells, β_2-AR activation had no effect on cell migration [114]. These findings suggested a model where exposure to β_2-AR agonists stimulates PP2A phosphatase

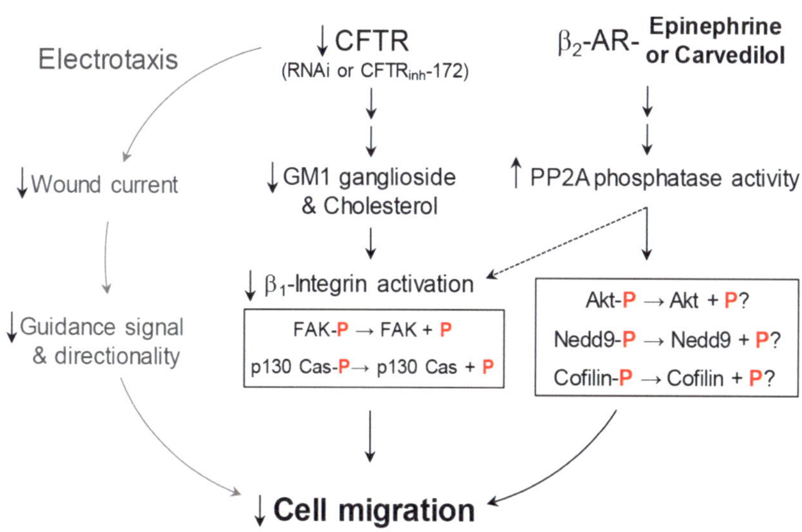

Figure 3. Summary of proposed interactions and pathways accounting for the decrease in cell migration and epithelial repair associated with loss of CFTR function and β_2-AR activation in airway epithelial cells. This model was adapted from Ref. [114].

activity to produce dephosphorylation of multiple proteins involved in the control of cell motility (see **Figure 3**). Moreover, CFTR inhibition or silencing and β_2-AR stimulation appear to converge on a common control point involving the activation of β_1 integrin, which is thought to be the reason why CFTR silencing and β_2-AR activation do not produce additive effects on cell migration.

4. Conclusions

This chapter has focused on the impact of CFTR dysfunction on cell migration and epithelial repair that has direct relevance to airway barrier function. This role for CFTR constitutes an important intrinsic deficit of the CF epithelium that contributes to disease progression. Other intrinsic deficits such as those linked to altered innate immune function appear to underlie abnormal regeneration and remodeling of the CF epithelium that occurs in the absence of infection. Delayed wound repair exacerbates intrinsic inflammation by providing opportunities for pathogen access to the airway submucosa, augmenting inflammation and tissue damage. Furthermore, dysregulation of the repair process establishes a chronic cycle of injury and inadequate restitution that intensifies remodeling, ultimately leading to deterioration of lung function. Further investigation is required to more clearly understand the molecular and cellular mechanisms by which CFTR expression and function affect cell motility. Results from these studies should aid in identifying pathways that could be targeted for development of novel pharmacotherapies to reduce airway infection and inflammation in CF.

Author details

Scott M. O'Grady

Address all correspondence to: ograd001@umn.edu

Departments of Animal Science, Integrative Biology and Physiology, University of Minnesota, St. Paul, MN, USA

References

[1] Stock C, Ludwig FT, Hanley PJ, Schwab A. Roles of ion transport in control of cell motility. Compr Physiol. 2013; 3:59–119.

[2] Schwab A, Stock C. Ion channels and transporters in tumour cell migration and invasion. Philos Trans R Soc Lond B Biol Sci. 2014; 369:1–8.

[3] Schwab A, Fabian A, Hanley PJ, Stock C. Role of ion channels and transporters in cell migration. Physiol Rev. 2012; 92:1865–913.

[4] Hoffmann EK. Ion channels involved in cell volume regulation: effects on migration, proliferation, and programmed cell death in non adherent EAT cells and adherent ELA cells. Cell Physiol Biochem. 2011; 28:1061–78.

[5] Chifflet S, Justet C, Hernandez JA, Nin V, Escande C, Benech JC. Early and late calcium waves during wound healing in corneal endothelial cells. Wound Repair Regen. 2012; 20:28–37.

[6] Rao JN, Platoshyn O, Li L, Guo X, Golovina VA, Yuan JX, Wang JY. Activation of K(+) channels and increased migration of differentiated intestinal epithelial cells after wounding. Am J Physiol Cell Physiol. 2002; 282:C885–98.

[7] Minns MS, Teicher G, Rich CB, Trinkaus-Randall V. Purinoreceptor P2X7 regulation of Ca(2+) mobilization and cytoskeletal rearrangement is required for corneal reepithelialization after injury. Am J Pathol. 2016; 186:285–96.

[8] Alvarez A, Lagos-Cabre R, Kong M, Cardenas A, Burgos-Bravo F, Schneider P, Quest AF, Leyton L. Integrin-mediated transactivation of P2X7R via hemichannel-dependent ATP release stimulates astrocyte migration. Biochim Biophys Acta. 2016; 1863:2175–88.

[9] Miyazaki A, Ohkubo T, Hatta M, Ishikawa H, Yamazaki J. Integrin alpha6beta4 and TRPV1 channel coordinately regulate directional keratinocyte migration. Biochem Biophys Res Commun. 2015; 458:161–7.

[10] Girault A, Chebli J, Prive A, Trinh NT, Maille E, Grygorczyk R, Brochiero E. Complementary roles of KCa3.1 channels and beta1-integrin during alveolar epithelial repair. Respir Res. 2015; 16:100.

[11] Chen JP, Luan Y, You CX, Chen XH, Luo RC, Li R. TRPM7 regulates the migration of human nasopharyngeal carcinoma cell by mediating Ca(2+) influx. Cell Calcium. 2010; 47:425–32.

[12] Veeravalli KK, Ponnala S, Chetty C, Tsung AJ, Gujrati M, Rao JS. Integrin alpha9beta1-mediated cell migration in glioblastoma via SSAT and Kir4.2 potassium channel pathway. Cell Signal. 2012; 24:272–81.

[13] Frizzell RA, Hanrahan JW. Physiology of epithelial chloride and fluid secretion. Cold Spring Harb Perspect Med. 2012; 2:a009563.

[14] Butler R, Hunt T, Smith NJ. ENaC inhibitors for the treatment of cystic fibrosis. Pharm Pat Anal. 2015; 4:17–27.

[15] Lu C, Jiang C, Pribanic S, Rotin D. CFTR stabilizes ENaC at the plasma membrane. J Cyst Fibros. 2007; 6:419–22.

[16] Wagner CJ, Schultz C, Mall MA. Neutrophil elastase and matrix metalloproteinase 12 in cystic fibrosis lung disease. Mol Cell Pediatr. 2016; 3:25.

[17] Cohen-Cymberknoh M, Kerem E, Ferkol T, Elizur A. Airway inflammation in cystic fibrosis: molecular mechanisms and clinical implications. Thorax. 2013; 68:1157–62.

[18] Voynow JA, Fischer BM, Zheng S. Proteases and cystic fibrosis. Int J Biochem Cell Biol. 2008; 40:1238-45.

[19] Tirouvanziam R. Neutrophilic inflammation as a major determinant in the progression of cystic fibrosis. Drug News Perspect. 2006; 19:609–14.

[20] Adam D, Roux-Delrieu J, Luczka E, Bonnomet A, Lesage J, Merol JC, Polette M, Abely M, Coraux C. Cystic fibrosis airway epithelium remodeling: involvement of inflammation. J Pathol. 2015; 235:408–19.

[21] Collawn JF, Matalon S. CFTR and lung homeostasis. Am J Physiol Lung Cell Mol Physiol. 2014; 307:L917–23.

[22] Iosifidis T, Garratt LW, Coombe DR, Knight DA, Stick SM, Kicic A. Airway epithelial repair in health and disease: orchestrator or simply a player? Respirology. 2016; 21:438–48.

[23] Ranganathan SC, Parsons F, Gangell C, Brennan S, Stick SM, Sly PD. Evolution of pulmonary inflammation and nutritional status in infants and young children with cystic fibrosis. Thorax. 2011; 66:408–13.

[24] Sly PD, Brennan S, Gangell C, de Klerk N, Murray C, Mott L, Stick SM, Robinson PJ, Robertson CF, Ranganathan SC. Lung disease at diagnosis in infants with cystic fibrosis detected by newborn screening. Am J Respir Crit Care Med. 2009; 180:146–52.

[25] Khan TZ, Wagener JS, Bost T, Martinez J, Accurso FJ, Riches DW. Early pulmonary inflammation in infants with cystic fibrosis. Am J Respir Crit Care Med. 1995; 151:1075–82.

[26] Gifford AM, Chalmers JD. The role of neutrophils in cystic fibrosis. Curr Opin Hematol. 2014; 21:16–22.

[27] Conese M, Copreni E, Di Gioia S, De Rinaldis P, Fumarulo R. Neutrophil recruitment and airway epithelial cell involvement in chronic cystic fibrosis lung disease. J Cyst Fibros. 2003; 2:129–35.

[28] Cantin AM, Hartl D, Konstan MW, Chmiel JF. Inflammation in cystic fibrosis lung disease: pathogenesis and therapy. J Cyst Fibros. 2015; 14:419–30.

[29] Voglis S, Quinn K, Tullis E, Liu M, Henriques M, Zubrinich C, Penuelas O, Chan H, Silverman F, Cherepanov V, Orzech N, Khine AA, Cantin A, Slutsky AS, Downey GP, Zhang H. Human neutrophil peptides and phagocytic deficiency in bronchiectatic lungs. Am J Respir Crit Care Med. 2009; 180:159–66.

[30] Elizur A, Cannon CL, Ferkol TW. Airway inflammation in cystic fibrosis. Chest. 2008; 133:489–95.

[31] Sly PD, Gangell CL, Chen L, Ware RS, Ranganathan S, Mott LS, Murray CP, Stick SM. Risk factors for bronchiectasis in children with cystic fibrosis. N Engl J Med. 2013; 368:1963–70.

[32] Pongnimitprasert N, El-Benna J, Foglietti MJ, Gougerot-Pocidalo MA, Bernard M, Braut-Boucher F. Potential role of the "NADPH oxidases" (NOX/DUOX) family in cystic fibrosis. Ann Biol Clin (Paris). 2008; 66:621–9.

[33] Townsend DM, Tew KD, Tapiero H. The importance of glutathione in human disease. Biomed Pharmacother. 2003; 57:145–55.

[34] Hudson VM. Rethinking cystic fibrosis pathology: the critical role of abnormal reduced glutathione (GSH) transport caused by CFTR mutation. Free Radic Biol Med. 2001; 30:1440–61.

[35] Linsdell P, Hanrahan JW. Glutathione permeability of CFTR. Am J Physiol. 1998; 275:C323–6.

[36] Shah VS, Meyerholz DK, Tang XX, Reznikov L, Abou Alaiwa M, Ernst SE, Karp PH, Wohlford-Lenane CL, Heilmann KP, Leidinger MR, Allen PD, Zabner J, McCray PB Jr, Ostedgaard LS, Stoltz DA, Randak CO, Welsh MJ. Airway acidification initiates host defense abnormalities in cystic fibrosis mice. Science. 2016; 351:503–7.

[37] Luckie DB, Van Alst AJ, Massey MK, Flood RD, Shah AA, Malhotra V, Kozel BJ. Chemical rescue of DeltaF508-CFTR in C127 epithelial cells reverses aberrant extracellular pH acidification to wild-type alkalization as monitored by microphysiometry. Biochem Biophys Res Commun. 2014; 451:535–40.

[38] Fischer H, Widdicombe JH. Mechanisms of acid and base secretion by the airway epithelium. J Membr Biol. 2006; 211:139–50.

[39] Machen TE. Innate immune response in CF airway epithelia: hyperinflammatory? Am J Physiol Cell Physiol. 2006; 291:C218–30.

[40] Coakley RD, Grubb BR, Paradiso AM, Gatzy JT, Johnson LG, Kreda SM, O'Neal WK, Boucher RC. Abnormal surface liquid pH regulation by cultured cystic fibrosis bronchial epithelium. Proc Natl Acad Sci U S A. 2003; 100:16083–8.

[41] Verkman AS, Song Y, Thiagarajah JR. Role of airway surface liquid and submucosal glands in cystic fibrosis lung disease. Am J Physiol Cell Physiol. 2003; 284:C2–15.

[42] Grassme H, Riethmuller J, Gulbins E. Ceramide in cystic fibrosis. Handb Exp Pharmacol. 2013; 216:265-74.

[43] Becker KA, Grassme H, Zhang Y, Gulbins E. Ceramide in *Pseudomonas aeruginosa* infections and cystic fibrosis. Cell Physiol Biochem. 2010; 26:57–66.

[44] Worgall TS. Lipid metabolism in cystic fibrosis. Curr Opin Clin Nutr Metab Care. 2009; 12:105–9.

[45] Grassme H, Carpinteiro A, Edwards MJ, Gulbins E, Becker KA. Regulation of the inflammasome by ceramide in cystic fibrosis lungs. Cell Physiol Biochem. 2014; 34:45–55.

[46] Becker KA, Tummler B, Gulbins E, Grassme H. Accumulation of ceramide in the trachea and intestine of cystic fibrosis mice causes inflammation and cell death. Biochem Biophys Res Commun. 2010; 403:368–74.

[47] Teichgraber V, Ulrich M, Endlich N, Riethmuller J, Wilker B, De Oliveira-Munding CC, van Heeckeren AM, Barr ML, von Kurthy G, Schmid KW, Weller M, Tummler B, Lang F, Grassme H, Doring G, Gulbins E. Ceramide accumulation mediates inflammation, cell death and infection susceptibility in cystic fibrosis. Nat Med. 2008; 14:382–91.

[48] Bartoszewski R, Rab A, Fu L, Bartoszewska S, Collawn J, Bebok Z. CFTR expression regulation by the unfolded protein response. Methods Enzymol. 2011; 491:3–24.

[49] Bartoszewski R, Rab A, Jurkuvenaite A, Mazur M, Wakefield J, Collawn JF, Bebok Z. Activation of the unfolded protein response by deltaF508 CFTR. Am J Respir Cell Mol Biol. 2008; 39:448–57.

[50] Rab A, Bartoszewski R, Jurkuvenaite A, Wakefield J, Collawn JF, Bebok Z. Endoplasmic reticulum stress and the unfolded protein response regulate genomic cystic fibrosis transmembrane conductance regulator expression. Am J Physiol Cell Physiol. 2007; 292:C756–66.

[51] Vij N, Fang S, Zeitlin PL. Selective inhibition of endoplasmic reticulum-associated degradation rescues DeltaF508-cystic fibrosis transmembrane regulator and suppresses interleukin-8 levels: therapeutic implications. J Biol Chem. 2006; 281:17369–78.

[52] Hajj R, Lesimple P, Nawrocki-Raby B, Birembaut P, Puchelle E, Coraux C. Human airway surface epithelial regeneration is delayed and abnormal in cystic fibrosis. J Pathol. 2007; 211:340–50.

[53] Trinh NT, Prive A, Maille E, Noel J, Brochiero E. EGF and K+ channel activity control normal and cystic fibrosis bronchial epithelia repair. Am J Physiol Lung Cell Mol Physiol. 2008; 295:L866–80.

[54] Maille E, Trinh NT, Prive A, Bilodeau C, Bissonnette E, Grandvaux N, Brochiero E. Regulation of normal and cystic fibrosis airway epithelial repair processes by TNF-alpha after injury. Am J Physiol Lung Cell Mol Physiol. 2011; 301:L945–55.

[55] Ransom CB, O'Neal JT, Sontheimer H. Volume-activated chloride currents contribute to the resting conductance and invasive migration of human glioma cells. J Neurosci. 2001; 21:7674–83.

[56] Ullrich N, Bordey A, Gillespie GY, Sontheimer H. Expression of voltage-activated chloride currents in acute slices of human gliomas. Neuroscience. 1998; 83:1161–73.

[57] Ullrich N, Gillespie GY, Sontheimer H. Human astrocytoma cells express a unique chloride current. Neuroreport. 1996; 7:1020–4.

[58] McFerrin MB, Sontheimer H. A role for ion channels in glioma cell invasion. Neuron Glia Biol. 2006; 2:39–49.

[59] Zierler S, Frei E, Grissmer S, Kerschbaum HH. Chloride influx provokes lamellipodium formation in microglial cells. Cell Physiol Biochem. 2008; 21:55–62.

[60] Leis JA, Bekar LK, Walz W. Potassium homeostasis in the ischemic brain. Glia. 2005; 50:407–16.

[61] Rappert A, Biber K, Nolte C, Lipp M, Schubel A, Lu B, Gerard NP, Gerard C, Boddeke HW, Kettenmann H. Secondary lymphoid tissue chemokine (CCL21) activates CXCR3 to trigger a Cl- current and chemotaxis in murine microglia. J Immunol. 2002; 168:3221–6.

[62] Schiller KR, Maniak PJ, O'Grady SM. Cystic fibrosis transmembrane conductance regulator is involved in airway epithelial wound repair. Am J Physiol Cell Physiol. 2010; 299:C912–21.

[63] Sun YH, Reid B, Fontaine JH, Miller LA, Hyde DM, Mogilner A, Zhao M. Airway epithelial wounds in rhesus monkey generate ionic currents that guide cell migration to promote healing. J Appl Physiol (1985). 2011; 111:1031–41.

[64] Trinh NT, Bardou O, Prive A, Maille E, Adam D, Lingee S, Ferraro P, Desrosiers MY, Coraux C, Brochiero E. Improvement of defective cystic fibrosis airway epithelial wound repair after CFTR rescue. Eur Respir J. 2012; 40:1390–400.

[65] Marino GI, Kotsias BA. Cystic fibrosis transmembrane regulator (CFTR) in human trophoblast BeWo cells and its relation to cell migration. Placenta. 2014; 35:92–8.

[66] Castro-Parodi M, Levi L, Dietrich V, Zotta E, Damiano AE. CFTR may modulate AQP9 functionality in preeclamptic placentas. Placenta. 2009; 30:642–8.

[67] Xu J, Yong M, Li J, Dong X, Yu T, Fu X, Hu L. High level of CFTR expression is associated with tumor aggression and knockdown of CFTR suppresses proliferation of ovarian cancer in vitro and in vivo. Oncol Rep. 2015; 33:2227–34.

[68] Dong J, Jiang X, Zhang X, Liu KS, Zhang J, Chen J, Yu MK, Tsang LL, Chung YW, Wang Y, Zhou WL, Chan HC. Dynamically regulated CFTR rxpression and its functional role in cutaneous wound healing. J Cell Physiol. 2015; 230:2049–58.

[69] Li J, Zhang JT, Jiang X, Shi X, Shen J, Feng F, Chen J, Liu G, He P, Jiang J, Tsang LL, Wang Y, Rosell R, Jiang L, He J, Chan HC. The cystic fibrosis transmembrane conductance regulator as a biomarker in non-small cell lung cancer. Int J Oncol. 2015; 46:2107–15.

[70] Qu Z, Yao W, Yao R, Liu X, Yu K, Hartzell C. The Ca(2+) -activated Cl(-) channel, ANO1 (TMEM16A), is a double-edged sword in cell proliferation and tumorigenesis. Cancer Med. 2014; 3:453–61.

[71] Jacobsen KS, Zeeberg K, Sauter DR, Poulsen KA, Hoffmann EK, Schwab A. The role of TMEM16A (ANO1) and TMEM16F (ANO6) in cell migration. Pflugers Arch. 2013; 465:1753–62.

[72] Oh U, Jung J. Cellular functions of TMEM16/anoctamin. Pflugers Arch. 2016; 468:443–53.

[73] Huang F, Wong X, Jan LY. International Union of Basic and Clinical Pharmacology. LXXXV: calcium-activated chloride channels. Pharmacol Rev. 2012; 64:1–15.

[74] Chenevert J, Duvvuri U, Chiosea S, Dacic S, Cieply K, Kim J, Shiwarski D, Seethala RR. DOG1: a novel marker of salivary acinar and intercalated duct differentiation. Mod Pathol. 2012; 25:919–29.

[75] Simon S, Grabellus F, Ferrera L, Galietta L, Schwindenhammer B, Muhlenberg T, Taeger G, Eilers G, Treckmann J, Breitenbuecher F, Schuler M, Taguchi T, Fletcher JA, Bauer S. DOG1 regulates growth and IGFBP5 in gastrointestinal stromal tumors. Cancer Res. 2013; 73:3661–70.

[76] Liu W, Lu M, Liu B, Huang Y, Wang K. Inhibition of Ca(2+)-activated Cl(-) channel ANO1/TMEM16A expression suppresses tumor growth and invasiveness in human prostate carcinoma. Cancer Lett. 2012; 326:41–51.

[77] Sauter DR, Novak I, Pedersen SF, Larsen EH, Hoffmann EK. ANO1 (TMEM16A) in pancreatic ductal adenocarcinoma (PDAC). Pflugers Arch. 2015; 467:1495–508.

[78] Ruffin M, Voland M, Marie S, Bonora M, Blanchard E, Blouquit-Laye S, Naline E, Puyo P, Le Rouzic P, Guillot L, Corvol H, Clement A, Tabary O. Anoctamin 1 dysregulation alters bronchial epithelial repair in cystic fibrosis. Biochim Biophys Acta. 2013; 1832:2340–51.

[79] Ridley AJ. Life at the leading edge. Cell. 2011; 145:1012–22.

[80] Bisi S, Disanza A, Malinverno C, Frittoli E, Palamidessi A, Scita G. Membrane and actin dynamics interplay at lamellipodia leading edge. Curr Opin Cell Biol. 2013; 25:565–73.

[81] Schaub S, Meister JJ, Verkhovsky AB. Analysis of actin filament network organization in lamellipodia by comparing experimental and simulated images. J Cell Sci. 2007; 120:1491–500.

[82] Svitkina TM, Borisy GG. Arp2/3 complex and actin depolymerizing factor/cofilin in dendritic organization and treadmilling of actin filament array in lamellipodia. J Cell Biol. 1999; 145:1009–26.

[83] Bugyi B, Carlier MF. Control of actin filament treadmilling in cell motility. Annu Rev Biophys. 2010; 39:449–70.

[84] Stock C, Cardone RA, Busco G, Krahling H, Schwab A, Reshkin SJ. Protons extruded by NHE1: digestive or glue? Eur J Cell Biol. 2008; 87:591–9.

[85] Stock C, Schwab A. Role of the Na/H exchanger NHE1 in cell migration. Acta Physiol (Oxf). 2006; 187:149–57.

[86] Martin C, Pedersen SF, Schwab A, Stock C. Intracellular pH gradients in migrating cells. Am J Physiol Cell Physiol. 2011; 300:C490–5.

[87] Ludwig FT, Schwab A, Stock C. The Na+ /H+ -exchanger (NHE1) generates pH nanodomains at focal adhesions. J Cell Physiol. 2013; 228:1351–8.

[88] Putney LK, Denker SP, Barber DL. The changing face of the Na+/H+ exchanger, NHE1: structure, regulation, and cellular actions. Annu Rev Pharmacol Toxicol. 2002; 42:527–52.

[89] Zhao M, Chalmers L, Cao L, Vieira AC, Mannis M, Reid B. Electrical signaling in control of ocular cell behaviors. Prog Retin Eye Res. 2012; 31:65–88.

[90] Tai G, Reid B, Cao L, Zhao M. Electrotaxis and wound healing: experimental methods to study electric fields as a directional signal for cell migration. Methods Mol Biol. 2009; 571:77–97.

[91] Liu CY, Kao WW. Corneal epithelial wound healing. Prog Mol Biol Transl Sci. 2015; 134:61–71.

[92] Liu Q, Song B. Electric field regulated signaling pathways. Int J Biochem Cell Biol. 2014; 55:264–8.

[93] Pu J, McCaig CD, Cao L, Zhao Z, Segall JE, Zhao M. EGF receptor signaling is essential for electric-field-directed migration of breast cancer cells. J Cell Sci. 2007; 120:3395–403.

[94] Zhao M, Pu J, Forrester JV, McCaig CD. Membrane lipids, EGF receptors, and intracellular signals colocalize and are polarized in epithelial cells moving directionally in a physiological electric field. FASEB J. 2002; 16:857–9.

[95] Wu D, Ma X, Lin F. DC electric fields direct breast cancer cell migration, induce EGFR polarization, and increase the intracellular level of calcium ions. Cell Biochem Biophys. 2013; 67:1115–25.

[96] Zhao M, Dick A, Forrester JV, McCaig CD. Electric field-directed cell motility involves up-regulated expression and asymmetric redistribution of the epidermal growth factor receptors and is enhanced by fibronectin and laminin. Mol Biol Cell. 1999; 10:1259–76.

[97] Wolf-Goldberg T, Barbul A, Ben-Dov N, Korenstein R. Low electric fields induce ligand-independent activation of EGF receptor and ERK via electrochemical elevation of H(+) and ROS concentrations. Biochim Biophys Acta. 2013; 1833:1396–408.

[98] Zhao M, Song B, Pu J, Wada T, Reid B, Tai G, Wang F, Guo A, Walczysko P, Gu Y, Sasaki T, Suzuki A, Forrester JV, Bourne HR, Devreotes PN, McCaig CD, Penninger JM. Electrical signals control wound healing through phosphatidylinositol-3-OH kinase-gamma and PTEN. Nature. 2006; 442:457–60.

[99] Cao L, Graue-Hernandez EO, Tran V, Reid B, Pu J, Mannis MJ, Zhao M. Downregulation of PTEN at corneal wound sites accelerates wound healing through increased cell migration. Invest Ophthalmol Vis Sci. 2011; 52:2272–8.

[100] Li F, Chen T, Hu S, Lin J, Hu R, Feng H. Superoxide mediates direct current electric field-induced directional migration of glioma cells through the activation of AKT and ERK. PLoS One. 2013; 8:e61195.

[101] Li F, Wang H, Li L, Huang C, Lin J, Zhu G, Chen Z, Wu N, Feng H. Superoxide plays critical roles in electrotaxis of fibrosarcoma cells via activation of ERK and reorganization of the cytoskeleton. Free Radic Biol Med. 2012; 52:1888–96.

[102] Itokazu Y, Pagano RE, Schroeder AS, O'Grady SM, Limper AH, Marks DL. Reduced GM1 ganglioside in CFTR-deficient human airway cells results in decreased beta1-integrin signaling and delayed wound repair. Am J Physiol Cell Physiol. 2014; 306:C819–30.

[103] Domingue JC,Rao MC. CFTR and GM1 "gangl-ing" up to heal thy wound. Focus on "Reduced GM1 ganglioside in CFTR-deficient human airway cells results in decreased beta1-integrin signaling and delayed wound repair". Am J Physiol Cell Physiol. 2014; 306:C789–91.

[104] Dosanjh A, Muchmore EA. Expression of DeltaF508 cystic fibrosis transmembrane regulator (CFTR) decreases membrane sialylation. Open Respir Med J. 2009; 3:79–84.

[105] Dosanjh A, Lencer W, Brown D, Ausiello DA, Stow JL. Heterologous expression of delta F508 CFTR results in decreased sialylation of membrane glycoconjugates. Am J Physiol. 1994; 266:C360–6.

[106] Regina Todeschini A, Hakomori SI. Functional role of glycosphingolipids and gangliosides in control of cell adhesion, motility, and growth, through glycosynaptic microdomains. Biochim Biophys Acta. 2008; 1780:421–33.

[107] Toledo MS, Suzuki E, Handa K, Hakomori S. Effect of ganglioside and tetraspanins in microdomains on interaction of integrins with fibroblast growth factor receptor. J Biol Chem. 2005; 280:16227–34.

[108] Kowalski MP, Pier GB. Localization of cystic fibrosis transmembrane conductance regulator to lipid rafts of epithelial cells is required for Pseudomonas aeruginosa-induced cellular activation. J Immunol. 2004; 172:418–25.

[109] Bryan R, Kube D, Perez A, Davis P, Prince A. Overproduction of the CFTR R domain leads to increased levels of asialoGM1 and increased Pseudomonas aeruginosa binding by epithelial cells. Am J Respir Cell Mol Biol. 1998; 19:269–77.

[110] Peitzman ER, Zaidman NA, Maniak PJ, O'Grady SM. Carvedilol binding to beta2-adrenergic receptors inhibits CFTR-dependent anion secretion in airway epithelial cells. Am J Physiol [Lung Cell Mol Physiol]. 2016; 310:L50–8.

[111] Pullar CE, Grahn JC, Liu W, Isseroff RR. Beta2-adrenergic receptor activation delays wound healing. FASEB J. 2006; 20:76–86.

[112] Pullar CE, Chen J, Isseroff RR. PP2A activation by beta2-adrenergic receptor agonists: novel regulatory mechanism of keratinocyte migration. J Biol Chem. 2003; 278:22555–62.

[113] Naren AP, Cobb B, Li C, Roy K, Nelson D, Heda GD, Liao J, Kirk KL, Sorscher EJ, Hanrahan J, Clancy JP. A macromolecular complex of beta 2 adrenergic receptor, CFTR, and ezrin/radixin/moesin-binding phosphoprotein 50 is regulated by PKA. Proc Natl Acad Sci U S A. 2003; 100:342–6.

[114] Peitzman ER, Zaidman NA, Maniak PJ, O'Grady SM. Agonist binding to β-adrenergic receptors on human airway epithelial cells inhibits migration and wound repair. Am J Physiol [Cell Physiol]. 2015; 309:C847–55.

[115] Zaidman NA, Panoskaltsis-Mortari A, O'Grady SM. Differentiation of human bronchial epithelial cells: role of hydrocortisone in development of ion transport pathways involved in mucociliary clearance. Am J Physiol [Cell Physiol]. 2016; 311:C225–36.

Chapter 2

Cystic Fibrosis–Related Diabetes

Bernadette Prentice, Shihab Hameed, Chee Y. Ooi,
Charles F. Verge and John Widger

Additional information is available at the end of the chapter

http://dx.doi.org/10.5772/66452

Abstract

Cystic fibrosis–related diabetes (CFRD) results in significant morbidity and mortality for patients with cystic fibrosis (CF). It is the endpoint of a spectrum of progressive insulin deficiency with resulting abnormalities of glucose tolerance. The consequence of glycaemic abnormalities in CF is poorer nutritional status, an increase in respiratory exacerbations with decline in lung function and ultimately greater morbidity and mortality. CFRD can be diagnosed by the standard oral glucose tolerance test (OGTT) usually performed from 10 years of age. However, this may miss early glycaemic abnormalities which appear to be clinically important. Early recognition of CFRD and treatment have been shown to improve outcomes in CF. Novel diagnostic methods such as 30-min sampled OGTT and continuous glucose monitoring (CGM) may prove to be useful in screening for this disorder and in the early identification of glycaemic abnormalities.

Keywords: cystic fibrosis–related diabetes, glucose, insulin, abnormal glucose tolerance, indeterminate glycaemia, impaired glucose tolerance, oral glucose tolerance test, continuous glucose monitoring

1. Introduction

Cystic fibrosis (CF) is the most common life-limiting autosomal recessive genetic condition seen in the Caucasian population, affecting approximately 1/2500 live births in Australia [1]. It is caused by mutations in the cystic fibrosis transmembrane regulator (CFTR) gene, located on the long arm of chromosome 7 [1] and expressed in the epithelial cells of lungs, pancreas and sweat glands and other organs. Cystic fibrosis–related diabetes (CFRD) is one of the most important complications of the disease as it is known to have a significant impact on morbidity and mortality [2]. Patients with CF ultimately die from recurrent respiratory tract infections and respiratory failure which may be hastened by abnormalities of glucose tolerance affecting respiratory function and nutrition.

2. Pathophysiology

The pathophysiology of CFRD is likely multifactorial and complex. Historically CFRD was thought to be the result of progressive pancreatic destruction by secretions of the exocrine pancreas, pancreatic autodigestion and replacement with nonfunctioning fatty tissue, amyloid deposits or fibrotic tissue [3, 4]. This theory was supported by ultrasound findings in patients with CF of an "echogenic" and atrophied pancreas which progresses with age. MRI has also been used to study the pancreas of patients with CF. Sequeiros et al. attempted to determine the pancreatic volume of patients with CF using MRI and compare with Type 1 diabetic patients and controls. In over 70% of patients with CF, the pancreas could not be visualised and this was irrespective of glycaemic status [5]. Pancreatic tissue on autopsies of patients with CF has also noted to have fewer islet cells and replacement with fibrotic tissue. Histologically, patients with CFRD have a relative decrease in the number of islet cells and insulin-containing cells within the islets, relative to the non-CFRD cohort [4, 6].

However, recent information supports the theory that destruction of the physical pancreas does not entirely explain the glycaemic abnormalities in patients with CF. Insulin deficiency has been shown to occur in young children and infants with CF [7], and even infants have been reported to have CFRD [8]. This has also been demonstrated in animal models of CF. In both the pig and ferret CF models, the animals demonstrate abnormal insulin secretion from birth, suggesting that CFTR may play a more direct role in insulin secretion [9, 10]. In the pig model, newborn pigs were noted to develop hyperglycaemia even when there was no significant islet cell destruction [10]. Recent studies of the CFTR potentiator ivacaftor (Kalydeco™), which improves gating defects and thus should not have any impact on fatty or fibrotic tissue, have demonstrated an improvement in glucose abnormalities [11, 12]. This suggests that the intrinsic abnormality in the CFTR protein may play a role in glycaemic control in CF.

The timeframe during which patients with CF develop glycaemic abnormalities and CFRD has significant variability, and the specific CFTR class abnormality does not entirely account for this unpredictability. Non-CFTR genetic modifiers may play a key role in determining this risk. Patients with CF who have a family history of Type 2 diabetes are known to have an increased risk of CFRD [13, 14]. Polymorphisms in *TCF7L2*, a "susceptibility gene" for Type 2 diabetes, are more common in patients with CFRD. The pathophysiology also appears to have similarities. Couce et al. noted that islet cell amyloidosis, which is characteristic of pancreatic histology of patients with Type 2 Diabetes mellitus, is also present in CF patients with CFRD and "borderline diabetes" but not in nondiabetic CF patients or controls [3]. Other genetic modifiers have been shown to modify CF phenotypes, including *SLC26A9* which has been demonstrated to be more common in patients who develop CFRD [15].

In normal insulin physiology, insulin secretion occurs in two phases—the first phase results from exocytosis of preformed insulin granules which is the result of a voltage-dependent calcium channel being triggered by blood glucose elevations [16–18]. The second phase requires maturation of insulin granules and lasts minutes to hours [19, 20]. Oral glucose ingestion results in a limited and delayed first-phase insulin peak when compared with intravenous administration [21, 22]. Overall, the amount of insulin secreted appears to be amplified when glucose is given orally, rather than intravenously. Incretins (glucagon-like peptide and gastric inhibitory peptide) are secreted from neuroendocrine cells of the gastrointestinal system and increase insulin secretion and decrease glucagon secretion. The secretion of incretins is hypothesised to be the result of the action of oral glucose within the gastrointestinal tract [21]. The role of incretins in CFRD has not yet been fully elucidated, and it is unclear whether or not patients with CFRD have abnormal levels of incretins. However, the diet of CF patients may play a role in the development of CFRD. In patients with Type 2 diabetes mellitus (DM), those prescribed orlistat, a lipase inhibitor, had diminished fat digestion which resulted in greater postprandial hyperglycaemia [23]. In a randomised crossover trial, Perano et al. demonstrated that adolescent patients with CF, who did not take appropriate pancreatic enzyme supplementation, experienced amplified postprandial hyperglycaemia [24]. Barrio postulates in her review that inadequate enzyme supplementation in patients with CF results in fat malabsorption, which may hasten gastric emptying, thereby inhibiting the normal augmentation of insulin response by the neuroendocrine cells [25]. Exogenous incretin therapy has proven beneficial in patients with Type 2 DM, but it has also been associated with weight loss in this cohort, an undesirable outcome for patients with CF [26]. Hyperglycaemia is known to promote beta-cell apoptosis, and as such, postprandial hyperglycaemia from dysfunctional incretin secretion in CF may potentiate the glycaemic abnormalities demonstrated and hasten the progression to CFRD.

CFRD is distinct from both Type 1 and Type 2 diabetes. CFRD is not an autoimmune condition like Type 1 DM and is not associated with autoantibodies found in Type 1 DM. Moreover, Type 2 DM is primarily a disorder of insulin resistance, whereas glucose abnormalities in CF are primarily the result of insulin deficiency, which is present even in CF patients with normal glucose tolerance on oral glucose tolerance test (OGTT) [7]. One of the features of CFRD that differentiates it from other forms of diabetes is the variation in glucose tolerance demonstrated over time [27]. Although abnormalities of glucose tolerance are known to progress and the complications of diabetes increase in the degree of abnormal glycaemia, some patients with the diagnosis of CFRD will have OGTT results that normalise [27]. The role of insulin resistance has been less well defined although there is emerging evidence of its importance. Ahmad et al. illustrated that patients with CF actually had an increase in peripheral insulin sensitivity compared to healthy controls matched for age and body mass index. They concluded that this increase in peripheral sensitivity in CF patients was a metabolic compensation for insulin deficiency [28]. Moran et al. replicated these findings in exocrine-insufficient CF patients without diabetes. However, once CFRD had developed, there was an increase in peripheral insulin resistance [29]. The mechanism by which this may occur could be the result of a downregulation of GLUT-4 insulin-sensitive channels secondary to chronic hyperglycaemia [30] ("glucose toxicity"). Insulin resistance is also thought to vary over time which could explain the variability of glucose tolerance seen in patients with CF, including a normalisation of previously abnormal glucose tolerance on OGTT. It is often cited that glucose abnormalities worsen during pulmonary exacerbations (due to cytokine and stress hormone release), but the data to support this suggestion is limited and was not found in the study by Widger et al. [31]. This group performed OGTT in patients with a pulmonary exacerbation and then repeated the OGTT when well. Although the sample size was small, 8/9 patients remained within their glycaemic category even when recovered from their pulmonary exacerbation. However insulin resistance is known to increase during periods of corticosteroid usage, overnight feeds [32, 33], pregnancy and during puberty [34–36]. In the latter case, insulin resistance is thought to increase as a result of a physiological elevation in growth hormone [34], and this may account for the increased detection of CFRD in this age group.

Chronic inflammation may play a key role in the development of glucose abnormalities in CF. Bismuth et al. demonstrated in their cohort of patients with CF that the erythrocyte sedimentation rate (ESR), a marker of inflammation, positively correlated with HbA_{1c} and the area under the curve (AUC) for glucose in patients undergoing OGTT [37]. Significant and ongoing oxidative stress is one mechanism hypothesised to result in an inflammatory state and beta-cell apoptosis [38, 39]. One review postulated that the imbalance in inflammatory T-cell lymphocytes known to play a role in the development of other forms of diabetes may contribute to lung inflammation and thereby a chronic inflammatory states resulting in glucose abnormalities [40]. T-helper 17 (Th-17) lymphocyte cells secrete a pro-inflammatory cytokine-IL-17 known to be involve in pulmonary inflammation in CF and is known to be present in higher levels compared to controls in patients with Type 2 diabetes. Furthermore, studies also suggest that IL-17 may play an important role in the development of Type 1 diabetes [41] and may contribute to β-cell destruction. It has also been postulated that cytokines such as TNF-α may act directly on the insulin receptor by inducing insulin resistance, thereby inhibiting the potential action of insulin [42].

The pathophysiology of CFRD is likely to be multifactorial but ultimately resulting from progressive insulin deficiency secondary to islet cell destruction and defective beta-cell secretion, combined with stressors that intermittently increase insulin resistance resulting in a further deterioration of glycaemic status. Certain patients may be more at risk if non-CFTR genetic modifiers are present [13, 14], and perhaps these patients are unable to compensate for the degree of histological pancreatic destruction and defective beta-cell functioning.

3. Epidemiology

3.1. Prevalence of glycaemic abnormalities in CF

CFRD is known to occur in up to 50% of patients with CF by the age of 30 years [43] and the prevalence increases with age. CFRD can occur in young children with CF but is rare [8]. Recent studies suggest that CFRD affects approximately 9% in the 5–9 year age group [44] and a smaller proportion of children under 5 may also meet the CFRD diagnostic criteria. Yi et al. recently reported a series that suggested 5% of their cohort between 6 months and 5 years had CFRD [45]. Although a small proportion of young children have CFRD, the average age of onset is 20 years [46]. CFRD occurs more commonly in females with a prevalence of 17% in young female adults compared with 12% in males previously described [47].

Children with CF are known to be insulin deficient from birth. Milner et al. demonstrated that children with CF in the first year of life had lower insulin levels than controls [7]. Insulin deficiency will progress over time and results in a gradual deterioration of glucose tolerance. As such, impaired glucose tolerance is much more common than CFRD and can affect up to 41% of children in the 6–9 year age group [48], compared with only 10% of this group being classified as CFRD. The risk of early CFRD is much higher in children with abnormal glucose tolerance on OGTT [48].

3.2. Screening

The prevalence of identified CFRD has been shown to increase after the introduction of screening [49]. Unlike Type 1 or Type 2 diabetes which are often symptomatic, CFRD does not often present with symptoms of hyperglycaemia although this can occur in approximately one third of patients. Symptoms can include polyuria and polydipsia, but CFRD is more likely to present insidiously with the catabolic complications of insulin deficiency such as nutritional deterioration or decline in pulmonary function. When routine screening was introduced in Australia, the incidence of CFRD increased from 2.0 to 22.1 per 1000 person years between 2000 and 2008, which represents a tenfold increase [50]. A decline in the age of diagnosis has also been demonstrated after the introduction of routine screening; Noronha et al. reported a reduction in the mean age of diagnosis from 22.3 years to 13.5 years [49]. Routine screening from at least 10 years of age with an OGTT is recommended by most guidelines [51, 52].

3.3. Risk factors for CFRD

The risk factors for the development of CFRD are closely linked to the specific CFTR genotype and the severity of the CFTR protein dysfunction [53]. CFTR mutations are classified according to the resulting functional deficit [54]. Class 1 and class 2 mutations result in the total or partial absence of CFTR protein at the surface membrane due to defective/non-functional protein (Class 1, e.g. stop codon mutations) or due to defective transfer of the protein to the cell membrane, i.e. defective "trafficking" (Class 2, e.g. F508) [25]. Classes 3, 4, 5 and 6 have irregularities in regulation, conductance, prevalence and stability of CFTR at the membrane [55]. Of the latter, 4 classes, all except class 3, which is known as a gating mutation, have partial function. Those classes with no action have a more severe phenotype and are associated with a greater risk of CFRD, such as homozygous F508 patients [46].

CFRD generally occurs in patients with pancreatic insufficiency. There have been reports of CFRD in patients who are pancreatic sufficient, but the diagnostic criteria for exocrine pancreatic function do not appear to be robust [47]. Some of these patients were classified as pancreatic sufficient because they were not taking replacement enzymes, but had not undergone any formal diagnostic testing such as faecal elastase or 3-day fat stool sampling. More recent studies have demonstrated that the degree of pancreatic exocrine function appears to correlate with the development of CFRD. Soave et al. demonstrated a causal relationship between the level of serum trypsinogen on the newborn screen (a marker of exocrine pancreatic function used to diagnose CF) and the development of CFRD over time [15]. Trypsinogen is an inactive pancreatic enzyme precursor required for protein digestion and absorption. It is converted to trypsin when secreted into the small intestine, but this process is inhibited in CF and results in an elevated serum trypsinogen. A significant elevation in the blood levels of immunoreactive trypsinogen (IRT) on newborn screening is used to identify neonates with CF. The IRT level is known to decline rapidly over Time with ongoing pancreatic destruction. Soave et al. postulated that patients with CF who had more significant pancreatic disease at birth would have IRT levels that had already started to decline and would be relatively lower than the rest of the CF cohort [15]. They also demonstrated that those children with relatively low IRT amongst the CF cohort had an increased risk of CFRD, thus confirming the relationship between exocrine pancreatic function and endocrine disease.

The presence of CF liver disease appears to be a significant risk factor in the development of CFRD. Leung et al. examined over 700 liver ultrasounds of patients with CF and found that patients with the features of heterogenous or cirrhotic liver disease on ultrasound were more likely to have abnormalities of glucose tolerance, including CFRD, than those with normal liver ultrasounds [56]. The relationship between liver disease and CFRD remains unclear. It could be a result of the more severe genotypes causing CFRD also increasing the risk of liver disease, or it could be the result of a non-CFTR genetic modifier.

Abnormal glucose tolerance is a known risk factor for progression to CFRD. CF patients with glucose abnormalities are up to 11 times more likely to develop early CFRD than other 6–9-year-old patients [48].

4. The clinical impact of glucose abnormalities in CF

Glucose abnormalities in CF are associated with significantly increased morbidity and mortality [2]. Prior to the introduction of routine screening for CFRD, less than 25% of CFRD patients survived to age 30, compared with 60% of patients without diabetes [57]. When Moran et al. examined female CF cohorts with and without CFRD in the 1990s and compared them with cohorts after the introduction of routine CFRD screening, mortality rates had halved: 6.9 per 100 patients years in patients with CFRD versus 3.2 per 100 patient years in CF without diabetes, with similar results seen in men were reported [58]. Although mortality rates for patients with CFRD have seen a marked improvement, a significant difference between CF patients with and without diabetes persists [59].

CFRD leads to a significant increase in respiratory exacerbations, increased infection with CF pathogens [60] (including *Pseudomonas aeruginosa*) and poorer lung function [57, 61]. The mechanism by which insulin deficiency resulting in CFRD has such a negative impact on lung function in CF is probably multifactorial. The hyperglycaemic environment is said to create a "pro-inflammatory" environment, optimal for bacterial growth and colonisation that allows CF pathogens to thrive [52]. In vitro studies have demonstrated an amplification of bacterial growth, in particular *Staphylococcus aureus* and *P. aeruginosa* with increasing glucose concentrations [62], and this evidence supports the hypothesis of glycaemic abnormalities playing a significant and direct role in the infection and colonisation of patients with CF.

http://dx.doi.org/10.5772/66452

Blood glucose levels >8 mmol/L correlate with increased airway glucose levels in patients with CF [62]. In non-CF patients, elevated airway glucose has been demonstrated to be a risk factor for respiratory infections, including MRSA (based on studies in patients intubated due to critical illness in the intensive care unit [63]). When Brennan et al. examined the airway glucose of patients with CF, they demonstrated that even patients with normal glucose tolerance on OGTT had glucose in their airway for longer periods of time than the control population. The duration of time spent with airway glucose levels >8 mmol/L correlated with the degree of glucose abnormality [62]. The level at which glucose appears in the airway is much lower than the 2-h OGTT glycaemic threshold for CFRD and also appears to be very close to the level of blood glucose level (BGL) which correlates with significant nutritional and respiratory decline [64].

Respiratory tract infections may not entirely account for the deterioration in lung function seen in patients with CF. Patients with diabetes mellitus from other causes have also been demonstrated to have poorer lung function than matched controls, even in the absence of respiratory disease [65, 66]. It is unclear whether this is a direct result of glucose in the airways or an indirect result of inflammation from relative insulin deficiency.

Nutrition in CF has a direct correlation with survival [67], and insulin, an anabolic hormone, plays an integral role in maintaining weight and building muscle [18]. When CF patients are insulin deficient, this manifests as poorer nutritional status. Multiple studies have demonstrated the impact of CFRD and insulin deficiency on nutrition and growth [37]. The data of over 8000 CF patients on the epidemiologic study of cystic fibrosis (ESCF) was analysed in 2005 and confirmed a greater impairment in nutrition in the CFRD group when compared with the nondiabetic group [47]. The CFRD cohort had statistically lower height for age percentiles, weight for age percentiles and BMI ($p < 0.001$ for all three parameters). A statistically significant difference in body weight and BMI has also been demonstrated in the "prediabetic" CF patients when compared with CF patients with normal glucose tolerance [61]. This decline was detected by Lanng et al. in some patients 4 years prior to the diagnosis of CFRD being. Given the insidious nature of glycaemic abnormalities and the inherent difficulties with nutrition in patients with CF, particularly those with exocrine pancreatic insufficiency, the impact of insulin deficiency is often not recognised until CFRD is diagnosed on routine screening.

5. The spectrum of glucose abnormalities in CF

Insulin deficiency is progressive and results in a deterioration of glucose tolerance over time. CFRD lies at the end of a spectrum of glucose abnormalities. Glycaemic categories in CF are determined based on the results of the oral glucose tolerance test (OGTT) [51]. To perform an OGTT, a glucose load of 1.75 g/kg (maximum 75 g) is consumed after fasting. Classically the blood glucose level (BGL) is measured at 0 and 120 min [68]. Additional information about glucose tolerance is gained by also checking the BGL at 30 min, 60 min and 90 min, i.e. a 30-min sampled OGTT [64].

The diagnosis of CFRD is made based on the American Diabetic Association (ADA) criteria [51] (see **Table 1**). CFRD is diagnosed when the 2-h OGTT level is ≥ 11.1 mmol/L and can

Category	Fasting level	Midpoint peak (1 h)	2-h plasma level
Normal glucose tolerance	<7 mmol/L	<11.1 mmol/L	<7.8 mmol/L
Indeterminate glycaemia (INDET)	<7 mmol/L	≥11.1 mmol/L	<7.8 mmol/L
Impaired glucose tolerance (IGT)	<7 mmol/L		≥7.8 and < 11.1 mmol/L
CFRD without fasting hyperglycaemia	<7 mmol/L		≥11.1 mmol/L
CFRD with fasting hyperglycaemia	≥7 mmol/L		≥11.1 mmol/L

Table 1. Classification of abnormalities of glucose tolerance in cystic fibrosis on OGTT.

occur with or without fasting hyperglycaemia (fasting BGL ≥ 7.0 mmol/L is defined as fasting hyperglycaemia). Fasting hyperglycaemia can also be considered diagnostic of CFRD, if still abnormal when repeated. One fasting BGL ≥ 7.0 mmol/L and another non-fasting level ≥ 11.1 mmol/L can also make a diagnosis of CFRD. If a patient is sick and glycaemic abnormalities persist for two days, then the diagnosis can also be made. Most guidelines recommend the OGTT/BGL is repeated before the diagnosis is confirmed. Some guidelines subclassify CFRD based on the fasting BGL, but this distinction does not alter management, as insulin treatment is recommended for those with and without fasting hyperglycaemia.

Additional criteria have been published to subclassify the patients into glycaemic categories based on 30-min samples (see **Table 1**) [1]. Patients with normal glucose tolerance have fasting BGL <7.0 mmol/L and 2-h level <7.8 mmol/L. Indeterminate glycaemia (INDET) is defined as normal fasting and 2-h levels with a midpoint level ≥ 11.1 mmol/L. Impaired glucose tolerance (IGT) is defined by a 2-h level <11.1 mmol/L but ≥7.8 mmol/L.

Children with abnormal glucose tolerance and CF may fluctuate between glycaemic categories because of increasing insulin requirements at times of illness or because of variable levels of resistance. In one study 18% of CF patients with abnormal glucose tolerance had glycaemic abnormalities that improved over time. Twenty-two percent of patients had a deterioration in their glucose tolerance [27]. This variability was replicated by Lanng et al. who saw a normalisation of the patient OGTT in 58% of adult patients with CF when followed up after 5 years [69]. Yi et al. examined glucose tolerance in young children (<6 years) and found that some of these children with abnormal glucose tolerance that normalised, including those that met CFRD criteria [45]. This variability adds to the difficulty seen in managing patients with CFRD, particularly younger children.

6. Issues with the OGTT in CFRD

The OGTT was not designed to diagnose diabetes in the CF population. The test was designed to determine the treatment threshold for Pima Native American population with Type 2 diabetes based on their risk of developing microvascular complications [70].

Although microvascular diabetes complications can occur in CF, the major concern for CFRD is its impact on nutrition and lung function. Complications from chronic intermediate hyperglycaemia may also result in microvascular disease prior to the patient meeting the criteria for CFRD [71]. More practical goals would include an initiation of treatment at a time that would alleviate significant respiratory morbidity such as recurrent infections and respiratory function decline. The drop in nutritional status and weight, or poor growth in younger children because of insulin deficiency catabolism, would be a more relevant CF-specific outcome to guide diagnostic targets.

The decrease in lung function and nutrition seen in CFRD actually precedes the diagnosis by several years and is often insidious. Lanng et al. noted that a decline was present up to four years prior to the OGTT 2-h criteria being met [61]. Furthermore, insulin therapy has been demonstrated to reverse some of the nutritional decline seen in patients with abnormal glycaemia [72, 73]. However, once patients meet the criteria for CFRD, recovery of lung function is not always possible. Widger et al. postulate that by waiting until the patient meets the CFRD criteria to start insulin, the conceded progression from abnormal glucose tolerance to CFRD allows irreversible structural remodelling of the lungs that cannot be corrected with insulin therapy [74].

Further evidence for insulin therapy at an earlier stage of the glycaemic spectrum is warranted, and initial data has highlighted which patients may benefit most. Schmid et al. demonstrated that in 1000 patients with CF, patients with midpoint level ≥11.1 mmol/L (INDET) were predictive for later development of CFRD [75]. Brodsky et al. were able to establish that the 1-h level on the OGTT correlated with poorer lung function [76]. They examined 101 patients with CF and these patients with higher 1-h levels had poorer respiratory status even when corrected for nutritional status. The 2-h "diagnostic" level in this group did not correlate with BMI or lung function. The findings of Coriati et al. [77] confirm that waiting for the 2-h BGL to be diagnostic of CFRD may be too late. Their cohort of patients with indeterminate glycaemia already had significant loss of lung function, equivalent to the lung function of patients with newly diagnosed CFRD. The criteria to start insulin in the future may be determined by the patient's own risk of developing CFRD or by early clinical signals in lung function and intermediate glucose abnormalities.

Hameed et al. used a 30-min sampled OGTT and found that a peak BGL ≥ 8.2 mmol/L was reliably predictive of a decline in lung function and nutrition in the preceding year [64]. Based

Proposed new criteria	Peak blood glucose (BG_{max}) mmol/L	Blood glucose at 120 min mmol/L
CFID1	≥8.2	<11.1
CFID2	≥11.1	<11.1
CFID3		≥11.1 Without fasting hyperglycaemia
CFID4		≥11.1 With fasting hyperglycaemia

CFID = cystic fibrosis insulin deficiency.

Table 2. Proposed new staging criteria for insulin deficiency and early glucose abnormalities in CF, based on the OGTT with samples every 30 min.

on these results, this group proposed a new staging criteria to identify insulin deficiency and early glucose abnormalities in patients with CF (see **Table 2**) [78]. Cystic fibrosis insulin deficiencies (CFID) 4 and 3 correspond to existing CFRD categories with and without fasting hyperglycaemia, respectively. CFID 1 and 2 are earlier stages of insulin deficiency that are distinct from impaired glucose tolerance (IGT) because they are based on the peak glucose level and have 2-h levels < 11.1. CFID 1 is defined by a midpoint peak glucose level ≥8.2 mmol/L, and CFID2 has a midpoint glucose peak ≥11.1 mmol/L.

7. Continuous glucose monitoring in CF

Continuous glucose monitoring (CGM) has been used for several years in the management of Type 1 diabetes although it is not licenced for use as a diagnostic device. CGM uses a small probe inserted into the subcutaneous space where it measures interstitial glucose levels. Inserting the device is a relatively simple procedure that can be done within a few minutes in a clinic environment. It is easy to remove at home by the patient or carer, without any specific medical training. The device averages the glucose readings every five minutes and can be worn for several days whilst the patient continues to participate in normal activities and consumes their normal diet. The CGM device has been validated in CF and non-CF populations and shown to correlate with plasma glucose measurements [79, 80]. When compared with OGTT, CGM appears to be reproducible and a reliable assessment of glycaemic abnormalities. When used in Type 1 diabetes, Bergenstal was able to demonstrate that children and adults on insulin pumps had improved glycaemic control, as measured by HbA_{1c} than those who did not use CGM [81].

CGM may be particularly useful in managing cystic fibrosis. CF patients frequently demonstrate early postprandial hyperglycaemia [79, 82, 83], reflected by elevations in readings on a 30-min sampled OGTT in the setting of a normal 2-h level. This intermittent postprandial hyperglycaemia may be reflected in the poor correlation of HbA_{1c} (glycated haemoglobin) with early glycaemic abnormalities in CF. HbA_{1c} represents an index of the average of blood glucose concentrations in the preceding 2–3-month period, and the result is influenced by the half-life of the red cells [84]. When measured in CF, it is a poor indicator of glycaemic abnormalities as it is often still normal by the time a diagnosis of CFRD has been made. The poor sensitivity of the test may result from the intermittent nature of hyperglycaemia in patients with CF, which is not revealed in the HbA_{1c} level when the glucose levels are "averaged", as well as increased red cell turnover in CF.

CGM provides a useful tool to guide insulin treatment once the diagnosis of CFRD has been made [79], but it may also offer a potential opportunity to capture the moments of postprandial hyperglycaemia in CF in the screening and diagnostic phase. In CF patients with normal glucose tolerance on OGTT, abnormalities on CGM have been detected [79, 82, 83]. This could reflect the fact that patients with CF undergo a period of fasting prior to their glucose load in the OGTT which will only measure two values. When a CGM is worn, patients can be at home and may consume their normal CF diet including a carbohydrate load that may exceed the glucose level consumed during an OGTT. In the same way that HbA_{1c} may not reflect a true picture of glycaemic abnormalities in CF, so too may the OGTT underestimate the hyperglycaemia in these patients, particularly in the early phase of glucose abnormalities.

CGM may be a useful device in predicting which children with CF will develop glycaemic abnormalities. Schiaffini et al. performed OGTT and CGM on children with CF and then repeated the OGTT after 2 years. Children who had diabetic excursions on CGM at baseline, even those with normal glucose tolerance on OGTT, developed impaired glucose tolerance or CFRD when the OGTT was repeated 2 years later [83]. Initial data on CGM does appear to suggest that this tool may be useful in identifying clinically significant glucose abnormalities in CF. Leclercq et al. demonstrated, in a CF population with normal OGTT, that patients who recorded glucose levels in the diabetic range (≥11.1 mmol/L) on CGM had poorer lung function and greater colonisation with CF respiratory pathogens such as *P. aeruginosa* [85].

Glycaemic abnormalities are known to have a significant impact on nutrition in patients with CF. CGM may provide an opportunity to highlight which children are at risk of nutritional decline secondary to abnormities of glucose tolerance as described in the study by Hameed et al. [64]. In this study of 25 children with CF undergoing CGM, if ≥ 4.5% of the study duration was spent with an interstitial glucose reading >7.8 mmol/L, this was predictive of a decline in weight standard deviation score. This CGM criterion had a sensitivity of 89% and a specificity of 86% in detecting this nutritional decline. CGM abnormalities do appear to be clinically significant, but there are not studies as yet demonstrating a benefit from treatment based on CGM recordings in CF, and the device is not yet licenced to make a diagnosis of diabetes.

8. Management of CFRD

The main aim of CFRD treatment is to correct the hyperglycaemia and its downstream effects on respiratory function and infections, in addition to reversing significant protein catabolism secondary to insulin deficiency. Optimal management has been shown to improve lung function and morbidity [72]. Although a drop in mortality from late CFRD diagnosis has been seen, the risk of early mortality is still higher in this population. The mainstay of treatment is exogenous insulin therapy, but studies are underway examining the benefits of dietary changes and the use of oral hypoglycaemic agents in CF.

8.1. Insulin

Insulin plays a major role in the management of CFRD. Insulin replacement by subcutaneous injection in CFRD has been shown to improve lung function and reduce pulmonary exacerbation frequency [86]. It has also been shown to benefit the nutritional status of the patient, with an improvement in growth seen in children with CF [73]. Recent studies have also demonstrated that insulin therapy in the prediabetic phase may also play a valuable role in the management of patients with CF. Hameed et al. were able to replicate previous studies demonstrating a benefit of insulin therapy on lung function and nutrition in patients with CF and revealed an improvement in weight standard deviation score ($p = 0.003$) and lung function (FEV1 improvement $p = 0.004$) with once daily insulin injections (detemir, Levemir™) [73].

Insulin is given via subcutaneous injection. Unlike Type 1 diabetes, a once daily dose of long-acting insulin may be all that is required to demonstrate a benefit for this population [73]. Insulin doses vary with each patient, but because of the important anabolic role insulin plays in growth and nutrition, the highest tolerated dose without hypoglycaemia or other side effects is generally recommended [52] (taking into account patient-specific factors such as ability to recognise hypoglycaemic symptoms). The dose prescribed may vary over time with increasing requirements during times of relative increase in insulin resistance such as with glucocorticoid use or during periods of growth and pregnancy. Given the progressive nature of insulin deficiency in CF, increasing requirements may be seen over time, particularly in the paediatric population with CF that have age- and weight-based doses.

Insulin pumps that continuously deliver a small amount of insulin into the subcutaneous space have been used in patients with CFRD [87] although the uptake in CF has been poor when compared with other forms of diabetes. When wearing a pump, patients are currently required to undertake much more intensive finger-prick blood glucose testing than that required with a once daily insulin injection. This may prove to be too onerous for patients with CFRD who already have a significant treatment burden with multiple oral and nebulised medications and physiotherapy. Future insulin pump devices may include closed loop systems, in which interstitial glucose levels measured by CGM calibrate the rate and amount of insulin secreted by the pump [88]. These devices are currently under investigation for Type 1 DM, but there are no data published about their use in CFRD to date.

8.2. Nutrition

Nutritional education and support are of utmost importance for patients with a diagnosis of CFRD. Children with CF require a higher caloric intake (may need up to 200% of usual recommendations [89]) to achieve optimal nutritional and growth targets. If nutritional targets are not met, there may be significant consequences as a lower BMI has been associated with increased mortality in CF [67]. These additional calories are best taken from fat and protein-based meals, but a significant proportion is taken from carbohydrates [90]. Patients with abnormalities of glucose tolerance and CFRD will be required to recognise carbohydrates in their diet, as the carbohydrate load will affect the glucose level and the resulting insulin requirements. This is usually done by educating the family and patient about carbohydrate-insulin ratios.

There are very limited data regarding the dietary management of CFRD. This is of particular significance given that hyperglycaemia has been demonstrated to worsen glycaemic abnormalities in CF, possibly by potentiating beta-cell apoptosis. As such, glycaemic control in CFRD needs to be tight, and diets that perpetuate postprandial hyperglycaemia may have a negative impact on glycaemic abnormalities in CF and increase insulin requirements. A low glycaemic diet is often recommended in Type 1 and Type 2 diabetes to optimise control of hyperglycaemia and has been shown to decrease insulin requirements and improve glucose homeostasis, without having a significant impact on quality of life for these patients. Whereas weight loss due to change in diet may be beneficial in Type 2 DM, this may have serious negative consequence in CF. There is not enough information in the literature to recommend any dietary changes that might improve glycaemic control or prevent or delay progression to CFRD if instituted at an earlier stage.

8.3. Oral hypoglycaemic agents

Oral agents do not play a role in the management of patients with CFRD. Many agents target insulin resistance (e.g. metformin), which is not a major feature in the early glycaemic abnormalities of CF where insulin deficiency plays the key role and as such will not be of significant benefit to CF patients. Significant side effects from oral hypoglycaemic agents such as hepatotoxicity are a serious complication for the CF population where a significant proportion may develop CF liver disease [91]. Insulin therapy in states of insulin deficiency such as Type 1 diabetes has been shown to preserve insulin secretion and "rest" the residual beta cells. Conversely, agents that stimulate insulin secretion may potentially hasten beta-cell loss. For example, agents such as repaglinide may be useful in the short term but ultimately have a negative long-term impact.

8.4. The role of potentiators in CFRD

Evidence for the use of potentiators in CFRD is limited, but a few pilot studies have been published that suggest a benefit on glucose homeostasis in CF. In a single pair of CF siblings with abnormal glucose tolerance (one with CFRD) and gating mutations, a reduction in the glucose AUC and an improvement in the insulin secretion profile was demonstrated after the introduction of ivacaftor (Kalydeco™). Bellin et al. also demonstrated improvements in glucose homeostasis after the introduction of ivacaftor. In this group of five CF patients with glucose abnormalities, four of five demonstrated improvements in insulin secretion. The patient whose insulin secretion did not improve had long-standing CFRD, whereas the others had earlier glycaemic abnormalities. Theoretically, the patient with long-standing CFRD could already have undergone such significant pancreatic destruction that the abnormalities of glucose tolerance could not be corrected at the level of the CFTR.

9. Complications of CFRD

Long-standing hyperglycaemia and insulin deficiency will result in an increase in respiratory exacerbations and morbidity and poorer nutrition. It will also result in complications from chronic hyperglycaemia seen in other forms of diabetes. Historically the life-limiting nature of CF and in particularly those with CFRD meant that CF patients were unlikely to live long enough to develop end-organ dysfunction from the macrovascular and microvascular complications seen in other forms of diabetes. With an improvement in life expectancy, these long-term issues need to be addressed, and routine screening needs to be a part of CF clinical care. This will include examination for neuropathy and retinopathy and urine screening for microalbuminuria. In one study, 10 years after the diagnosis of CFRD has been made, subjects with fasting glycaemia demonstrated rates of microalbuminuria of approximately 14%, retinopathy 16%, neuropathy 55% and autonomic gastropathy 50% [51]. Gilchrist et al. reported retinopathy in three patients with abnormal glucose tolerance but not meeting criteria for CFRD [71] which further supports the proposition that the OGTT may not be the ideal test for significant glycaemic abnormalities in patients with CF.

10. Conclusion

Cystic fibrosis–related diabetes continues to pose a significant risk of increased morbidity and mortality to the CF population. However, CFRD lies at the endpoint of spectrum of glucose abnormalities, and increasing evidence implies that earlier glycaemic abnormalities may also be clinically significant. The standard OGTT does not appear to be sensitive enough to pick up early, clinically significant abnormalities of glucose tolerance secondary to insulin deficiency and the dysregulation of insulin secretion detected in CF patients. Hyperglycaemia in CF affects lung function, risk of respiratory pathogens, nutrition and growth in young children, and treating teams need to be proactive in the screening and diagnosis of glycaemic abnormalities that may be insidious and potentially irreversible if recognised late. Early recognition of hyperglycaemia in CF is required to prevent significant morbidity. Novel techniques such as continuous glucose monitoring may play a role in screening and early identification of at risk patients, as they have been shown to be predictive of significant glucose abnormalities in the future such as CFRD, but there is not enough evidence as yet to recommend their routine use in diagnosis. Future directions may include the use of potentiators and correctors in CF which appear to have potential to correct abnormalities of glucose tolerance but may be limited if instituted late and once significant pancreatic destruction has occurred.

Acknowledgements

SH and CFV are grateful for funding assistance from the National Health and Medical Research Council of Australia, Australasian Cystic Fibrosis Research Trust, Regional Diabetes Support Scheme, Sydney Children's Hospital Foundation and Australasian Paediatric Endocrine Care Grant from Pfizer and for industry support from Novo Nordisk, Medtronic and Abbott Diagnostics. BP has been awarded a scholarship from the Thoracic Society of Australia and New Zealand and Vertex.

Author details

Bernadette Prentice[1,2*], Shihab Hameed[2,3], Chee Y. Ooi[2,4], Charles F. Verge[2,3] and John Widger[1,2]

*Address all correspondence to: bernadette.prentice@health.nsw.gov.au

1 Department of Respiratory Medicine, Sydney Children's Hospital, Randwick, NSW, Australia

2 Discipline of Paediatrics, School of Women's and Children's Health, The University of New South Wales, Sydney, NSW, Australia

3 Department of Endocrinology, Sydney Children's Hospital, Randwick, NSW, Australia

4 Department of Gastroenterology, Sydney Children's Hospital, Randwick, NSW, Australia

References

[1] Hameed, S., Jaffe, A., and Verge, C.F., *Advances in the detection and management of cystic fibrosis related diabetes*. Curr Opin Pediatr, 2015. **27**(4): pp. 525-33.

[2] Chamnan, P., et al., *Diabetes as a determinant of mortality in cystic fibrosis*. Diabetes Care, 2010. **33**(2): pp. 311-6.

[3] Couce, M., et al., *Diabetes mellitus in cystic fibrosis is characterized by islet amyloidosis*. J Clin Endocrinol Metab, 1996. **81**(3): pp. 1267-72.

[4] Iannucci, A., et al., *Endocrine pancreas in cystic fibrosis: an immunohistochemical study*. Hum Pathol, 1984. **15**(3): pp. 278-84.

[5] Sequeiros, I., et al., *MRI appearance of the pancreas in patients with cystic fibrosis: a comparison of pancreas volume in diabetic and non-diabetic patients*. British J Radiol, 2014.

[6] Abdul-Karim, F.W., et al., *Islets of Langerhans in adolescents and adults with cystic fibrosis. A quantitative study*. Arch Pathol Lab Med, 1986. **110**(7): pp. 602-6.

[7] Milner, A.D., *Blood glucose and serum insulin levels in children with cystic fibrosis*. Arch Dis Child, 1969. **44**(235): pp. 351-5.

[8] Gelfand, I.M., Eugster, E.A., and Haddad, N.G., *Infancy-onset cystic fibrosis-related diabetes*. Diabetes Care, 2005. **28**(10): pp. 2593-4.

[9] Olivier, A.K., et al., *Abnormal endocrine pancreas function at birth in cystic fibrosis ferrets*. J Clin Invest, 2012. **122**(10): pp. 3755-68.

[10] Uc, A., et al., *Glycaemic regulation and insulin secretion are abnormal in cystic fibrosis pigs despite sparing of islet cell mass*. Clin Sci (Lond), 2015. **128**(2): pp. 131-42.

[11] Bellin, M.D., et al., *Insulin secretion improves in cystic fibrosis following ivacaftor correction of CFTR: a small pilot study*. Pediatr Diabetes, 2013. **14**(6): pp. 417-21.

[12] Tsabari, R., et al., *CFTR potentiator therapy ameliorates impaired insulin secretion in CF patients with a gating mutation*. J Cyst Fibros, 2015.

[13] Blackman, S.M., et al., *A susceptibility gene for type 2 diabetes confers substantial risk for diabetes complicating cystic fibrosis*. Diabetologia, 2009. **52**(9): pp. 1858-65.

[14] Blackman, S.M., et al., *Genetic modifiers play a substantial role in diabetes complicating cystic fibrosis*. J Clin Endocrinol Metab, 2009. **94**(4): pp. 1302-9.

[15] Soave, D., et al., *Evidence for a causal relationship between early exocrine pancreatic disease and cystic fibrosis-related diabetes: a Mendelian randomization study*. Diabetes, 2014. **63**(6): pp. 2114-9.

[16] Gold, G., Gishizky, M.L., and Grodsky, G.M., *Evidence that glucose "marks" beta cells resulting in preferential release of newly synthesized insulin*. Science, 1982. **218**(4567): pp. 56-8.

[17] Daniel, S., et al., *Identification of the docked granule pool responsible for the first phase of glucose-stimulated insulin secretion*. Diabetes, 1999. **48**(9): pp. 1686-90.

[18] Newsholme, P., et al., *Nutrient regulation of insulin secretion and action*. J Endocrinol, 2014. **221**(3): pp. R105-20.

[19] Del Prato, S., Marchetti, P., and Bonadonna, R.C., *Phasic insulin release and metabolic regulation in type 2 diabetes*. Diabetes, 2002. **51**(1): pp. S109-16.

[20] Jing, X., et al., *Ca V 2.3 calcium channels control second-phase insulin release*. J Clin Invest, 2005. **115**(1): pp. 146-54.

[21] Kelly, A., and Moran, A., *Update on cystic fibrosis-related diabetes*. J Cyst Fibros, 2013. **12**(4): pp. 318-31.

[22] Caumo, A., and Luzi, L., *First-phase insulin secretion: does it exist in real life? Considerations on shape and function*. Am J Physiol Endocrinol Metab, 2004. **287**(3): pp. E371-85.

[23] O'Donovan, D., et al., *Effects of lipase inhibition on gastric emptying of, and on the glycaemic, insulin and cardiovascular responses to, a high-fat/carbohydrate meal in type 2 diabetes*. Diabetologia, 2004. **47**(12): pp. 2208-14.

[24] Perano, S., et al., *Cystic fibrosis related diabetes--a new perspective on the optimal management of postprandial glycemia*. J Diabetes Complications, 2014. **28**(6): pp. 904-11.

[25] Barrio, R., *Management of endocrine disease: cystic fibrosis-related diabetes: novel pathogenic insights opening new therapeutic avenues*. Eur J Endocrinol, 2015. **172**(4): pp. R131-41.

[26] Amori, R.E., Lau, J., and Pittas, A.G., *Efficacy and safety of incretin therapy in type 2 diabetes: systematic review and meta-analysis*. JAMA, 2007. **298**(2): pp. 194-206.

[27] Milla, C.E., Warwick, W.J., and Moran, A., *Trends in pulmonary function in patients with cystic fibrosis correlate with the degree of glucose intolerance at baseline*. Am J Respir Crit Care Med, 2000. **162**(3 Pt 1): pp. 891-5.

[28] Ahmad, T., Nelson, R., and Taylor, R., *Insulin sensitivity and metabolic clearance rate of insulin in cystic fibrosis*. Metabolism, 1994. **43**(2): pp. 163-7.

[29] Moran, A., et al., *Insulin sensitivity in cystic fibrosis*. Diabetes, 1994. **43**(8): pp. 1020-6.

[30] Hardin, D.S., et al., *Mechanisms of insulin resistance in cystic fibrosis*. Am J Physiol Endocrinol Metab, 2001. **281**(5): pp. E1022-8.

[31] Widger, J., et al., *Glucose tolerance during pulmonary exacerbations in children with cystic fibrosis*. PLoS One, 2012. **7**(9): pp. e44844.

[32] MacDonald, A., *Nutritional management of cystic fibrosis*. Arch Dis Child, 1996. **74**(1): pp. 81-7.

[33] Smith, D., Clarke, J., and Stableforth, D., *A nocturnal nasogastric feeding programme in cystic fibrosis adults*. J Hum Nutr Diet, 1994. **7**(4): pp. 257-62.

[34] Amiel, S.A., et al., *Impaired insulin action in puberty. A contributing factor to poor glycemic control in adolescents with diabetes.* N Engl J Med, 1986. **315**(4): pp. 215-9.

[35] Hardin, D.S., et al., *The metabolic effects of pregnancy in cystic fibrosis.* Obstet Gynecol, 2005. **106**(2): pp. 367-75.

[36] Moran, A., *Endocrine complications of cystic fibrosis.* Adolesc Med Clin, 2002. **13**(1): p. 145.

[37] Bismuth, E., et al., *Glucose tolerance and insulin secretion, morbidity, and death in patients with cystic fibrosis.* The Journal of Pediatrics, 2008. **152**(4): pp. 540-5.e1.

[38] Ntimbane, T., et al., *Cystic fibrosis-related diabetes: from CFTR dysfunction to oxidative stress.* Clin Biochem Rev, 2009. **30**(4): pp. 153-77.

[39] Galli, F., et al., *Oxidative stress and antioxidant therapy in cystic fibrosis.* Biochim Biophys Acta, 2012. **1822**(5): pp. 690-713.

[40] Ziai, S., et al., *Could T cells be involved in lung deterioration and hyperglycemia in cystic fibrosis?* Diabetes Res Clin Pract, 2014. **105**(1): pp. 22-9.

[41] Roep, B.O., and Peakman, M., *Diabetogenic T lymphocytes in human type 1 diabetes.* Curr Opin Immunol, 2011. **23**(6): pp. 746-53.

[42] Hotamisligil, G.S., et al., *IRS-1-mediated inhibition of insulin receptor tyrosine kinase activity in TNF-alpha- and obesity-induced insulin resistance.* Science, 1996. **271**(5249): pp. 665-8.

[43] Lanng, S., et al., *Diabetes mellitus in Danish cystic fibrosis patients: prevalence and late diabetic complications.* Acta Paediatr, 1994. **83**(1): pp. 72-7.

[44] Moran, A., et al., *Abnormal glucose metabolism in cystic fibrosis.* J Pediatr, 1998. **133**(1): pp. 10-7.

[45] Yi, Y., et al., *Abnormal glucose tolerance in infants and young children with cystic fibrosis.* American Journal of Respiratory and Critical Care Medicine, 2016.

[46] Rosenecker, J., et al., *Genetic determination of diabetes mellitus in patients with cystic fibrosis. Multicenter Cystic Fibrosis Study Group.* J Pediatr, 1995. **127**(3): pp. 441-3.

[47] Marshall, B.C., et al., *Epidemiology of cystic fibrosis-related diabetes.* J Pediatr, 2005. **146**(5): pp. 681-7.

[48] Ode, K.L., et al., *Oral glucose tolerance testing in children with cystic fibrosis.* Pediatr Diabetes, 2010. **11**(7): pp. 487-92.

[49] Noronha, R.M., et al., *Importance of screening with oral glucose tolerance test for early diagnosis of cystic fibrosis-related diabetes mellitus.* Pediatr Diabetes, 2014. **15**(4): pp. 309-12.

[50] Rana, M., et al., *Increased detection of cystic-fibrosis-related diabetes in Australia.* Arch Dis Child, 2011. **96**(9): pp. 823-6.

[51] Moran, A., et al., *Clinical care guidelines for cystic fibrosis-related diabetes: a position statement of the American Diabetes Association and a clinical practice guideline of the Cystic Fibrosis*

Foundation, endorsed by the Pediatric Endocrine Society. Diabetes Care, 2010. **33**(12): pp. 2697-708.

[52] Moran, A., et al., *ISPAD Clinical Practice Consensus Guidelines 2014. Management of cystic fibrosis-related diabetes in children and adolescents*. Pediatric Diabetes, 2014. **15** (20): pp. 65-76.

[53] Adler, A.I., et al., *Genetic determinants and epidemiology of cystic fibrosis-related diabetes: results from a British cohort of children and adults*. Diabetes Care, 2008. **31**(9): pp. 1789-94.

[54] Boyle, M.P., and De Boeck, K., *A new era in the treatment of cystic fibrosis: correction of the underlying CFTR defect*. Lancet Respir Med, 2013. **1**(2): pp. 158-63.

[55] De Boeck, K., et al., *The relative frequency of CFTR mutation classes in European patients with cystic fibrosis*. J Cyst Fibros, 2014. **13**(4): pp. 403-9.

[56] Leung, D.H., et al., *Baseline ultrasound and clinical correlates in children with cystic fibrosis*. J Pediatr, 2015. **167**(4): pp. 862-8 e2.

[57] Finkelstein, S.M., et al., *Diabetes mellitus associated with cystic fibrosis*. J Pediatr, 1988. **112**(3): pp. 373-7.

[58] Moran, A., et al., *Cystic fibrosis-related diabetes: current trends in prevalence, incidence, and mortality*. Diabetes Care, 2009. **32**(9): pp. 1626-31.

[59] Lewis, C., et al., *Diabetes-related mortality in adults with cystic fibrosis. Role of genotype and sex*. Am J Respir Crit Care Med, 2015. **191**(2): pp. 194-200.

[60] Campbell, J., et al., *328 Use of an insulin pump combined with the FreeStyle Libre interstitial glucose monitor in a needle-phobic adolescent with cystic fibrosis-related diabetes*. J Cyst Fibros, 2015. **14**: p. S142.

[61] Lanng, S., et al., *Influence of the development of diabetes mellitus on clinical status in patients with cystic fibrosis*. Eur J Pediatr, 1992. **151**(9): pp. 684-7.

[62] Brennan, A.L., et al., *Airway glucose concentrations and effect on growth of respiratory pathogens in cystic fibrosis*. J Cyst Fibros, 2007. **6**(2): pp. 101-9.

[63] Philips, B.J., et al., *Glucose in bronchial aspirates increases the risk of respiratory MRSA in intubated patients*. Thorax, 2005. **60**(9): pp. 761-4.

[64] Hameed, S., et al., *Early glucose abnormalities in cystic fibrosis are preceded by poor weight gain*. Diabetes Care, 2010. **33**(2): pp. 221-6.

[65] van den Borst, B., et al., *Pulmonary function in diabetes: a metaanalysis*. Chest, 2010. **138**(2): pp. 393-406.

[66] Mohamad, I.L., et al., *Evaluation of pulmonary function changes in children with type 1 diabetes mellitus in Upper Egypt*. Therapeutic Adv Endocrinol Metab, 2015: p. 2042018815580514.

[67] Kraemer, R., et al., *Relative underweight in cystic fibrosis and its prognostic value*. Acta Paediatr Scand, 1978. **67**(1): pp. 33-7.

[68] Moran, A., et al., *Diagnosis, screening and management of cystic fibrosis related diabetes mellitus: a consensus conference report*. Diabetes Res Clin Pract, 1999. **45**(1): pp. 61-73.

[69] Lanng, S., et al., *Glucose tolerance in patients with cystic fibrosis: five year prospective study*. BMJ, 1995. **311**(7006): pp. 655-9.

[70] Bennett, P.H., Burch, T.A., and Miller, M., *Diabetes mellitus in American (Pima) Indians*. Lancet, 1971. **2**(7716): pp. 125-8.

[71] Gilchrist, F.J., et al., *Diabetic retinopathy in patients who do not meet the diagnostic criteria for cystic fibrosis related diabetes*. Practical Diabetes, 2015. **32**(9): pp. 333-335a.

[72] Lanng, S., et al., *Diabetes mellitus in cystic fibrosis: effect of insulin therapy on lung function and infections*. Acta Paediatr, 1994. **83**(8): pp. 849-53.

[73] Hameed, S., et al., *Once daily insulin detemir in cystic fibrosis with insulin deficiency*. Arch Dis Child, 2012. **97**(5): pp. 464-7.

[74] Widger, J., Ranganathan, S., and Robinson, P.J., *Progression of structural lung disease on CT scans in children with cystic fibrosis related diabetes*. J Cyst Fibros, 2013. **12**(3): pp. 216-21.

[75] Schmid, K., et al., *Predictors for future cystic fibrosis-related diabetes by oral glucose tolerance test*. J Cyst Fibros, 2014. **13**(1): pp. 80-5.

[76] Brodsky, J., et al., *Elevation of 1-hour plasma glucose during oral glucose tolerance testing is associated with worse pulmonary function in cystic fibrosis*. Diabetes Care, 2011. **34**(2): pp. 292-5.

[77] Coriati, A., et al., *Characterization of patients with cystic fibrosis presenting an indeterminate glucose tolerance (INDET)*. J Cyst Fibros, 2016. **15**(1): pp. 127-32.

[78] Hameed, S., Jaffe, A., and Verge, C.F., *Cystic fibrosis related diabetes (CFRD)--the end stage of progressive insulin deficiency*. Pediatr Pulmonol, 2011. **46**(8): pp. 747-60.

[79] O'Riordan, S.M., et al., *Validation of continuous glucose monitoring in children and adolescents with cystic fibrosis: a prospective cohort study*. Diabetes Care, 2009. **32**(6): pp. 1020-2.

[80] Dobson, L., Sheldon, C.D., and Hattersley, A.T., *Validation of interstitial fluid continuous glucose monitoring in cystic fibrosis*. Diabetes Care, 2003. **26**(6): pp. 1940-1.

[81] Bergenstal, R.M., et al., *Effectiveness of sensor-augmented insulin-pump therapy in type 1 diabetes*. N Engl J Med, 2010. **363**(4): pp. 311-20.

[82] Moreau, F., et al., *Continuous glucose monitoring in cystic fibrosis patients according to the glucose tolerance*. Horm Metab Res, 2008. **40**(7): pp. 502-6.

[83] Schiaffini, R., et al., *Abnormal glucose tolerance in children with cystic fibrosis: the predictive role of continuous glucose monitoring system*. Eur J Endocrinol, 2010. **162**(4): pp. 705-10.

[84] Bennett, C., Guo, M., and Dharmage, S., *HbA1c as a screening tool for detection of type 2 diabetes: a systematic review*. Diabet Med, 2007. **24**(4): pp. 333-43.

[85] Leclercq, A., et al., *Early assessment of glucose abnormalities during continuous glucose monitoring associated with lung function impairment in cystic fibrosis patients*. J Cyst Fibros, 2014. **13**(4): pp. 478-84.

[86] Moran, A., et al., *Epidemiology, pathophysiology, and prognostic implications of cystic fibrosis-related diabetes: a technical review*. Diabetes Care, 2010. **33**(12): pp. 2677-83.

[87] Hardin, D.S., et al., *Use of the insulin pump in treat cystic fibrosis related diabetes*. J Cyst Fibros, 2009. **8**(3): pp. 174-8.

[88] Thabit, H., et al., *Home use of an artificial beta cell in type 1 Diabetes*. N Engl J Med, 2015. **373**(22): pp. 2129-40.

[89] Stallings, V.A., et al., *Evidence-based practice recommendations for nutrition-related management of children and adults with cystic fibrosis and pancreatic insufficiency: results of a systematic review*. J Am Diet Assoc, 2008. **108**(5): pp. 832-9.

[90] Wilson, D., et al., *Challenges in the dietary treatment of cystic fibrosis related diabetes mellitus*. Clin Nutr, 2000. **19**(2): pp. 87-93.

[91] Colombo, C., et al., *Liver disease in cystic fibrosis: a prospective study on incidence, risk factors, and outcome*. Hepatology, 2002. **36**(6): pp. 1374-82.

Chapter 3

The Cystic Fibrosis Airway Microbiome and Pathogens

Ibrahim A. Janahi and Abdul Rehman

Additional information is available at the end of the chapter

http://dx.doi.org/10.5772/67846

Abstract

Cystic fibrosis (CF) is an autosomal recessive genetic disorder resulting from genetic defects in the gene coding for the cystic fibrosis transmembrane conductance regulator (CFTR) protein. CFTR dysfunction in patients with CF leads to a number of pleiotropic manifestations with the prime pathology being mucus plugging in the airways and paranasal sinuses. Patients with CF are prone to polymicrobial infections and the airway microbiome in such patients changes continuously and evolves over time. The composition of the airway microbiome in CF patients is dependent on a number of factors including geographic variation, type of genetic mutation (e.g., ΔF508), antibiotic exposures, and chronic infection with certain pathogenic bacteria (e.g., *Pseudomonas aeruginosa*). Proteomic and genomic approaches to understanding the microbiome of patients with CF have provided new insights into the pathogenesis of this disease. High-throughput pyrosequencing, Sanger sequencing, and phylogenetic microarray analysis have enabled the recognition of multiple lineages and clonal populations of a single bacterial species within the same patient. This provides a unique opportunity to explore novel therapeutic approaches to this disease (for instance, use of probiotics and environmental manipulation) and potentially translate them into bedside clinical interventions.

Keywords: cystic fibrosis, microbiome, dysbiosis, *Pseudomonas aeruginosa*, burkholderia cenocepacia

1. Introduction

Cystic fibrosis (CF) is an autosomal recessive genetic disease caused by mutations in the CFTR (cystic fibrosis transmembrane conductance regulator) gene [1]. CF is most prevalent in the Caucasian population and is a common life-limiting disease [2]. CFTR is expressed on the apical surface of epithelial cells of the respiratory, gastrointestinal, pancreatic and reproductive tracts, and sweat glands [3]. The prime function of CFTR ion channel is to transport chloride ions across epithelial surfaces in order to maintain the osmotic gradient. Chloride ions are actively pumped out into the luminal side of the gastrointestinal and respiratory tracts, which decrease water potential on the luminal side. Subsequently, water molecules move from a higher osmotic potential to a lower osmotic potential (down the osmotic gradient) and combine with mucin glycoproteins to keep them adequately hydrated. This in turn helps to maintain the thin consistency of the mucus layer, which is essential for optimal mucociliary function [4]. Thick and viscid mucus caused by a defect in chloride-conducting transmembrane channel results in stagnation of mucus. Moreover, CFTR channel also plays an important role in regulating the transepithelial transport of sodium and bicarbonate ions [5]. Defective CFTR functioning leads to an increase in pH of the mucus layer, which compromises the innate immune system and promotes inflammation. Defects in innate immunity and chronic inflammation predispose patients to recurrent pulmonary infections, which result in permanent lung damage—the prime cause of morbidity and mortality [6]. Pulmonary system is not the only organ-system affected in CF; endocrine, gastrointestinal, and reproductive systems are also involved in this multisystem disorder [3].

The human microbiome project aims to identify and characterize microbial flora of healthy and diseased individuals [7]. Understanding the role of infectious pathogens in the pathogenesis of CF in general and pulmonary exacerbations and lung damage in particular has enabled the scientific community to devise new treatment modalities for CF patients, which can potentially improve outcomes and survival in such patients. In patients with CF, different bacteria inhabit different parts of the lung at various stages of the disease and persistent inflammation in the lungs can change and modify the composition of the microbiome [8]. For instance, methicillin-sensitive *Staphylococcus aureus* (MSSA) and *Hemophilus influenzae* are common pathogens early in life of such patients [9]. As the disease progresses, more virulent pathogens—such as *Pseudomonas aeruginosa* and methicillin-resistant *S. aureus* (MRSA)—invade the lung and cause pulmonary damage [10]. By understanding the evolution of the CF microbiome, we can gain further insights into the natural course of CF. This in turn can have important implications for developing interventions that can halt or reverse the course of progressive pulmonary damage and prolong survival and quality of life in CF patients [11]. In the following pages, we discuss the CF microbiome, its evolution and heterogeneity in CF patients, interaction between different bacteria within the CF lung and the factors that potentially affect the CF microbiome.

2. The microbiome

As mentioned previously, the human microbiome project aims to identify and characterize microbial flora of healthy and diseased individuals [7]. There is a diversity of microbes in every single human being i.e., diversity being defined as the number and distribution of a particular type of organism in a body habitat. Every human has particular and distinct microbes; dysbiosis (alteration in composition and balance) of these microbes is now thought to underlie the pathogenesis of many diseases, such as inflammatory bowel disease, *Clostridium difficile* (CD) colitis, bacterial vaginosis, obesity, and CF [12]. The human microbiome plays a very important role in human biology, defense mechanisms, metabolic processes (such as digestion, absorption, and assimilation) and even pathogenesis of acute and chronic diseases [13]. For instance, CD colitis is a disease that arises as a consequence of interaction of bacterial virulence factors, host immune mechanism and the intestinal microbiome [14]. Research studies have shown that variability in the innate host response may also impact upon the severity of CD colitis, and this variation may be accounted for by alterations in the gut microbiota [15]. Based on improved understanding of the pathogenesis of CD colitis, fecal microbiota transplantation (FMT) and other novel types of bacteriotherapy have become potentially effective treatment options for this deadly disease [16].

Another example of a disease where microbiota plays a major role in pathogenesis is Crohn's disease. The exact cause of Crohn's disease is unknown; however, evidence suggests that microbiota contribute to the underlying pathology and disease development [17]. No single bacterium has been convincingly shown to contribute to the overall pathogenesis of Crohn's disease. Instead, dysbiosis (bacterial imbalance) is more widely accepted as a leading factor in the disrupted host immune system cross-talk that results in subsequent intestinal inflammation [18]. Depletion of symbiont (beneficial) microbes (including Firmicutes, Bifidobacteriaceae, and Clostridia) in conjunction with an increase in pathobiont (harmful) microbes (such as Bacteroidetes and Enterobacteriaceae) is a striking feature observed in Crohn's disease. No single factor has been definitely identified as driving this dysbiosis; instead, a host of environmental factors—such as the diet, antibiotic exposures and possible early life infections—in the presence of underlying genetic susceptibilities may contribute to the overall pathogenesis of Crohn's disease [17].

In CF patients, composition of the microbiome of pulmonary and gastrointestinal tracts changes over time, presumably as a consequence of inflammation [19]. Most research studies have demonstrated the influence of inflammation in negatively selecting against potential pathogens. Moreover, some bacterial species may also have the ability to exploit inflammatory byproducts for their benefit, which may promote their natural selection in inflamed habitats [20]. Reactive nitrogen species produced during inflammatory responses can be exploited by pathogens for their growth. Moreover, inflammatory mediators can provide an environment for some bacteria to grow and use these inflammatory mediators for their survival [21]. Examples of such bacteria include *Escherichia coli* and *P. aeruginosa* in the gastrointestinal and respiratory tracts of CF patients, respectively. *P. aeruginosa* uses nitric oxide produced in the process of inflammation for its anaerobic respiration and promotes its growth in inflammatory environments. Likewise, *E. coli* uses increased nitrate in the environment for its anaerobic respiration and enhances its growth in the inflamed gut of CF patients [19].

3. Heterogeneity of the CF airway microbiome

Due to defects in innate immunity, CF patients are prone to polymicrobial infections and their airway microbiome changes continuously and evolves over time. The primary cause of death in CF patients is respiratory failure due to persistent and recurrent pulmonary infections with different pathogenic organisms [22]. Over the past decade, the median survival for such patients stands at 37 years despite increases in life expectancy [23]. MSSA and *H. influenzae* are one of the most common pathogens cultured from sputum samples of affected children. *P. aeruginosa* has been associated with increased morbidity as most strains of this organism are multidrug resistant. Infections with bacteria of the Bukholderia cepacia complex (BCC) are associated with a worse prognosis [24]. Likewise, other multidrug resistant organisms, such as *Achromobacter xylosoxidans* and *Stenotrophomonas maltophilia*, can also be isolated from CF patients with end-stage pulmonary disease [25]. Nontuberculous mycobacterium (NTM) has also been identified as emerging causes of infections in patients with CF and their incidence may have been underestimated in the past [26]. More recently, research studies have shown that when sputum samples obtained from adults with CF are cultured, a significantly high density of anaerobic bacteria can be isolated—the most common of which are *Streptococcus milleri*, *Prevotella* spp., *Actinomyces*, and *Veillonella* [27].

Microbes of the lower airways in all humans exist in a dynamic state. Literature published on microbiome of CF patients has shown a complex and dynamic interaction between different organisms in the airways of such patients [28]. Organisms within a single patient are genetically and phenotypically diverse and heterogeneity is detectable even in different parts of the same lung. Over a period of time, community diversity of bacteria declines in CF patients as pulmonary function declines and lung disease progressively worsens. Studies have shown that diversity of microbial communities correlates positively with pulmonary function and outcome [29]. Such diversity was previously unrecognized as most studies relied solely on culture-based methods of culturing bacteria. However, novel state-of-the-art molecular techniques (such as Sanger sequencing of clone libraries, terminal restriction fragment length polymorphism [RFLP] analysis and microarray hybridization) have enabled the detection of subtle molecular diversity among seemingly similar bacterial species [30]. This diversity may be influenced by a number of factors including the patient's age, sex, type of CFTR mutation, antibiotic exposures, environmental factors, and extent and severity of lung disease. In a study by Zhao et al., sputum samples were collected from six CF patients over a period of 10 years. Of a total of 126 sputum samples, 662 operational taxonomic units (OTU) were identified and each patient had 5–114 different OTUs [29]. Similarly, in another observational study, sputum samples of patients with acute infective exacerbation of non-CF related bronchiectasis were collected. Sputum cultures from each patient contained large quantities of multiple bacterial species with a single predominant pathogenic species [31]. In one study, polymerase chain reaction (PCR)-temporal temperature gel electrophoresis (PCR-TTGE) was used to evaluate intraspecific and intragenomic 16S rDNA variability among commonly isolated respiratory pathogens from CF patients [32]. Significant discordance in intraspecific and intragenomic variability was noted among different bacterial species with *H. influenzae* displaying the highest level of intraspecific variability.

4. Composition of the CF microbiome and its determinants

The composition of the airway microbiome in CF patients is dependent on a number of factors including geographic variation (more common in white population), type of genetic

http://dx.doi.org/10.5772/67846

mutation (e.g., ΔF508), antibiotic exposures, and chronic infection with certain pathogenic bacteria (e.g., *P. aeruginosa*) [8]. Fetal lungs are sterile, just like fetal gastrointestinal tract, but they soon become colonized after birth. Fetal skin becomes colonized with microbes present in maternal reproductive and gastrointestinal tracts and lungs become colonized from gut flora of the child [33]. The common phyla found in healthy lungs include Bacteroides, Firmicutes, and Proteobacterium. Other genera include Prevotella, Veillonella, Streptococcus and Pseudomonas [34]. Many techniques have been used for the detection of microbes in CF patients. Some of these techniques include terminal RFLP profiling, microarray analysis, clone library sequencing, and pyrosequencing. The most frequently used samples from CF patients for analysis are expectorated sputum, tracheal aspirates, bronchial washings, and bronchoalveolar lavage (BAL).

The microbiome in patients with CF evolves as patients grow older, and this is a consequence of the wide adaptability of pathogenic bacteria. Clustering of phylogenetically similar bacterial communities and loss of the architectural diversity of the airway microbiome is a key feature of late-stage CF airway disease. Moreover, the type of bacterial species predominating at a particular age group is also of immense importance. In one study, phylogenetic diversity of CF airway microbiota in patients of different age groups was studied using microarray analysis [35]. *S. aureus* was detected in 65% of sputum samples and was more common in the pediatric population (72% of the pediatric sample). *Pseudomonas* spp. was found in 73% of samples and were most common in adults (91% of the adult sample). In the same study, older CF patients had reduced airway bacterial diversity and aggregation of relatively similar organisms; this process occurred in conjunction with a progressive decline in pulmonary function. *H. influenzae* was most prevalent in the pediatric population when the bacterial diversity was highest. Conversely, *P. aeruginosa* was most common in older individuals with a lower level of bacterial diversity. Likewise, members of the Mycobacteriaceae family and obligate intracellular pathogens (such as Chlamydia and Mycoplama spp.) were more prevalent in younger CF patients. Certain known or potential pathogens of CF patients, such as members of the Burkholderiaceae and Thermoactinomycetaceae families, were almost exclusively observed among adult patients.

In another study [29], CF patients with progressive lung disease were noted to have a decrease in bacterial diversity with increasing age, but the total bacterial density remained stable over time. Antibiotic exposures in conjunction with recurrent pulmonary exacerbations were proposed as a possible contributing factor toward this observation. In a study by Tunney et al., several anaerobic species (including a number of Veillonella and Prevotella species) constituted a significant portion of the CF airway microbiota [36]. In a unique study, next generation sequencing was used to study the microorganisms of gastric juice among patients with CF and non-CF controls [37]. CF gastric juice was noted to have an abundance of Pseudomonas spp. and a relative paucity of normal gut bacteria (such as Bacteroides and Faecalibacterium), which was in contrast with normal gastric juice samples. These results suggest that CF patients possess a unique aerodigestive microbiome that is inter-related. This explanation seems plausible as the factors that influence the airway microbiome (for instance, antibiotic exposures) are also likely to influence the microbiota of gut and other organ-systems of the body [38].

In patients with CF, different bacterial colony morphotypes can be isolated from a single sputum sample. There is some evidence to suggest that these different morphotypes arise from a single bacterial strain [39]. Microbes in the lungs of CF patients are capable of constantly adapting to selection pressures. Some of the mechanisms that enable the evolution of microbes include motility, type III secretion systems, lipopolysaccharide, plasmids (encoding for antibiotic resistance), biofilm formation, small colony variants, quorum sensing, and hypermutability. As a consequence of these mechanisms, different phenotypes arise from a single bacterial species and, over time, a single bacterial strain with dominating features may evolve [40]. Given that different bacterial strains have differing capacities to evolve, multiple lineages of bacterial colonies evolve and coexist [41]. Some studies have shown that complexity of bacterial communities inversely correlates with patient age, antibiotic exposures, and presence of *P. aeruginosa* [42]. In one study, heterozygosity for the ΔF508 mutation and presence of mutations other than the ΔF508 was associated with relative preservation of airway bacterial diversity over time [35]. This shows that apart from environmental exposures (such as antibiotic pressures), patients' genotype (type of mutation) also plays an important role in determining the composition of the CF airway microbiome. In terms of environmental exposures, antibiotic use has been shown to be the prime factor that adversely affects microbial diversity among CF patients [29]. Loss of bacterial diversity (under the selection pressure of antibiotics) has been associated with an increased risk of pneumonia in mechanically ventilated patients colonized with *P. aeruginosa* [43]. Smith et al. studied this further by performing whole genomic analysis of a single species of *P. aeruginosa* isolated from a patient with CF. Whole genomic sequencing was repeated multiple times during the course of the patient's illness, which enabled the detection of an overwhelming number of mutations. Based on these analyses, it was found that the strain of *P. aeruginosa* that inhabits patients with advanced CF differs significantly from wild-type *P. aeruginosa* [40].

The interaction among different bacterial colonies has also become a subject of intense research and genomic and proteomic approaches are currently being used to understand their interrelationships. In an experimental study, production of 4-hydroxy-2-heptylquinoline-N-oxide (HQNO) by a strain of *P. aeruginosa* enhanced the aminoglycoside resistance of *S. aureus* [44]. This study provided some evidence of how bacterial interspecies interaction can alter the airway microbiome by selecting for resistant strains of a bacterial species. Previous studies have shown that HQNO is detectable in the sputum of infected CF patients. Therefore, an interaction between *P. aeruginosa* and *S. aureus* may account for the increased incidence of small colony variant (SCV) of *S. aureus* species in CF patients with advanced lung disease.

In the recent literature, an increasing number of unusual microbes have been reported as the cause of infective exacerbations of CF. Such bacteria include multidrug resistant pathogens like *S. maltophilia*, multidrug resistant *P. aeruginosa*, MRSA, *Burkholderia cenocepacia* and even NTM [45]. The emergence of such bacteria as members of the CF airway microbiome can have important implications for management and prognosis for patients. For instance, studies have shown that in CF patients with an acute exacerbation, there is discordance between the results of microbial sensitivity testing and response to antibacterial therapy [46]. Polymicrobial infections and presence of fastidious organisms may account for this observation. Moreover, such pathogenic bacteria can interact with other less virulent bacterial species and lead to architectural distortion of the entire CF microbiome. In the following lines, we discuss common members of the CF airway microbiome, some of which are commonly implicated in infective exacerbations.

4.1. Methicillin-sensitive *Staphylococcus aureus*

S. aureus is a common colonizer of the anterior nares of adolescent and adult patients [47]. Among patients with CF, MSSA is one of the most common pathogens isolated from sputum samples obtained for culture and sensitivity testing. In the CF Foundation (CFF) patient registry (Bethesda, Maryland, USA), *S. aureus* was most commonly isolated from children and adolescents accounting for approximately 51% of the total samples. Moreover, the overall prevalence of *S. aureus* has been increasing over the past few decades. Infection with *S. aureus* has been associated with increased bronchial inflammation and decreasing pulmonary function [48]. Moreover, when coinfection with *P. aeruginosa* and MSSA occurs, mortality is increased manifold. Interestingly, studies have shown that MSSA is associated with more severe disease in children as compared to adults.

With the widespread use of antistaphylococcal antibiotics, incidence of Gram-negative infections among CF patients has increased and MSSA has become less common among adult patients. Overall, the most common cause of chronic lung infections in CF patients is *P. aeruginosa*, an oxidase-positive Gram-negative bacillus. Moreover, as CF patients grow older, MRSA becomes a more frequent cause of infective exacerbation than MSSA. Over the past few years, the incidence of MRSA infections has been steadily increasing, owing to increasing use of antistaphylococcal penicillins (such as oxacillin and nafcillin) [49]. More recently, a subtype of *S. aureus* species (viz. small colony variant) has been isolated more frequently from CF patients. The small colony variant of *S. aureus* species is fastidious and slow-growing, and it has also been associated with rapid decline in pulmonary function. As mentioned previously, selection of small colony variant species is promoted by HQNO—a product synthesized and secreted by *P. aeruginosa* species [44]. Increasing use of broad-spectrum antibiotics that select for multidrug resistant pathogens can explain this distortion in the composition of the airway microbiome in patients with CF.

4.2. Methicillin-resistant *Staphylococcus aureus*

S. aureus is typically the first bacterial pathogen to invade the pulmonary parenchyma in patients with CF. Chronic infection with this organism can persist in the airways of CF patients for several years. Acquisition of mecA gene mediates methicillin resistance in community-acquired MRSA by encoding for a mutated penicillin binding protein-2A (PBP-2A) [50]. The prevalence of MRSA has increased substantially over the past several years from an estimated 7.3% in 2001 to 22.6% in the year 2008 and 25.7% in 2012 [10]. This increase in prevalence of MRSA was noticed across CF patients of all age groups with the highest increase being in the adolescent age bracket. This increase in the prevalence of MRSA in CF patients has been directly linked to the increase in overall incidence of community-acquired MRSA in the general population [51]. In a study by Glikman et al., 22 of 34 (64.7%) MRSA isolates from patients with CF contained the gene SCCmec II—a typical feature of health-care associated

MRSA strains. On the other hand, 9 of 34 (26.5%) MRSA strains harbored the SCCmec IV gene, which characterizes them as community-acquired MRSA strains. Most patients with community-acquired MRSA were newly colonized with the strain. Additionally, children with CF were more likely to harbor MRSA isolates that were resistant to clindamycin and ciprofloxacin compared with strains from non-CF patients [52]. Other studies have reported persistent infections in CF patients with both hospital-acquired and community-acquired MRSA strains (including Panton-Valentine leukocidin-positive strains) with an overall prevalence of 7.8% [53]. In these studies, persistence was due to presence of different clones over time or identical clones that underwent minor modifications in their toxin content. Moreover, isolation of MRSA from CF patients aged 7–24 years has been associated with an increased severity of the disease. Alarmingly, some of these strains may be vancomycin-intermediate *S. aureus* (VISA), which implies that treatment with glycopeptides (such as vancomycin) may also be ineffective. Highly virulent strains, such as vancomycin-resistant *S. aureus* (VRSA), have also been reported to cause necrotizing pneumonia in a small number of CF patients [54]. Persistent infection with virulent strains of *S. aureus* has been associated with a rapid decline in pulmonary function [55]. In a case-control study, CF patients who were colonized with MRSA had a significantly higher rate of decline in FEV_1 (forced expiratory volume in first second) as compared to those who were not colonized with MRSA [56]. Moreover, MRSA-infected CF patients have been shown to have longer hospital stays than age- and sex-matched controls [57]. Serious manifestations of MRSA infections have also been described in various reports. Cavitary lesions have been described in two CF patients infected with Panton-Valentine leukocidin-positive MRSA strains [54]. This observation was consistent with other reports of serious pulmonary manifestations of community acquired MRSA infection [54, 58]. In a cohort study of longitudinal data, risk of death among CF patients who had at least one culture positive for MRSA was 1.27 times greater than for CF patients in whom MRSA was never detected [55]. In a meta-analysis of 76 studies, a clear and strong association was noted between exposure to antibiotics and isolation of MRSA [59]. The risk of acquiring MRSA was increased by 1.8-fold in patients who had taken antibiotics as compared to others. The risk ratios for quinolones, glycopeptides, cephalosporins, and other beta-lactam antibiotics were 3, 2.9, 2.2, and 1.9, respectively.

4.3. Hemophilus influenzae

H. influenzae is a facultative, anaerobic, Gram-negative bacillus. In many patients, this organism begins to colonize the upper respiratory tract since infancy. Approximately 20% of infants with CF are colonized by the end of first year of life and the rate is even higher for patients of older ages [60]. By the age of 5–6 years, more than 50% of children are colonized with this bacterium [61]. *H. influenzae* is a common pathogen of chronic lung infections and is frequently implicated in infective exacerbations of CF [62]. In children with CF, about 32% are colonized with this microorganism. However, as these patients grow older and are exposed to a wide range of broad-spectrum antibiotics, more virulent bacteria inhabit their respiratory tracts. Consequently, in adults with CF, the rate of colonization with *H. influenzae* is reported to be only 10–15%. Having said this, the prevalence of *H. influenzae* has increased from 10.3% in the year 1995 to 16.3% in the year 2008.

Similar to the general population, colonization of the upper respiratory tract of CF patients with *H. influenzae* is quite a dynamic process. Children will typically carry multiple strains of this bacterium simultaneously, whilst adults will be colonized with only one strain [63]; again, this is a natural consequence of the loss of microbial diversity induced by antibiotic selection pressures. Even in most healthy adults, the upper airway is colonized with *H. influenzae*; most strains in such healthy subjects are nontypeable. In particular, the nasopharynx is an area of the respiratory tract that serves as a potential reservoir of this bacterium. Eventually, the organism may spread from the nasopharynx to the lower respiratory tract and cause an infection of the pulmonary parenchyma [64]. Studies have shown that most CF patients are cocolonized with two or more distinct strains of *H. influenzae* [65].

H. influenzae is not considered a virulent pathogen in patients with CF. Interestingly, some studies have shown that colonization with *H. influenzae* is associated with a relatively preserved lung function. This is in sharp contrast to other microorganisms like *P. aeruginosa* and MRSA, whose colonization of the pulmonary parenchyma is strongly associated with a rapid decline in lung function [66]. In a prospective study, 27 patients with CF (under the age of 12 years) and 27 matched patients with asthma were followed up for 1 year [67]. The isolation rate of noncapsulated (nontypeable) strains of *H. influenzae* was significantly higher in the CF group as compared to that of the asthma group. During exacerbations, the isolation rate of *H. influenzae* in the CF group was significantly greater than at other times, whereas there was no significant difference in the control group. The distribution of biotypes of *H. influenzae* and *Hemophilus parainfluenzae* was similar in the two groups. In the CF group, biotype I was commonly detected and was associated with infective exacerbations of CF. In contrast, biotype V was more common in the asthma group, although it had no association with the development of infective exacerbations [67].

4.4. Pseudomonas aeruginosa

P. aeruginosa is an obligate aerobic, oxidase-positive, nonlactose fermenting Gram-negative rod. *P. aeruginosa* is the most common organism implicated in infective exacerbations in patients with CF. In the CFF patient registry (Bethesda, Maryland, USA), more than half of the patients (52.5%) were reported to be infected with *P. aeruginosa* in 1995. The risk of chronic infection with *P. aeruginosa* increased proportionately with increasing age. Moreover, the incidence of *P. aeruginosa* has been reported to be increasing in infants. Despite changes in the management of patients with CF, the frequency of persistent infection with *P. aeruginosa* has remained relatively stable over time [68]. In a study based on the CFF patient registry, prevalence of colonization with *P. aeruginosa* was 60% in 1995 and 56.1% in 2005 [69]. However, recent data suggest that the prevalence of P. aeruginosa is slowly decreasing over time and has been estimated to be 30.4% in the year 2015 [70].

The main reservoir of *P. aeruginosa* is the environment surrounding CF patients. It has been thought that among siblings with CF, prolonged exposure of young children to their older siblings with CF is a potential risk factor for acquisition of *P. aeruginosa*. A study published in 1991 reported that *P. aeruginosa* may be acquired by patients at CF recreation camps, clinics, and/or rehabilitation centers [71]. Studies on genotypes of *P. aeruginosa* performed using conventional pyocin typing and DNA probe analysis reported that most CF patients harbored a persistent strain of *P. aeruginosa* in their lungs [72]. These studies suggested that cross-colonization possibly could occur among patients. Another study showed that 59% of CF patients harbored a clonal strain of *P. aeruginosa* and the dominant pulsotype was indistinguishable from nonclonal strains with respect to both colony morphology and resistance patterns [73]. Wolz et al. used DNA probe amplification assays and demonstrated that 46% of CF patients (who were initially uninfected) acquired P. aeruginosa infection at the end of a CF recreation camp [74]. Clear evidence of a cross-infection among patients attending a CF clinic was published in 2001 [75]. In this study, 22 of 154 patients attending an adult CF clinic were chronically infected with similar isolates (based on pyocin typing and pulsed-field gel electrophoresis [PFGE] analysis) of *P. aeruginosa* that shared unusual phenotypic features: lack of motility and pigmentation along with a remarkable resistance to many antibiotics. In another study from a large pediatric CF clinic from Australia, 65 patients (55%) were found to be infected with a similar strain of *P. aeruginosa*. These patients were more likely to have been hospitalized in the preceding 1 year for respiratory exacerbations [76]. On the other hand, a study conducted by Speert et al. in Vancouver (Canada) reported a low rate of transmission of *P. aeruginosa* from one CF patient to the other [77]. In this study, a total of 157 genetic types of *P. aeruginosa* were identified, of which 123 were unique to individual patients. These apparently conflicting findings may be accounted for by the highly adaptable nature of *P. aeruginosa* and its ability to evolve. In a study by Mahenthiralingam et al., different strains of *P. aeruginosa* were studied using genomic fingerprinting and random DNA amplification assays [78]. A total of 385 isolates from 20 patients were grouped into 35 random amplified polymorphic DNA (RAPD) strain types. Secretion of mucoid exopolysaccharide, loss of expression of RpoN-dependent surface factors and acquisition of serum-susceptible phenotypes in Pseudomonas were shown to be a specific adaptation to infection, rather than being acquired from a new bacterial strain. This explanation is also in congruence with observations from other studies that found different strains of *P. aeruginosa* in unrelated CF patients and identical or closely related strains among siblings [79]. The presence of distinct strains of *P. aeruginosa* in these studies reflects an absence of nosocomial transmission of organisms at respective CF centers [80]. This may be a consequence of strict hygiene measures and microbiologic surveillance instituted at most CF centers across the world following reports of nosocomial spread [75, 76].

The effects of *P. aeruginosa* infection on the CF lung are deleterious. In one observational study, outcomes of CF children colonized with *P. aeruginosa* were compared with those of noncolonized patients. Children colonized with *P. aeruginosa* had a worse outcome and experienced rapid decline in pulmonary function as measured by FEV_1 and FEF_{25} (forced expiratory flow at 25% of vital capacity) [81]. In another longitudinal observational study, the temporal relationship between *P. aeruginosa* infection and pulmonary damage (as measured by FEV_1 and Wisconsin additive chest radiograph score) was explored. Acquisition of *P. aeruginosa* was independently associated with a worsening pulmonary status in children with CF [82]. Moreover, in these studies, decline in pulmonary function after colonization with *P. aeruginosa* was observed to be gradual. This decline in pulmonary function associated with *P. aeruginosa* infection is noted across all age groups. In another study, acquisition of mucoid

http://dx.doi.org/10.5772/67846

strains of *P. aeruginosa* was associated with an unfavorable prognosis [83]. From a pathologic perspective, *P. aeruginosa* causes repeated airway infections with eventual progression to chronic airway infection. This organism can also lead to necrotizing pneumonia, chronic bronchopneumonia, and chronic parenchymal lung disease. While the aggressive use of antipseudomonal antibiotics has been shown to delay the onset of chronic infection, prevalence rates of *P. aeruginosa* colonization have remained relatively stable over the past two decades [84, 85].

The CF airway provides a pathological milieu and a scaffold for chronic infection with resistant organisms, the most notable of them being *P. aeruginosa*. A number of virulent factors enable this resilient organism to establish it within the CF airways. One such virulence factor—overproduction of alginate slime capsule—characterizes the mucoid type of *P. aeruginosa*, which allows it to adhere firmly to the airway epithelium. Being encoded by the AlgT gene, alginate negatively regulates flagella, fimbriae, and quorum sensing. TTSS (injectosome) positively regulates alginate production indirectly through heat shock, osmotic, and oxidative stress responses [86]. In the inflamed CF airway, polymorphonuclear leukocytes (PMN) lead to the production of reactive oxygen species (ROS) and reactive nitrogen intermediates (RNI) [87]. Moreover, mutated CF epithelial cells are unable to efflux glutathione (a potent free radical scavenger) and unable to absorb other dietary antioxidants. Production of ROS and RNI by PMN leads to DNA damage, lipid peroxidation and denaturation of proteins. At the same time, RNI and ROS lead to upregulation of alginate production by *P. aeruginosa*. The alginate slime capsule enables the bacterium to adhere firmly to the airway epithelial cells and results in persistence of this organism within the airways. At the same time, other virulence factors produced by *P. aeruginosa* (such as exotoxins) incur progressive pulmonary damage and help it to evade the (already impaired) host immune response. Over time, ROI and RNI lead to loss of microbial diversity and disruption of the airway microbiota. Simultaneously, such an environment favors the survival and selection of *P. aeruginosa* within the CF airway and leads to persistent infection with this organism [88, 89]. Moreover, antibiotic exposures select for multidrug resistant variants of the organism and allow them to predominate and colonize the airways [24, 90]. Alarmingly, recent reports from CF centers across the world have described certain strains of *P. aeruginosa* that exhibit resistance to all clinically relevant classes of antimicrobials ("pan-resistant" *P. aeruginosa*) [91]. This can explain the worse prognosis associated with this organism in most studies of CF patients.

4.5. Burkholderia cepacia complex

More than 60 species belonging to the genus Burkholderia are not pathogenic to humans, but some of the remaining species are implicated in serious infections in CF patients. Using 16S rDNA and recA gene analysis, 17 species of this genus have been grouped together as the Burkholderia cepacia complex (BCC). BCC is a group of virulent pathogens that are frequently implicated in infective exacerbations in CF patients with end-stage lung disease. Colonization with BCC in CF patients indicates a poor prognosis and has been shown to be associated with a requirement for lung transplantation. This worse prognosis is due to the inherent antibiotic resistance possessed by these organisms and their ability to rapidly spread from patient to patient. In some cases, infection with BCC can lead to the development of cepacia syndrome—a rapid fulminating pneumonia that often leads to bacteremia and sepsis. Given their virulent nature, strict infection control measures are essential to prevent outbreaks of BCC in CF clinics and centers [92]. A report of rapid spread and outbreak of BCC infection was reported in a CF center in Toronto [93]. This center reported the development of cepacia syndrome in many patients, being characterized by rapidly deteriorating pulmonary function, fever, leukocytosis, elevated markers of inflammation, and BCC bacteremia. Furthermore, in another report, cepacia syndrome occurred in approximately 20% of infected patients and had a case fatality rate of 62% [93].

Outside of the BCC group, a few other species of the Burkholderia genus are also implicated in infective exacerbations. These species include *Burkholderia gladioli, Burkholderia fungorum, Burkholderia multivorans* and *Burkholderia pseudomallei* [94]. Of these, *B. gladioli* now accounts for a significant proportion of Burkholderia infections in CF patients [95]. In the United States, *B. multivorans* and *B. gladioli* together account for more than 50% of Burkholderia infections in CF patients.

Most infected CF patients harbor genotypically distinct strains of the BCC. Strains of Burkholderia spp. that are shared by multiple CF patients are very uncommon. This suggests that most Burkholderia infections in CF patients result from acquisition of strains from the natural environment [92, 96]. In this regard, *B. gladioli* and *B. cepacia* have been described as recognized plant pathogens. In one study, multilocus sequence typing of Burkholderia spp. revealed that more than 20% of CF isolates were identical to strains recovered from the environment [97].

In the CFF patient registry, prevalence of BCC was reported to have declined from 9% in 1985 to 4% in 2005. Incidence of BCC was also found to be reduced from 1.3% in 1995 to 0.8% in 2005 [69]. This has not changed significantly over the past decade as shown by data published in 2016 [70]. Ramette et al. analyzed 285 confirmed isolates of BCC using restriction analysis of recA and identified seven different BCC species in the environment [98]. Healthcare-associated outbreaks of BCC infections as a consequence of contaminated medical devices and products (such as mouthwashes, ultrasound gels, skin antiseptics, and medications) have been reported previously. While most of these outbreaks have generally involved non-CF patients, the potential for developing such outbreaks among CF patients remains a hazard [99]. Infection of the respiratory tract with BCC species in CF patients often results in a chronic persistent infection [100]. In most such cases, a single strain of Burkholderia spp. colonizes the respiratory tract.

Infection with BCC species has been associated with a worse prognosis. In one study, CF patients who were infected with *Burkholderia dolosa* had a rapid decline in FEV_1 over time [101]. In another study, patients colonized with *B. cenocepacia* had a worse outcome in terms of body mass index (BMI) and FEV_1 as compared to those colonized with *P. aeruginosa* or *B. multivorans* [102].

4.6. Anaerobic bacteria

Anaerobic bacteria have been described in the airways of people with healthy lungs and are generally not considered to be pathogenic. In patients with CF, anaerobic bacteria are persistent members of the lower airway community as the anaerobic conditions (and steep oxygen gradients) in the lower airways provide an ideal environment for their growth [88, 103].

However, in the CF lung, anaerobic bacteria can produce virulence factors and damage the lung parenchyma (perhaps as a consequence of impaired innate immunity), which may worsen pulmonary function and exacerbate the inflammatory response. Short-chain fatty acids produced by anaerobic bacteria can increase production of interleukin-8 (IL-8) by upregulating expression of the short-chain fatty acid receptor GPR41 [104]. Moreover, in the CF microbiome, anaerobic bacteria can interact with other established pathogens and lead to progressive pulmonary damage [105]. Previously, anaerobic bacteria were thought to be an infrequent cause of CF exacerbation; however, with the advent of novel (culture-independent) microbial detection methods [106–109], anaerobes have been isolated from more frequently. In one study, 23.8% of sputum specimens from CF patients grew more than 10^5 colony forming units (CFU) per milliliter of anaerobic bacteria [110]. In another study, 15 genera of obligate anaerobes were identified in 91% of CF patients with counts (CFU/ml) being comparable to that of *P. aeruginosa* and *S. aureus* [111]. The most common anaerobes were *Staphylococcus saccharolyticus* and *Peptostreptococcus prevotii*. Some studies suggest that patients with lower aerobic and anaerobic bacterial load have worse pulmonary function and higher levels of inflammatory markers [112]. From a biological standpoint, lower quantity of aerobes and anaerobes may reflect disruption of the CF microbiota. Studies have shown that antibiotic therapy directed against *P. aeruginosa* during acute exacerbations does not affect anaerobes [111]. This observation could be explained by considering the resistance patterns of anaerobes. In 58% of patients, obligate anaerobes detected during acute infective exacerbations were resistant to antibiotics used for treatment. The chief obligate anaerobes in such cases were *Bacteroides* spp., *Porphyromonas* spp., *Prevotella* sp., *Veillonella, anaerobic Streptococcus* spp., *Proprionibacterium, Actinomyces, S. saccharolyticus* and *P. prevotii* [36, 111, 113]. Interestingly, infection with *P. aeruginosa* significantly increases the likelihood of isolating anaerobic bacteria from CF patients [36]. Some of these anaerobic bacteria (such as S. milleri) are now known to be associated with worse clinical outcomes. Furthermore, new anaerobic organisms have been detected for the first time from samples of CF patients. Such bacteria, for instance Gemella and Rothia mucilaginosa, have been found to be associated with dismal pulmonary outcomes. Most such patients are often coinfected with *P. aeruginosa* as well [114, 115].

4.7. Nontuberculous mycobacteria

Traditionally, the frequency of CF patients infected with NTM has been reportedly low. In the CFF patient registry, the prevalence of NTM infections among CF patients has been estimated to be 2.2%. Nevertheless, the prevalence of NTM has been increasing slowly over the past few decades. The prevalence of NTM infection in 1999 among CF patients was 0.85%, which increased to 2.18% in 2008 [116]. More recent data published in 2016 shows that the prevalence of NTM may be as high as 11.9% [70]. The most common NTM species have been reported to be Mycobacterium avium-intracellulare (MAI) complex and *Mycobacterium abscessus*. Factors associated with a culture positive for NTM are older age, greater FEV_1, higher frequency of MSSA colonization and lower frequency of *P. aeruginosa* infection [117]. In most patients, unique strains of NTM are detected by molecular typing, which suggests that neither person-to-person transmission nor nosocomial acquisition is implicated. In one study, the prevalence of NTM infection among 385 patients in three Parisian centers was 8.1%. *M. abscessus* was isolated in all age groups. About 4.1% (16/385) of the study cohort met the American Thoracic Society (ATS) criteria for NTM-related lung disease [118]. In another multicenter study done in Israel [119], prevalence of NTM-related lung disease (as defined by the 2007 ATS criteria) was 10.8%. This study further suggested that the incidence of NTM infections is increasing over time. Other studies have demonstrated that the incidence of MAI complex infections in CF patients is decreasing with time, while that of *M. abscessus* complex is increasing [120]. Alarmingly, infection with *M. abscessus* complex has been associated with a worse impact on pulmonary function. Some researchers have proposed that eradication of *M. abscessus* complex may provide a significant improvement in terms of pulmonary outcome [121]. However, *M. abscessus* is difficult to manage, commonly affects younger children, and requires prolonged courses of intravenous antibiotics [122].

4.8. *Stenotrophomonas maltophilia*

S. maltophilia is a Gram-negative bacillus that is commonly implicated in nosocomial infections in non-CF patients. However, in patients with CF, *S. maltophilia* has been recognized as a cause of acute infective exacerbation. The medical importance of this pathogen is that it is inherently resistant to a wide range of broad-spectrum antibiotics (most notably carbapenems). The prevalence of infection with this organism has increased from 1 to 4% over a period of 20 years (1985–2005) [68]. In the CFF patient registry, the prevalence of *S. maltophilia* increased from 4.0% in 1996 to 12.4% in 2005 [69]. From 2005 till 2015, the prevalence of *S. maltophilia* seems to have plateaued [70]. *S. maltophilia* infections of the respiratory tract in CF patients tend to be acute and, in most cases, the organism does not persist in the lower airways (although recurrent infections can occur). Most isolates of this organism have been shown to be transmitted from patient-to-patient, especially among siblings, or those who are otherwise epidemiologically linked [123]. One-third of CF patients who experience recurrent infections with *S. maltophilia* harbor more than one strain of the organism [124]. The most important risk factors for acquiring *S. maltophilia* infections are therapy with carbapenems and central venous catheterization [125]. In one study, history of treatment with imipenem was 10 times more frequent among cases (who contracted *S. maltophilia*) than among controls [125]. Furthermore, all fatal infections with *S. maltophilia* occurred in patients who had received imipenem. Based on these results, it is advisable to cover *S. maltophilia* empirically in CF patients who develop super-infection while receiving imipenem therapy. In a report by Sanyal and Mokaddas [126], most strains of *S. maltophilia* were susceptible to ciprofloxacin and trimethoprim-sulfamethoxazole. Moreover, some evidence shows that CF patients infected with *S. maltophilia* were more likely to have been hospitalized for many days in the past one year [127]. Other factors associated with *S. maltophilia* acquisition were more than two courses of intravenous antibiotics, isolation of *Aspergillus fumigatus* or *P. aeruginosa* in sputum and oral steroid use [128]. *S. maltophilia* is also more common among CF patients who develop allergic bronchopulmonary aspergillosis (ABPA) [129]. While chronic infection with *S. maltophilia* is infrequent, it can occur in certain patients and requires repeated courses of antibiotics [130]. Chronic infection with *S. maltophilia* confers a threefold higher risk of mortality or the need for lung transplantation [131].

4.9. *Achromobacter xylosoxidans*

A. xylosoxidans has been recognized as a pathogen and cause of infective exacerbation in patients with CF [132]. In the CFF patient registry, the prevalence of *A. xylosoxidans* infection was 1.9% in 1995 [69]. In 2015, the prevalence had increased almost three-folds to 6.1% [70]. *A. xylosoxidans* is a ubiquitous organism that occurs widely in natural habitats. This organism is an opportunistic pathogen that affects only immunocompromised patients and those with CF. *A. xylosoxidans* is mostly implicated in nosocomial infections, such as hospital acquired pneumonia, catheter-associated urinary tract infection, and wound infections. Lung infections with this fastidious organism are difficult to eradicate. Most patients respond to antipseudomonal penicillins (such as piperacillin–tazobactam) and third- or fourth-generation cephalosporins [133]. In one report, two cases of *Achromobacter ruhlandii* developed after indirect contact between CF patients [134]. Another study from a French CF center reported that most isolates of Achromobacter spp. were resistant to fluoroquinolones and carbapenems [135]. In a retrospective study, CF patients who were chronically infected with *A. xylosoxidans* were more likely to have impaired pulmonary function. Additionally, the frequency of hospitalization was higher among such patients than others [136].

5. Implications for further research

Cystic fibrosis is a monogenetic multisystem disorder, but, pulmonary disease is the leading cause of morbidity and mortality. Recurrent pulmonary infections with pathogenic bacteria can lead to progressive pulmonary damage and eventually lead to death. Therefore, understanding the CF airway microbiome has immense importance for understanding the overall pathology of the disease. Disruption of the CF airway microbiome under the influence of environmental factors and antibiotic exposures is a crucial step in the development of end-stage pulmonary disease in such patients [40]. Colonization of the lower airways with pathogenic bacteria, such as *P. aeruginosa* [82] and *B. cenocepacia* [101], has been associated with end-stage pulmonary disease.

As the CF airway microbiome evolves under the influence of antibiotic exposures, microbes undergo a number of mutations and changes in their genome [137]. While these genetic mutations are an evolutionary mechanism for microorganisms (for instance, to acquire resistance to antibiotics), they create potential vulnerabilities that may be exploited in unique therapeutic approaches. Traditionally, the approach to management of CF pulmonary exacerbations has been through employment of antibiotics. While antibiotics are useful in the short run, multidrug resistant microbes eventually evolve and become a challenge to tackle. In view of this, novel approaches to the management of CF pulmonary disease have been proposed, which involve manipulating patients' microbial consortia [8]. From a theoretical perspective, such an approach aims to maintain the architecture of the CF airway microbiome and avoids the use of antimicrobials, thereby circumventing the problem of destroying the community structure of a patient's microbiome. Such a novel treatment approach is based on the principles of personalized medicine and aims to tailor treatment according to each patient's individual microbiome [138]. By manipulating and restoring the structure of a patient's airway microbiome, the complex metabolomic profile of the patient's sputum (and other body fluids) can be altered, which may have long-lasting and pleiotropic consequences [139].

Novel treatment approaches for the treatment of CF patients hold theoretical promise, but their practical applicability and clinical efficacy remains to be established [140]. A recent pilot study compared the use of a probiotic (*Lactobacillus* spp.) versus placebo in pediatric CF patients. Patients receiving the probiotic demonstrated a significant reduction in hospitalization for pulmonary exacerbation and a beneficial effect on the gut in terms of reducing gastrointestinal inflammation [141]. Another clinical trial examined the efficacy of enteric probiotics in reducing the frequency and severity of pulmonary exacerbations in CF patients. Both studies reported that the use of enteric probiotics provided a significant reduction in the frequency of pulmonary exacerbations when compared to the placebo group [142]. Larger randomized controlled studies are needed to more fully evaluate the effect of probiotics on hard clinical endpoints [143]. Other treatment options based on these novel concepts need to be developed further, and they may help to improve the overall outcomes of patients with CF [144].

Abbreviations

ABPA	Allergic bronchopulmonary aspergillosis
ATS	American Thoracic Society
BAL	Bronchoalveolar lavage
BCC	Burkholderia cepacia complex
CD	Clostridium difficile
CF	Cystic fibrosis
CFF	Cystic Fibrosis Foundation
CFTR	Cystic fibrosis transmembrane conductance regulator
CFU	Colony forming units
FAFLP	Fluorescent amplified fragment length polymorphism
FEF_{25}	Forced expiratory flow at 25% of vital capacity
FEV_1	Forced expiratory volume in first second
FMT	Fecal microbiota transplantation
HQNO	4-Hydroxy-2-heptylquinoline-N-oxide
IL-8	Interleukin-8
MAI	Mycobacterium avium-intracellulare
MRSA	Methicillin-resistant Staphylococcus aureus
MSSA	Methicillin-sensitive Staphylococcus aureus

NTM	Non-tuberculous mycobacteria
OTU	Operational taxonomic units
PCR	Polymerase chain reaction
PBP-2A	Penicillin binding protein-2A
PFGE	Pulsed-field gel electrophoresis
PMN	Polymorphonuclear leukocyte
RAPD	Random amplified polymorphic DNA
RFLP	Restriction fragment length polymorphism
RNI	Reactive nitrogen intermediates
ROS	Reactive oxygen species
VISA	Vancomycin-intermediate Staphylococcus aureus

Author details

Ibrahim A. Janahi[1]* and Abdul Rehman[2]

*Address all correspondence to: ijanahi@hamad.qa

1 Pediatric Pulmonology, Department of Pediatrics, Hamad Medical Corporation, Doha, Qatar

2 Internal Medicine Section, Department of Medicine, Hamad Medical Corporation, Doha, Qatar

References

[1] Dalemans W, Barbry P, Champigny G, *et al.* Altered chloride ion channel kinetics associated with the ΔF508 cystic fibrosis mutation. *Nature* 1991;**354**(6354):526-8.

[2] Elborn JS, Shale DJ, Britton JR. Cystic fibrosis: current survival and population estimates to the year 2000. *Thorax* 1991;**46**(12):881-5.

[3] Elborn JS. Cystic fibrosis. *The Lancet* 2016;**388**(10059):2519-2531.

[4] Sheppard DN, Welsh MJ. Structure and function of the CFTR chloride channel. *Physiological Reviews* 1999;**79**(1):S23-45.

[5] Stutts MJ, Canessa CM, Olsen JC, Hamrick M. CFTR as a cAMP-dependent regulator of sodium channels. *Science* 1995;**269**(5225):847-50.

[6] de Koff EM, Groot KM, Bogaert D. Development of the respiratory tract microbiota in cystic fibrosis. *Current Opinion in Pulmonary Medicine* 2016;**22**(6):623-8.

[7] Cho I, Blaser MJ. The human microbiome: at the interface of health and disease. *Nature Reviews Genetics* 2012;**13**(4):260-70.

[8] Zemanick ET, Sagel SD, Harris JK. The airway microbiome in cystic fibrosis and implications for treatment. *Current Opinion in Pediatrics* 2011;**23**(3):319-24.

[9] Busquets NP, Baroni MR, Ochoteco MC, Zurbriggen ML, Virgolini S, Meneghetti FG. Bacterial isolates from respiratory samples of pediatric patients with cystic fibrosis and their distribution by ages. *Revista Argentina de Microbiologia* 2012;**45**(1):44-9.

[10] Salsgiver EL, Fink AK, Knapp EA, *et al.* Changing epidemiology of the respiratory bacteriology of patients with cystic fibrosis. *CHEST Journal* 2016;**149**(2):390-400.

[11] Paganin P, Fiscarelli EV, Tuccio V, *et al.* Changes in cystic fibrosis airway microbial community associated with a severe decline in lung function. *PLoS ONE* 2015;**10**(4): e0124348.

[12] Fredricks DN. The human microbiota: How microbial communities affect health and disease. Hoboken, NJ: John Wiley & Sons; 2013. pp. 3-4.

[13] Schnorr SL, Sankaranarayanan K, Lewis CM, Warinner C. Insights into human evolution from ancient and contemporary microbiome studies. *Current Opinion in Genetics & Development* 2016;**41**:14-26.

[14] von Müller L. New aspects on Clostridium difficile infection. *Deutsche medizinische Wochenschrift* 2016;**141**(16):1144-7.

[15] Gallo A, Passaro G, Gasbarrini A, Landolfi R, Montalto M. Modulation of microbiota as treatment for intestinal inflammatory disorders: an uptodate. *World Journal of Gastroenterology* 2016;**22**(32):7186-202.

[16] Schenck LP, Beck PL, MacDonald JA. Gastrointestinal dysbiosis and the use of fecal microbial transplantation in *Clostridium difficile* infection. *World Journal of Gastrointestinal Pathophysiology* 2015;**6**(4):169-80.

[17] Alhagamhmad MH, Day AS, Lemberg DA, Leach ST. An overview of the bacterial contribution to Crohn disease pathogenesis. *Journal of Medical Microbiology* 2016;**65**(10):1049-1059.

[18] Carding S, Verbeke K, Vipond DT, Corfe BM, Owen L. Dysbiosis of the gut microbiota in disease. *Microbial Ecology in Health and Disease* 2015;**26**:26191. doi: 10.3402/mehd.v26.26191

[19] Scales BS, Dickson RP, Huffnagle GB. A tale of two sites: how inflammation can reshape the microbiomes of the gut and lungs. *Journal of Leukocyte Biology* 2016;**100**(5):943-50.

[20] Lawley TD, Walker AW. Intestinal colonization resistance. *Immunology* 2013;**138**(1):1-11.

[21] Spooner R, Yilmaz Ö. The role of reactive-oxygen-species in microbial persistence and inflammation. *International Journal of Molecular Sciences* 2011;**12**(1):334-52.

[22] Lyczak JB, Cannon CL, Pier GB. Lung infections associated with cystic fibrosis. *Clinical Microbiology Reviews* 2002;**15**(2):194-222.

[23] Nathan K, Shteinberg M, Rivlin J. Cystic fibrosis survival trends in carmel medical center. *Harefuah* 2015;**154**(6):373-6.

[24] Hauser AR, Jain M, Bar-Meir M, McColley SA. Clinical significance of microbial infection and adaptation in cystic fibrosis. *Clinical Microbiology Reviews* 2011;**24**(1):29-70.

[25] Vu-Thien H, Moissenet D, Valcin M, Dulot C, Tournier G, Garbarg-Chenon A. Molecular epidemiology of Burkholderia cepacia, Stenotrophomonas maltophilia, and Alcaligenes xylosoxidans in a cystic fibrosis center. *European Journal of Clinical Microbiology and Infectious Diseases* 1996;**15**(11):876-9.

[26] Johnson MM, Odell JA. Nontuberculous mycobacterial pulmonary infections. *Journal of Thoracic Disease* 2014;**6**(3):210-20.

[27] Fodor AA, Klem ER, Gilpin DF, *et al.* The adult cystic fibrosis airway microbiota is stable over time and infection type, and highly resilient to antibiotic treatment of exacerbations. *PLoS ONE* 2012;**7**(9):e45001.

[28] Filkins LM, O'Toole GA. Cystic fibrosis lung infections: polymicrobial, complex, and hard to treat. *PLoS Pathogens* 2015;**11**(12):e1005258.

[29] Zhao J, Schloss PD, Kalikin LM, *et al.* Decade-long bacterial community dynamics in cystic fibrosis airways. *Proceedings of the National Academy of Sciences* 2012;**109**(15):5809-14.

[30] DeAngelis KM, Wu CH, Beller HR, *et al.* PCR amplification-independent methods for detection of microbial communities by the high-density microarray PhyloChip. *Applied and Environmental Microbiology* 2011;**77**(18):6313-22.

[31] Rogers GB, Zain NM, Bruce KD, *et al.* A novel microbiota stratification system predicts future exacerbations in bronchiectasis. *Annals of the American Thoracic Society* 2014;**11**(4):496-503.

[32] Michon AL, Jumas-Bilak E, Imbert A, *et al.* Intragenomic and intraspecific heterogeneity of the 16S rRNA gene in seven bacterial species from the respiratory tract of cystic fibrosis patients assessed by PCR-Temporal Temperature Gel Electrophoresis. *Pathologie Biologie* 2012;**60**(3):e30-5.

[33] Madan JC, Koestler DC, Stanton BA, *et al.* Serial analysis of the gut and respiratory microbiome in cystic fibrosis in infancy: interaction between intestinal and respiratory tracts and impact of nutritional exposures. *mBio* 2012;**3**(4):e00251-12.

[34] Dickson RP, Erb-Downward JR, Huffnagle GB. The role of the bacterial microbiome in lung disease. *Expert Review of Respiratory Medicine* 2013;**7**(3):245-57.

[35] Cox MJ, Allgaier M, Taylor B, *et al.* Airway microbiota and pathogen abundance in age-stratified cystic fibrosis patients. *PLoS ONE* 2010;**5**(6):e11044.

[36] Tunney MM, Field TR, Moriarty TF, *et al.* Detection of anaerobic bacteria in high numbers in sputum from patients with cystic fibrosis. *American Journal of Respiratory and Critical Care Medicine* 2008;**177**(9):995-1001.

[37] Al-Momani H, Perry A, Stewart CJ, *et al*. Microbiological profiles of sputum and gastric juice aspirates in Cystic Fibrosis patients. *Scientific Reports* 2016;**6**:26985.

[38] Rodríguez JM, Murphy K, Stanton C, *et al*. The composition of the gut microbiota throughout life, with an emphasis on early life. *Microbial Ecology in Health and Disease* 2015;**26**:26050. doi: 10.3402/mehd.v26.26050

[39] Häussler S. Multicellular signalling and growth of *Pseudomonas aeruginosa*. *International Journal of Medical Microbiology* 2010;**300**(8):544-8.

[40] Smith EE, Buckley DG, Wu Z, Saenphimmachak C, Hoffman LR, D'Argenio DA, *et al*. Genetic adaptation by *Pseudomonas aeruginosa* to the airways of cystic fibrosis patients. *Proceedings of the National Academy of Sciences* 2006;**103**(22):8487-92.

[41] Kussmann M, van Bladeren P. The extended nutrigenomics–understanding the interplay between the genomes of food, gut microbes, and human host. *Frontiers in Genetics* 2011;**2**:21.

[42] Klepac-Ceraj V, Lemon KP, Martin TR, *et al*. Relationship between cystic fibrosis respiratory tract bacterial communities and age, genotype, antibiotics and *Pseudomonas aeruginosa*. *Environmental Microbiology* 2010;**12**(5):1293-303.

[43] Flanagan JL, Brodie EL, Weng L, *et al*. Loss of bacterial diversity during antibiotic treatment of intubated patients colonized with *Pseudomonas aeruginosa*. *Journal of Clinical Microbiology* 2007;**45**(6):1954-62.

[44] Hoffman LR, Déziel E, D'Argenio DA, *et al*. Selection for *Staphylococcus aureus* small-colony variants due to growth in the presence of *Pseudomonas aeruginosa*. *Proceedings of the National Academy of Sciences* 2006;**103**(52):19890-5.

[45] De Vrankrijker AM, Wolfs TF, van der Ent CK. Challenging and emerging pathogens in cystic fibrosis. *Paediatric Respiratory Reviews* 2010;**11**(4):246-54.

[46] Smith AL, Fiel SB, Mayer-Hamblett N, Ramsey B, Burns JL. Susceptibility testing of *Pseudomonas aeruginosa* isolates and clinical response to parenteral antibiotic administration: lack of association in cystic fibrosis. *CHEST Journal* 2003;**123**(5):1495-502.

[47] Tenover FC, McAllister S, Fosheim G, *et al*. Characterization of Staphylococcus aureus isolates from nasal cultures collected from individuals in the United States in 2001 to 2004. *Journal of Clinical Microbiology* 2008;**46**(9):2837-41.

[48] Rosenfeld M, Gibson RL, McNamara S, *et al*. Early pulmonary infection, inflammation, and clinical outcomes in infants with cystic fibrosis. *Pediatric Pulmonology* 2001;**32**(5):356-66.

[49] Aldridge KE. Methicillin-resistant Staphylococcus aureus: clinical and laboratory features. *Infection Control* 1985;**6**(11):461-5.

[50] Hiramatsu K, Cui L, Kuroda M, Ito T. The emergence and evolution of methicillin-resistant Staphylococcus aureus. *Trends in Microbiology* 2001;**9**(10):486-93.

[51] Lo DKH, Hurley MN, Muhlebach MS, Smyth AR. Interventions for the eradication of methicillin-resistant Staphylococcus aureus (MRSA) in people with cystic fibrosis. *Cochrane Database System Review* 2015;**2015**(2):CD009650.

http://dx.doi.org/10.5772/67846

[52] Glikman D, Siegel JD, David MZ, *et al.* Complex molecular epidemiology of methicillin-resistant Staphylococcus aureus isolates from children with cystic fibrosis in the era of epidemic community-associated methicillin-resistant *S. aureus*. *CHEST Journal* 2008;**133**(6):1381-7.

[53] Cafiso V, Bertuccio T, Spina D, *et al.* Methicillin resistance and vancomycin heteroresistance in Staphylococcus aureus in cystic fibrosis patients. *European Journal of Clinical Microbiology & Infectious Diseases* 2010;**29**(10):1277-85.

[54] Elizur A, Orscheln RC, Ferkol TW, *et al.* Panton-Valentine Leukocidin-positive methicillin-resistant Staphylococcus aureus lung infection in patients with cystic fibrosis. *CHEST Journal* 2007;**131**(6):1718-25.

[55] Dasenbrook EC, Merlo CA, Diener-West M, Lechtzin N, Boyle MP. Persistent methicillin-resistant Staphylococcus aureus and rate of FEV_1 decline in cystic fibrosis. *American Journal of Respiratory and Critical Care Medicine* 2008;**178**(8):814-21.

[56] Cox DW, Kelly C, Rush R, O'Sullivan N, Canny G, Linnane B. The impact of MRSA infection in the airways of children with cystic fibrosis; a case-control study. *Irish Medical Journal* 2011;**104**(10):305-8.

[57] Nadesalingam K, Conway SP, Denton M. Risk factors for acquisition of methicillin-resistant Staphylococcus aureus (MRSA) by patients with cystic fibrosis. *Journal of Cystic Fibrosis* 2005;**4**(1):49-52.

[58] Francis JS, Doherty MC, Lopatin U, *et al.* Severe community-onset pneumonia in healthy adults caused by methicillin-resistant Staphylococcus aureus carrying the Panton-Valentine leukocidin genes. *Clinical Infectious Diseases* 2005;**40**(1):100-7.

[59] Tacconelli E, De Angelis G, Cataldo MA, Pozzi E, Cauda R. Does antibiotic exposure increase the risk of methicillin-resistant Staphylococcus aureus (MRSA) isolation? A systematic review and meta-analysis. *Journal of Antimicrobial Chemotherapy* 2008;**61**(1):26-38.

[60] Howard AJ, Dunkin KT, Millar GW. Nasopharyngeal carriage and antibiotic resistance of Haemophilus influenzae in healthy children. *Epidemiology and Infection* 1988;**100**(02):193-203.

[61] Brawnwald E, Fauci AS, Kasper DL, Hauser SL, Longo DL, Jameson J. Harrison's principles of internal medicine, 11th edition. New York City, NY: McGraw Hillbook Company; pp. 1995-2001.

[62] Rajan S, Saiman L. Pulmonary infections in patients with cystic fibrosis. *Seminars in Respiratory Infections* 2002;**17**(1):47-56.

[63] Murphy TF, Sethi S, Klingman KL, Brueggemann AB, Doern GV. Simultaneous respiratory tract colonization by multiple strains of nontypeable Haemophilus influenzae in chronic obstructive pulmonary disease: implications for antibiotic therapy. *Journal of Infectious Diseases* 1999;**180**(2):404-9.

[64] King P. Haemophilus influenzae and the lung (Haemophilus and the lung). *Clinical and Translational Medicine* 2012;**1**(1):10.

[65] Román F, Cantón R, Pérez-Vázquez M, Baquero F, Campos J. Dynamics of long-term colonization of respiratory tract by Haemophilus influenzae in cystic fibrosis patients shows a marked increase in hypermutable strains. *Journal of Clinical Microbiology* 2004;**42**(4):1450-9.

[66] Hector A, Kirn T, Ralhan A, *et al.* Microbial colonization and lung function in adolescents with cystic fibrosis. *Journal of Cystic Fibrosis* 2016;**15**(3):340-9.

[67] Rayner RJ, Hiller EJ, Ispahani P, Baker M. Haemophilus infection in cystic fibrosis. *Archives of Disease in Childhood* 1990;**65**(3):255-8.

[68] Millar FA, Simmonds NJ, Hodson ME. Trends in pathogens colonising the respiratory tract of adult patients with cystic fibrosis, 1985-2005. *Journal of Cystic Fibrosis* 2009;**8**(6):386-91.

[69] Razvi S, Quittell L, Sewall A, Quinton H, Marshall B, Saiman L. Respiratory microbiology of patients with cystic fibrosis in the United States, 1995 to 2005. *CHEST Journal* 2009;**136**(6):1554-60.

[70] Cystic Fibrosis Foundation Patient Registry. 2015 Annual Data Report. Cystic Fibrosis Foundation (Bethesda, Maryland); pp. 29-34.

[71] Tümmler B, Koopmann U, Grothues D, Weissbrodt H, Steinkamp G, von der Hardt H. Nosocomial acquisition of *Pseudomonas aeruginosa* by cystic fibrosis patients. *Journal of Clinical Microbiology* 1991;**29**(6):1265-7.

[72] Fegan M, Francis P, Hayward AC, Fuerst JA. Heterogeneity, persistence, and distribution of *Pseudomonas aeruginosa* genotypes in cystic fibrosis patients. *Journal of Clinical Microbiology* 1991;**29**(10):2151-7.

[73] O'Carroll MR, Syrmis MW, Wainwright CE, *et al.* Clonal strains of *Pseudomonas aeruginosa* in paediatric and adult cystic fibrosis units. *European Respiratory Journal* 2004;**24**(1):101-6.

[74] Wolz C, Kiosz G, Ogle JW, *et al. Pseudomonas aeruginosa* cross-colonization and persistence in patients with cystic fibrosis. Use of a DNA probe. *Epidemiology and Infection* 1989;**102**(02):205-14.

[75] Jones AM, Govan JR, Doherty CJ, *et al.* Spread of a multiresistant strain of *Pseudomonas aeruginosa* in an adult cystic fibrosis clinic. *The Lancet* 2001;**358**(9281):557-8.

[76] Armstrong DS, Nixon GM, Carzino R, *et al.* Detection of a widespread clone of *Pseudomonas aeruginosa* in a pediatric cystic fibrosis clinic. *American Journal of Respiratory and Critical Care Medicine* 2002;**166**(7):983-7.

[77] Speert DP, Campbell ME, Henry DA, *et al.* Epidemiology of *Pseudomonas aeruginosa* in cystic fibrosis in British Columbia, Canada. *American Journal of Respiratory and Critical Care Medicine* 2002;**166**(7):988-93.

[78] Mahenthiralingam E, Campbell ME, Foster J, Lam JS, Speert DP. Random amplified polymorphic DNA typing of *Pseudomonas aeruginosa* isolates recovered from patients with cystic fibrosis. *Journal of Clinical Microbiology* 1996;**34**(5):1129-35.

[79] Grothues D, Koopmann U, von der Hardt H, Tümmler B. Genome fingerprinting of *Pseudomonas aeruginosa* indicates colonization of cystic fibrosis siblings with closely related strains. *Journal of Clinical Microbiology* 1988;**26**(10):1973-7.

[80] Scott FW, Pitt TL. Identification and characterization of transmissible *Pseudomonas aeruginosa* strains in cystic fibrosis patients in England and Wales. *Journal of Medical Microbiology* 2004;**53**(7):609-15.

[81] Pamukcu A, Bush A, Buchdahl R. Effects of *Pseudomonas aeruginosa* colonization on lung function and anthropometric variables in children with cystic fibrosis. *Pediatric Pulmonology* 1995;**19**(1):10-5.

[82] Kosorok MR, Zeng L, West SE, *et al.* Acceleration of lung disease in children with cystic fibrosis after *Pseudomonas aeruginosa* acquisition. *Pediatric Pulmonology* 2001;**32**(4):277-87.

[83] Henry RL, Mellis CM, Petrovic L. Mucoid *Pseudomonas aeruginosa* is a marker of poor survival in cystic fibrosis. *Pediatric Pulmonology* 1992;**12**(3):158-61.

[84] Johansen HK, Høiby N. Seasonal onset of initial colonisation and chronic infection with *Pseudomonas aeruginosa* in patients with cystic fibrosis in Denmark. *Thorax* 1992;**47**(2):109-11.

[85] Høiby N, Frederiksen B, Pressler T. Eradication of early *Pseudomonas aeruginosa* infection. *Journal of Cystic Fibrosis* 2005;**4**:49-54.

[86] Folkesson A, Jelsbak L, Yang L, *et al.* Adaptation of *Pseudomonas aeruginosa* to the cystic fibrosis airway: an evolutionary perspective. *Nature Reviews Microbiology* 2012;**10**(12):841-51.

[87] Hull J, Vervaart P, Grimwood K, Phelan P. Pulmonary oxidative stress response in young children with cystic fibrosis. *Thorax* 1997;**52**(6):557-60.

[88] Worlitzsch D, Tarran R, Ulrich M, *et al.* Effects of reduced mucus oxygen concentration in airway Pseudomonas infections of cystic fibrosis patients. *The Journal of Clinical Investigation* 2002;**109**(3):317-25.

[89] Kolpen M, Hansen CR, Bjarnsholt T, *et al.* Polymorphonuclear leucocytes consume oxygen in sputum from chronic *Pseudomonas aeruginosa* pneumonia in cystic fibrosis. *Thorax* 2010;**65**(1):57-62.

[90] Johansen HK, Nørregaard L, Gøtzsche PC, Pressler T, Koch C, Høiby N. Antibody response to *Pseudomonas aeruginosa* in cystic fibrosis patients: a marker of therapeutic success?—A 30-year Cohort study of survival in Danish CF patients after onset of chronic *P. aeruginosa* lung infection. *Pediatric Pulmonology* 2004;**37**(5):427-32.

[91] Siegel JD, Rhinehart E, Jackson M, and Chiarello L. 2007 Guideline for isolation precautions and preventing transmission of infectious agents in healthcare settings. *American Journal of Infection Control* 2007;**35**(10 Suppl 2):S65-S164.

[92] Govan JR, Brown AR, Jones AM. Evolving epidemiology of *Pseudomonas aeruginosa* and the Burkholderia cepacia complex in cystic fibrosis lung infection. *Future Medicine* 2007;**2**(2):153-64.

[93] Isles A, Maclusky I, Corey M, *et al*. Pseudomonas cepacia infection in cystic fibrosis: an emerging problem. *The Journal of Pediatrics* 1984;**104**(2):206-10.

[94] Coenye T, Goris J, Spilker T, Vandamme P, LiPuma JJ. Characterization of unusual bacteria isolated from respiratory secretions of cystic fibrosis patients and description of *Inquilinus limosus* gen. nov., sp. nov. *Journal of Clinical Microbiology* 2002;**40**(6):2062-9.

[95] Coenye T, Laevens S, Willems A, *et al*. Burkholderia fungorum sp. nov. and Burkholderia caledonica sp. nov., two new species isolated from the environment, animals and human clinical samples. *International Journal of Systematic and Evolutionary Microbiology* 2001;**51**(3):1099-107.

[96] Mortensen JE, Fisher MC, LiPuma JJ. Recovery of *Pseudomonas cepacia* and other *Pseudomonas species* from the environment. *Infection Control & Hospital Epidemiology* 1995;**16**(1):30-2.

[97] Baldwin A, Mahenthiralingam E, Drevinek P, *et al*. Environmental Burkholderia cepacia complex isolates in human infections. *Emerging Infectious Diseases* 2007;**13**(3):458-61.

[98] Spilker T, Baldwin A, Bumford A, Dowson CG, Mahenthiralingam E, LiPuma JJ. Expanded multilocus sequence typing for Burkholderia species. *Journal of Clinical Microbiology* 2009;**47**(8):2607-10.

[99] Pegues CF, Pegues DA, Ford DS, *et al*. Burkholderia cepacia respiratory tract acquisition: epidemiology and molecular characterization of a large nosocomial outbreak. *Epidemiology and Infection* 1996;**116**(3):309-17.

[100] Yang JH, Spilker T, LiPuma JJ. Simultaneous coinfection by multiple strains during Burkholderia cepacia complex infection in cystic fibrosis. *Diagnostic Microbiology and Infectious Disease* 2006;**54**(2):95-8.

[101] Kalish LA, Waltz DA, Dovey M, *et al*. Impact of Burkholderia dolosa on lung function and survival in cystic fibrosis. *American Journal of Respiratory and Critical Care Medicine* 2006;**173**(4):421-5.

[102] Courtney JM, Dunbar KE, McDowell A, *et al*. Clinical outcome of Burkholderia cepacia complex infection in cystic fibrosis adults. *Journal of Cystic Fibrosis* 2004;**3**(2):93-8.

[103] Yoon SS, Hennigan RF, Hilliard GM, *et al*. *Pseudomonas aeruginosa* anaerobic respiration in biofilms: relationships to cystic fibrosis pathogenesis. *Developmental Cell* 2002;**3**(4):593-603.

[104] Mirković B, Murray MA, Lavelle GM, *et al*. The role of short-chain fatty acids, produced by anaerobic bacteria, in the cystic fibrosis airway. *American Journal of Respiratory and Critical Care Medicine* 2015;**192**(11):1314-24.

[105] Sherrard LJ, Bell SC, Tunney MM. The role of anaerobic bacteria in the cystic fibrosis airway. *Current Opinion in Pulmonary Medicine* 2016;**22**(6):637-43.

[106] Bittar F, Richet H, Dubus JC, *et al*. Molecular detection of multiple emerging pathogens in sputa from cystic fibrosis patients. *PLoS ONE* 2008;**3**(8):e2908.

[107] Kolak M, Karpati F, Monstein HJ, Jonasson J. Molecular typing of the bacterial flora in sputum of cystic fibrosis patients. *International Journal of Medical Microbiology* 2003;**293**(4):309-17.

[108] Rogers GB, Carroll MP, Serisier DJ, Hockey PM, Jones G, Bruce KD. Characterization of bacterial community diversity in cystic fibrosis lung infections by use of 16S ribosomal DNA terminal restriction fragment length polymorphism profiling. *Journal of Clinical Microbiology* 2004;**42**(11):5176-83.

[109] Rogers GB, Carroll MP, Serisier DJ, *et al*. Bacterial activity in cystic fibrosis lung infections. *Respiratory Research* 2005;**6**(1):49.

[110] Jewes LA, Spencer RC. The incidence of anaerobes in the sputum of patients with cystic fibrosis. *Journal of Medical Microbiology* 1990;**31**(4):271-4.

[111] Worlitzsch D, Rintelen C, Böhm K, *et al*. Antibiotic-resistant obligate anaerobes during exacerbations of cystic fibrosis patients. *Clinical Microbiology and Infection* 2009;**15**(5):454-60.

[112] O'Neill K, Bradley JM, Johnston E, *et al*. Reduced bacterial colony count of anaerobic bacteria is associated with a worsening in lung clearance index and inflammation in cystic fibrosis. *PLoS ONE* 2015;**10**(5):e0126980.

[113] Harris JK, de Groote MA, Sagel SD, *et al*. Molecular identification of bacteria in bronchoalveolar lavage fluid from children with cystic fibrosis. *Proceedings of the National Academy of Sciences* 2007;**104**(51):20529-33.

[114] Carmody LA, Zhao J, Schloss PD, *et al*. Changes in cystic fibrosis airway microbiota at pulmonary exacerbation. *Annals of the American Thoracic Society* 2013;**10**(3):179-87.

[115] Lim YW, Schmieder R, Haynes M, *et al*. Mechanistic model of Rothia mucilaginosa adaptation toward persistence in the CF lung, based on a genome reconstructed from metagenomic data. *PLoS ONE* 2013;**8**(5):e64285.

[116] LiPuma JJ. The changing microbial epidemiology in cystic fibrosis. *Clinical Microbiology Reviews* 2010;**23**(2):299-323.

[117] Olivier KN, Weber DJ, Wallace Jr RJ, *et al*. Nontuberculous mycobacteria: I: multicenter prevalence study in cystic fibrosis. *American Journal of Respiratory and Critical Care Medicine* 2003;**167**(6):828-34.

[118] Pierre-Audigier C, Ferroni A, Sermet-Gaudelus I, *et al*. Age-related prevalence and distribution of nontuberculous mycobacterial species among patients with cystic fibrosis. *Journal of Clinical Microbiology* 2005;**43**(7):3467-70.

[119] Levy I, Grisaru-Soen G, Lerner-Geva L, *et al*. Multicenter cross-sectional study of nontuberculous mycobacterial infections among cystic fibrosis patients, Israel. *Emerging Infectious Diseases* 2008;**14**(3):378-84.

[120] Samra Z, Kaufman L, Pitlik S, Shalit I, Bishara J. Emergence of Mycobacterium simiae in respiratory specimens. *Scandinavian Journal of Infectious Diseases* 2005;**37**(11-12):838-41.

[121] Qvist T, Taylor-Robinson D, Waldmann E, *et al*. Comparing the harmful effects of nontuberculous mycobacteria and Gram negative bacteria on lung function in patients with cystic fibrosis. *Journal of Cystic Fibrosis* 2016;**15**(3):380-5.

[122] Park IK, Olivier KN. Nontuberculous mycobacteria in cystic fibrosis and non-cystic fibrosis bronchiectasis. *Seminars in Respiratory and Critical Care Medicine* 2015;**36**(2): 217-224.

[123] Krzewinski JW, Nguyen CD, Foster JM, Burns JL. Use of random amplified polymorphic DNA PCR to examine epidemiology of *Stenotrophomonas maltophilia* and *Achromobacter* (*Alcaligenes*) *xylosoxidans* from patients with cystic fibrosis. *Journal of Clinical Microbiology* 2001;**39**(10):3597-602.

[124] Marzuillo C, de Giusti M, Tufi D, *et al*. Molecular characterization of Stenotrophomonas maltophilia isolates from cystic fibrosis patients and the hospital environment. *Infection Control & Hospital Epidemiology* 2009;**30**(08):753-8.

[125] Elting LS, Khardori N, Bodey GP, Fainstein V. Nosocomial infection caused by Xanthomonas maltophilia: a case-control study of predisposing factors. *Infection Control & Hospital Epidemiology* 1990;**11**(3):134-8.

[126] Sanyal SC, Mokaddas EM. The increase in carbapenem use and emergence of *Stenotrophomonas maltophilia* as an important nosocomial pathogen. *Journal of Chemotherapy* 1999; **11**(1):28-33.

[127] Denton M, Todd NJ, Littlewood J. Role of anti-pseudomonal antibiotics in the emergence of *Stenotrophomonas maltophilia* in cystic fibrosis patients. *European Journal of Clinical Microbiology and Infectious Diseases* 1996;**15**(5):402-5.

[128] Marchac V, Equi A, Le Bihan-Benjamin C, Hodson M, Bush A. Case-control study of *Stenotrophomonas maltophilia* acquisition in cystic fibrosis patients. *European Respiratory Journal* 2004;**23**(1):98-102.

[129] Ritz N, Ammann RA, Casaulta-Aebischer C, Schoeni-Affolter F, Schoeni MH. Risk factors for allergic bronchopulmonary aspergillosis and sensitisation to Aspergillus fumigatus in patients with cystic fibrosis. *European Journal of Pediatrics* 2005;**164**(9):577-82.

[130] Waters V, Yau Y, Prasad S, *et al*. *Stenotrophomonas maltophilia* in cystic fibrosis: serologic response and effect on lung disease. *American Journal of Respiratory and Critical Care Medicine* 2011;**183**(5):635-40.

[131] Waters V, Atenafu EG, Lu A, Yau Y, Tullis E, Ratjen F. Chronic *Stenotrophomonas maltophilia* infection and mortality or lung transplantation in cystic fibrosis patients. *Journal of Cystic Fibrosis* 2013;**12**(5):482-6.

[132] Klinger JD, Thomassen MJ. Occurrence and antimicrobial susceptibility of gram-negative nonfermentative bacilli in cystic fibrosis patients. *Diagnostic Microbiology and Infectious Disease* 1985;**3**(2):149-58.

[133] Swenson CE, Sadikot RT. Achromobacter respiratory infections. *Annals of the American Thoracic Society* 2015;**12**(2):252-8.

[134] Hansen CR, Pressler T, Ridderberg W, Johansen HK, Skov M. Achromobacter species in cystic fibrosis: cross-infection caused by indirect patient-to-patient contact. *Journal of Cystic Fibrosis* 2013;**12**(6):609-15.

[135] Amoureux L, Bador J, Siebor E, Taillefumier N, Fanton A, Neuwirth C. Epidemiology and resistance of Achromobacter xylosoxidans from cystic fibrosis patients in Dijon, Burgundy: first French data. *Journal of Cystic Fibrosis* 2013;**12**(2):170-6.

[136] Firmida MC, Pereira RH, Silva EA, Marques EA, Lopes AJ. Clinical impact of Achromobacter xylosoxidans colonization/infection in patients with cystic fibrosis. *Brazilian Journal of Medical and Biological Research* 2016;**49**(4):e5097.

[137] Price KE, Hampton TH, Gifford AH, *et al.* Unique microbial communities persist in individual cystic fibrosis patients throughout a clinical exacerbation. *Microbiome* 2013;**1**:27.

[138] Quinn RA, Lim YW, Mak TD, *et al.* Metabolomics of pulmonary exacerbations reveals the personalized nature of cystic fibrosis disease. *PeerJ* 2016;**4**:e2174.

[139] Quinn RA, Phelan VV, Whiteson KL, *et al.* Microbial, host and xenobiotic diversity in the cystic fibrosis sputum metabolome. *The ISME Journal* 2016;**10**:1483-98.

[140] Anderson JL, Miles C, Tierney AC. Effect of probiotics on respiratory, gastrointestinal and nutritional outcomes in patients with cystic fibrosis: a systematic review. *Journal of Cystic Fibrosis* 2016; Epub ahead of print. doi: 10.1016/j.jcf.2016.09.004

[141] Bruzzese E, Raia V, Spagnuolo MI, *et al.* Effect of Lactobacillus GG supplementation on pulmonary exacerbations in patients with cystic fibrosis: a pilot study. *Clinical Nutrition* 2007;**26**(3):322-8.

[142] Weiss B, Bujanover Y, Yahav Y, Vilozni D, Fireman E, Efrati O. Probiotic supplementation affects pulmonary exacerbations in patients with cystic fibrosis: a pilot study. *Pediatric Pulmonology* 2010;**45**(6):536-40.

[143] Ananthan A, Balasubramanian H, Rao S, Patole S. Probiotic supplementation in children with cystic fibrosis—a systematic review. *European Journal of Pediatrics* 2016;**175**(10): 1255-66.

[144] Janahi IA, Rehman A. Clinical manifestations of cystic fibrosis and their management. In: *Cystic and Idiopathic Pulmonary Fibrosis: Risk Factors, Management and Long-Term Health Outcomes.* Robertson L (ed). Hauppauge, NY: Nova Publishers, Inc. 2016; pp.1-56.

Chapter 4

Burkholderia cepacia Complex Infections Among Cystic Fibrosis Patients: Perspectives and Challenges

Jorge H. Leitão, Joana R. Feliciano, Sílvia A. Sousa,
Tiago Pita and Soraia I. Guerreiro

Additional information is available at the end of the chapter

http://dx.doi.org/10.5772/67712

Abstract

The *Burkholderia cepacia* complex (Bcc) is a group of closely related bacterial species that emerged in the 1980s as the etiological agents of severe and often lethal respiratory infections among cystic fibrosis (CF) patients. After several outbreaks in CF centers in Europe and North America, segregation measures were introduced to avoid patient-to-patient transmission. Presently, the prevalence of Bcc infections among CF patients worldwide is below 5% in the majority of CF centers, although exceptions are registered in some European countries. Infections by these pathogens remain problematic due to the high resistance to antimicrobials, the easy patient-to-patient transmission, and the unpredictable outcome of infections that range from asymptomatic carriage to the cepacia syndrome, a fulminating pneumonia often associated with septicemia that can lead to the decease of patients within a period of time as short as 1 week. In this chapter, we review the evolving epidemiology of Bcc infections in CF patients, the virulence traits and mechanisms used by these bacteria, and the recent developments in vaccine and vaccine components research to prevent Bcc infections.

Keywords: *Burkholderia cepacia* complex, emerging species, evolving epidemiology, virulence determinants, immunoreactive proteins, vaccine development

1. Introduction

The *Burkholderia cepacia* complex (hereafter referred to as Bcc) is a group of closely related bacteria that emerged in the 1980s as problematic pathogens to cystic fibrosis (CF) patients [1]. Infections by Bcc are particularly feared due to (1) the easy patient-to-patient transmission of specific strains; (2) the ability to resist to multiple antibiotics; and (3) the unpredictable outcome of infections, which ranges from asymptomatic carriage to the so-called cepacia syndrome, an often lethal necrotizing pneumonia accompanied with septicemia [1, 2]. Initially described in the 1950s by Burkholder [3] as the cause of soft rot in onions, the species then named *Pseudomonas cepacia* was moved into the new genus *Burkholderia* after the work of Yabuuchi and colleagues in 1992 [4]. However, the most impressive developments on the taxonomy of this group of bacteria have been achieved after the seminal work of Vandamme and colleagues who proposed the division of the species into distinct genomovars [5]. Presently, the Bcc comprises 20 species (**Table 1**), and the genome sequence of several strains is publicly available in databases such as the Burkholderia Genome DB and the Integrated Microbial Genomes & Microbiomes [6, 7].

Bcc species	Genome sequence availability	Reference
B. ambifaria	4 complete genomes (strains AMMD, MC40-6, MEX-5, IOP-120)	[8]
B. anthina	In progress	[9]
B. arboris	In progress	[10]
B. cenocepacia	18 complete genomes (strains J2315, H111, AU1054, B1, MCO-3, PC184, HI2424, DDS 22E-1, DWS 37E-2, ST32, 842, 895, MSMB384 WGS, 6, 7, CEIB, 869T2, TAtl-371)	[11]
B. cepacia	8 complete genomes (strains 383, AMMD, ATCC 25416; Bu72, DDS 7H-2, GG4, JBK9, LO6)	[4]
B. contaminans	1 complete genome (strain MS14)	[12]
B. diffusa	In progress	[10]
B. dolosa	1 complete genome (strain AU0158)	[13]
B. lata	1 complete genome (strain 383)	[12]
B. latens	In progress	[10]
B. metallica	No information	[10]
B. multivorans	3 complete genomes (ATCC17616, ATCC BAA-247, DDS 15A-1)	[5]
B. pseudomultivorans	In progress	[14]
B. pyrrocinia	1 complete genome (strain DSM 10685)	[9]
B. seminalis	In progress	[10]
B. stabilis	No information	[15]
B. stagnalis	In progress	[16]
B. territorii	In progress	[16]
B. ubonensis	1 complete genome (strain MSMB22)	[17]
B. vietnamiensis	3 complete genomes (strains G4, LMG10929, WPB)	[18]

Databases were assessed by the end of July 2016.

Table 1. *Burkholderia cepacia* complex species names and genome sequence availability in the databases Burkholderia Genome DB and Integrated Microbial Genomes & Microbiomes [6, 7].

2. Evolving epidemiology of Bcc infections

All Bcc species are virtually potential pathogens to CF patients. However, epidemiology studies have shown an uneven geographical and regional distribution of clinical isolates among the Bcc species, with the predominance of *Burkholderia cenocepacia,* followed by *Burkholderia multivorans*. Early studies performed during the 1980s and 1990s have shown that in addition to cases of chronic infection due to specific strains, many outbreaks reported in Europe and North America were due to the spread of particularly virulent strains that easily disseminated within a given CF center [1]. Although the environment is thought to be the natural reservoir of these strains, a definitive proof is still lacking.

A few particularly epidemic strains became notorious for the worst reasons. Perhaps, the best-known strain is the Edinburgh-Toronto lineage also known as the ET12 clone, an intercontinental clone responsible for several infections and fatalities in CF centers in the UK and Canada [19]. The best-known representative strain of this highly transmissible clone is the *B. cenocepacia* J2315 strain, the first Bcc strain with its genome sequence publicly available (**Table 1**) and one of the best studied Bcc strains [20]. Another example of a strain that disseminated within centers and even among centers is the PHDC strain. The strain, responsible for almost 20% prevalence in one CF center in the USA, was later found in another CF center, where an increase in Bcc prevalence was experienced. The dissemination of the strain was associated with the transfer of an infected patient from the initial center to the second one [21]. A later study by Coenye et al. [22] showed that the PHDC strain was also present in European patients (namely in France, Italy, and the UK), concluding that the PHDC strain was the second-identified Bcc transatlantic clone. Interestingly, both intercontinental clones belong to the *B. cenocepacia* species, although the ET12 belongs to subgroup IIIA and the PHDC belongs to subgroup IIIB. The *B. cenocepacia* species includes other clones that spread among CF centers, namely the Midwest American clone and the CZI Czech epidemic clone [23, 24]. Evidence of transmission of particularly epidemic strains of *B. cenocepacia* led to the introduction of segregation measures in CF centers in Europe and America, with a significant reduction of prevalence of infections [1, 25–27]. However, these segregation policies had a devastating impact on patients infected with Bcc due to social isolation and stigma and negative psychological impacts [28]. Although effective in interrupting strain transmission, segregation measures do not prevent new acquisitions. Nevertheless, these measures led to a reduction of prevalence of Bcc infections from more than 20% in several centers to less than 5% both in the USA and the majority of European countries [29, 30]. However, prevalence of chronic Bcc infections is still ranging 5–10% in Denmark, Portugal, Slovak Republic, Russian Federation, and Latvia, reaching values of 15 and 23% in Serbia and Lithuania, respectively [30].

Although the Bcc strains responsible for the vast majority of infections both in Europe and North America belong to the *B. cenocepacia* species, recent evidence indicates a changing epidemiology. *B. multivorans* emerged as the dominant species in France by 2004 and as the second most important species in the USA [31, 32]. Recent reports also indicate *Burkholderia contaminans* as an emerging Bcc species associated with CF infections. Early reports of a high incidence of the species among CF patients came from Portugal and Argentina [33–35].

Interestingly, in the case of the Portuguese CF population, two *B. contaminans* clones infecting CF patients were found as indistinguishable from two *B. contaminans* strains isolated from nonsterile nasal saline solutions of commercial origin during routine surveillance by the Portuguese Medicines and Health Products Authority [36]. A recent work by Medina-Pascual and colleagues on the surveillance of Bcc infections in Spanish CF patients also reported a *B. contaminans* overall incidence of 36.5% in the period 2008–2012, surpassing the previously dominant species *B. cenocepacia* and *B. multivorans* [37]. The emergence of *B. contaminans* among Spanish CF patients was hypothesized to be due to unspecified ecological advantages that enable the species to increase its presence in hospitals or in the environment [37]. In the case of Swiss CF-patients, *B. cenocepacia* was the most frequently isolated species in the period 1998–2013, but *B. multivorans* and *B. contaminans* emerged during the last years of the study period [38]. A 30-year study of Bcc infections among CF patients from British Columbia (Canada) evidenced a major impact of segregation measures in Bcc epidemiology; while *B. cenocepacia* was dominant before the introduction of these measures, *B. multivorans* strains became dominant after implementation of novel infection control measures in 1995 [39]. This study and others highlight the impact of infection control measures on Bcc species recovered from CF patients. It is now apparent that while epidemic *B. cenocepacia* strains dominated in early years, nonclonal *B. multivorans* and *B. contaminans* strains are emerging.

3. Bcc virulence factors and traits

Over the last 20 years, substantial progress has been achieved on the knowledge of Bcc virulence factors and determinants, although the exact contribution of some of them to the success of infection remains to be fully understood. It is currently accepted that Bcc virulence does not rely on a single virulence factor, being multifactorial. Bacterial structures such as flagella, the cable pili, and the 22-kDa adhesin are considered virulence factors since they play important roles in the initial steps of interaction with the host cell, promoting the adherence to the lung surface and the invasion of lung epithelial cells [39–41]. In addition, the majority of *B. cenocepacia* strains are able to survive and replicate intracellularly in airway epithelial cells and macrophages, evading the primary cellular defense mechanisms of the lung and avoiding clearance. The factors involved in this ability, exopolysaccharide (EPS) biosynthesis, biofilm formation, resistance to antibiotics, and oxidative stress resistance, as well as the iron acquisition ability are also among virulence determinants described for Bcc [20, 42, 43]. Some of these virulence factors are further detailed below.

3.1. Alternative sigma factors

RpoE and RpoN are two alternative sigma factors involved in the regulation of the ability of intracellular *B. cenocepacia* to delay phagolysosomal fusion in murine macrophages [44, 45]. RpoE is the extra-cytoplasmic stress response regulator required by *B. cenocepacia* to grow under conditions of high osmolarity and high temperature [44]. RpoN, or sigma factor σ^{54}, is best known for its involvement in nitrogen-related gene regulation. In *B. cenocepacia*, σ^{54} is involved in motility and biofilm formation [45]. Results from the mapping of σ^{54} regulon and the characterization of a *B. cenocepacia* H111-derived σ^{54} mutant suggest that this alternative sigma factor plays an important role in the control of nitrogen metabolism, in the metabolic adaptation of *B. cenocepacia* H111 to stressful and nutrient-limited environments and in virulence toward the nematode *Caenorhabditis elegans* [46]. In addition, it was also reported that RpoN regulates genes involved in exopolysaccharide production, biofilm formation, motility, and virulence [46]. A *B. cenocepacia* mutant defective in a gene encoding a putative σ^{54}-related transcription regulator (BCAL1536) was found as attenuated in the rat agar bead infection model [47].

3.2. Lipopolysaccharides and extracellular polysaccharides

One of the central components of the outer membrane in Gram-negative bacteria is the lipopolysaccharide (LPS), a complex molecule composed by the lipid A, the core oligosaccharide, and the O-antigen moieties (reviewed in Ref. [48]). The genes involved in LPS production by *B. cenocepacia* are located in chromosome I, organized in three main clusters, one for each LPS component (lipid A: *BCAL1929* to *BCAL1935*; core: *BCAL2402* to *BCAL2408*; O antigen: *BCAL3110* to *BCAL3125*) together with additional genes encoding sugar modification enzymes [49, 50]. Bcc bacteria LPS differs from other Gram-negative bacteria LPS due to the complete lack of negatively charged residues and the presence of the heterodimeric disaccharide D-glycero-D-talo-oct-2-ulosonic acid-(2–4)-3-deoxy-D-manno-oct-2-ulosonic acid (Ko-(2–4)-Kdo) in the core region; the presence of a 4-amino-4-deoxyarabinose (Ara4N) residue, either in the core or in lipid A; and the structure of O-antigen [50, 51]. This particular composition changes the bacterial surface charge, inhibiting the binding and successful action of antibiotics, contributing to the persistence of bacterial infection [51]. Recently, it was demonstrated that although L-Ara4N modifications do not affect recognition, they are critical for the establishment of infection [52]. Several studies have demonstrated that when neutrophils interact with Bcc LPS, the expression of CD11b on their surface increases, stimulating neutrophil respiratory burst response [53]. In addition, macrophages and human blood cells are also stimulated by Bcc LPS, producing pro-inflammatory cytokines such as TNF-α, IL-6, and IL-8 [54, 55].

B. cenocepacia J2315 is unable to produce the O-antigen. In this particular strain, this is due to an interruption in the *wbcE* gene-encoding BCAL 3125 [56]. The expression of O-antigen by Bcc strains was demonstrated to reduce phagocytosis by macrophages without interfering with the intracellular survival of bacteria [56].

The production of exopolysaccharides (EPSs) was described for several *Burkholderia* species. EPS production by Bcc is regarded as playing an important role in the chronicity of Bcc infections [57–62]. Cepacian is the most common EPS produced by Bcc and non-Bcc species, both from clinical and environmental sources [59, 63]. Cepacian interferes with phagocytosis by human neutrophils, facilitating the bacterial persistence in a mouse model of infection [64, 65]. The EPS was shown to inhibit the production of ROS by neutrophils and to scavenge reactive oxygen species (ROS), playing a role in the survival of cepacian-producing strains in different environments [64–67]. As a result of a frameshift mutation in the *bceB* gene (*BCAM0856*) encoding a putative glycosyltransferase, Cepacian is not produced by the *B. cenocepacia* ET12 representative strain J2315 [49, 62].

3.3. Biofilms

Bcc bacteria were found to persist in biofilms *in vitro*. Biofilm formation and maturation depend on many factors, including EPS production, motility, iron availability, and multiple gene regulatory systems, such as quorum sensing, alternative sigma factors, or global regulators such as the ShvR and AtsR [45, 58, 68–73]. In addition, Bcc can form small colony variants *in vitro*, a colony morphology that is associated with enhanced biofilm formation, antibiotic resistance, and persistence [74].

Several studies have been performed to understand the importance and relevance of biofilm formation in Bcc biology. Bcc bacteria growing in biofilms are usually more tolerant to multiple antibiotics, although similar susceptibilities were reported for plancktonic and biofilm cells to the antibiotics kanamycin, amikacin, and ciprofloxacin [75, 76]. Recently, Bcc biofilms were shown to contain persister cells that are able to survive in the presence of high concentrations of antibiotics by avoiding production of reactive oxygen species [77]. In addition, using neutrophil-like dHL60 cells, it was shown that the presence of these immune system cells enhanced biofilm formation that protected Bcc bacteria against neutrophils by inducing their necrosis, acting as a barrier to the migration of neutrophils, and masking the bacteria from being recognized by neutrophils [78]. Although some evidence suggests that biofilm formation plays a role in bacterial persistence in the CF airways, this topic needs to be further studied.

3.4. Quorum sensing

Quorum sensing is a mode of regulation of gene expression that is dependent on the density of the bacterial population. Bcc bacteria have at least four quorum sensing systems. The CepIR quorum sensing system is homologous to the LuxIR system of *Vibrio fischeri* (reviewed in Ref. [79]). The CepIR system positively regulates the virulence of *B. cenocepacia* toward model organisms like *C. elegans*, *Galleria mellonella*, rodents, zebrafish, alfalfa, and onions [80–83]. In addition to the CepIR, *B. cenocepacia* encodes the CciIR, the CepR2, and the BDSF quorum sensing systems [84, 85]. While the CepIR and CciR quorum sensing systems rely on acyl homoserine lactones as signaling molecules, the BDSF system uses cis-2-dodecenoic acid as the signaling molecule, and the CepR2 is an orphan quorum sensing system [85]. An arsenal of genes regulated by quorum sensing in Bcc bacteria was described, including the negatively regulated siderophore synthesis and the positively regulated expression of the genes encoding zinc metalloproteases (Zmps), swarming motility and biofilm formation, all thought to have an impact when the bacterium is infecting the CF patient [71, 80, 86, 87].

3.5. Protein secretion systems

Both Gram-negative and positive bacteria use protein secretion systems to secrete toxins or other proteins, either directly into the environment or into host cells. These systems are particularly well studied in the CF pathogens Bcc and *Pseudomonas aeruginosa*. For instance, Bcc strains of the ET12 lineage and *Burkholderia vietnamiensis* harbor type I and II secretion systems (T1SS, T2SS) implicated, for instance, in the secretion of hemolytic proteins [88, 89]. The T2SS is also involved in *B. cenocepacia* secretion of two zinc metalloproteases, ZmpA and ZmpB, which play a role in virulence [80, 90]. Two T4SSs are encoded by *B. cenocepacia*; the T4SS-1 encoded in a plasmid, and the T4SS-2 encoded in chromosome 2 [91]. Until now, only the T4SS-1 was identified in *B. cenocepacia* strains as necessary for virulence in onions and intracellular survival in phagocytes [92].

In a mouse agar bead infection model, the T3SS has been shown to be important for bacterial pathogenesis [93]. Although the precise mechanism is still not clear, T3SS seems to play no role in intracellular survival of *B. cenocepacia* [94].

Four type V secretion systems are encoded within the genome of *B. cenocepacia* J2315 [49]. Proteins transported by this type of transporters contain pertactin and hemagglutinin domains and are thought to play a role in bacterial adhesion [49].

B. cenocepacia also encodes a T6SS, which was shown to affect the actin cytoskeleton of macrophages and the assembly of the reduced nicotinamide adenine dinucelotide phosphate (NADPH) oxidase complex in *B. cepacia*-containing vacuoles (BcCV's) by inactivation of Rac1 and Cdc42 [73, 95, 96]. *B. cenocepacia* was found to efficiently activate the inflammasome by a yet uncharacterized T6SS effector [97]. Consequently, monocytes and THP-1 cells release IL-1β in a pyrin-, Asc-, and T6SS-dependent manner [97]. The T6SS also enhances caspase-1 activation, negatively regulated by the sensor kinase-response regulator AtsR [73]. In addition, a recent paper suggests that the T6SS might be important for the secretion of T2SS effectors into the host cytoplasm, such as ZmpA and ZmpB, revealing an unanticipated role for type II secretion systems in intracellular survival and replication of *B. cenocepacia* [96]. Although membrane vesicles cannot be considered a canonical secretion system, they can effectively allow the secretion of several hydrolytic enzymes and toxins [98]. **Table 2** summarizes and compares the most relevant information available about secretion systems of Bcc bacteria and their counterparts in the major CF pathogen *P. aeruginosa*.

3.6. Iron uptake

In order to carry out iron chelation and uptake, members of the Bcc can produce up to four distinct siderophores: ornibactin, pyochelin, cepabactin, and cepaciachelin [122]. Ornibactin appears to be the most important and abundant siderophore produced by *B. cenocepacia* strains [123, 124]. The pathways and regulatory mechanisms of ornibactin synthesis and uptake are relatively well known [87, 125–127]. The requirement of this siderophore for *B. cenocepacia* virulence was demonstrated in different infection models, including the rat agar bead, *G. mellonella*, and *C. elegans* [82, 125, 127].

The competition for available iron by Bcc bacteria and other CF lung colonizing organisms such as *P. aeruginosa* was reported to occur in the CF lung, although it is not completely clear how Bcc organisms acquire iron from host proteins [128, 129].

Secretion system	***Burkholderia cepacia* complex**	***P. aeruginosa***
T1SS	Hemolytic proteins [88, 89]	HasAp (heme-binding) [99]; AprA and AprX (alkaline proteases) [100, 101]
T2SS	ZmpA and ZmpB [80, 90]	LasB (Major extracellular protease) [102], Staphylolysin LasA [102], Aminopeptidase PaAP [103], Protease IV [104], Lipases LipA, LipC, phospholipase C, PlcH, and PlcN [105, 106], CbpD Chitin-binding protein CbpD [107]; Exotoxin A [108]
T3SS	No effector described yet, plays a role in evasion of the host immune system [93, 94]	GTPase-activator ExoS and ADP-ribosyltransferase ExoT [109], adenylate cyclase ExoY [110], phospholipase A2 ExoU and ExoS [111]
T4SS	T4SS-1: Plant cytotoxic proteins, T4SS-2: Plasmid mobilization [91]	Integrative and conjugative elements (ICEs): ICE*clc* [112], Pathogenicity islands: pKLC102 (includes the type IV sex pili-encoding pil cluster and the *chvB* gene encoding a virulence factor) [113], and PAP-I (includes several virulence factors, such as CupD type fimbriae, and the PvrSR/RcsCB regulatory system) [114]
T5SS	Four T5SS: two containing pertactin domains involved in adhesion, other two contain haemagglutinin repeats [49]	Autotransporter: EstA (esterase activity) [115]; Two-partner secretion systems LepA/LepB [116] and CupB [117], and the PdtA/PdtB system [118]
T6SS	Hcp and VgrGs [73, 95, 96]	Hcp and VgrGs [119, 120]
Membrane vesicles (MV)	MV-associated (metallo)proteases, (phospho)lipases, peptidoglycan-degrading enzymes [98]	Multiple virulence factors: Alkaline phosphatase, hemolytic phospholipase C; the Cif toxin that inhibits CFTR-mediated chloride secretion in the airways [121]

Table 2. Summary of secretion systems from Bcc and the respective counterparts from the CF major pathogen *P. aeruginosa*.

3.7. Resistance to antimicrobials

Difficulties in eradicating Bcc infections mainly result from their intrinsic resistance to multiple antibiotics, including polymyxins, aminoglycosides, and most β-lactams. In addition, these bacteria have the ability to develop *in vivo* resistance to virtually all classes of antibiotics [20, 130, 131]. Antibiotics administration to CF patients was also reported to affect resistance profiles of Bcc bacteria [132]. Various mechanisms involved in the resistance of Bcc to multiple antibiotics have been described and include enzymatic inactivation (β-lactamases, aminoglycoside-inactivating enzymes, dihydrofolate reductase), alteration of drug targets, integrons, cell wall impermeability, and active efflux pumps [88, 133–140]. However, major contributions to intrinsic and acquired multidrug resistance by Bcc seem to be due to efflux pumps of the resistance nodulation cell division (RND) family. In fact, the *B. cenocepacia* J2315 genome encodes at least 16 efflux systems of the RND family [141]. At least six of these RND efflux pumps were implicated in drug resistance—RND-1, RND-3, RND-4, RND-8, RND-9, and RND-10 [138–140, 142,

143]. RND-3 and RND-4 efflux pumps were described as being involved in the resistance to various antimicrobial drugs including tobramycin and ciprofloxacin; the RND-3, RND-8, and RND-9 efflux systems protect biofilm-grown cells against tobramycin; the RND-8 and RND-9 efflux pumps are not involved in ciprofloxacin resistance; and RND-10 efflux pump seems to confer resistance to chloramphenicol, fluoroquinolones, and trimethoprim [140, 143]. It was suggested that mutations in the RND-3 regulator-encoding gene may be responsible for the prevalent overexpression of this efflux pump in clinical Bcc isolates, contributing to their high levels of antibiotics resistance [144].

3.8. Motility

Genes involved in the synthesis and assembly of *B. cenocepacia* flagella are located in chromosome I, distributed within five clusters, with two additional genes found on chromosomes 2 and 3 [49]. These genes were found as being upregulated when the organism was incubated in CF sputum, contributing to its virulence in a murine agar bead infection model [145, 146]. More recently, flagellin expression and flagellar morphology of *B. cenocepacia* grown in a medium mimicking the CF sputum was analyzed [147]. Those nutritional conditions led to increased motility and flagellin expression, by inducing the synthesis of multiple flagella on the cell surface of *B. cenocepacia* K56-2 [147]. A link between the loss of bacterial motility and the development of the cepacia syndrome was recently established based on a transcriptomics analysis comparing the *B. cenocepacia* ST32 CF isolates recovered from bloodstream, at the time of cepacia syndrome, with their sputum counterparts, recovered prior to the development of this syndrome, revealing that flagellar genes were downregulated in isolates recovered from the bloodstream [148].

3.9. Intracellular survival

Infection assays using free-living amoeba demonstrated that *B. cenocepacia* can survive in an acidified intracellular compartment [94, 149]. These bacteria were also demonstrated to have the ability to delay the maturation of phagolysosomes in murine macrophages [94–96, 150]. Although the *B. cenocepacia* containing vacuoles (BcCVs) progress normally to the early phagosomal stage, the fusion of the BcCV's with late endosomes and subsequent maturation is significantly delayed comparing with vacuoles containing heat-killed bacteria [94]. In contrast to heat-killed bacteria that ended up in phagolysosomes with a pH of 4.5, BcCVs did not acidify normally maintaining a luminal pH around 6.4 [94]. This ability of *B. cenocepacia* to alter the acidification of the vacuole seems to be correlated with the delay in recruitment or assembly on the BcCV membrane of both the 16-kDa subunit of the phagosomal vacuolar ATPase (vATPase) and the NADPH phagocyte oxidase [96, 151]. In contrast, Al-Khodor and colleagues demonstrated that *B. cenocepacia* J2315 only transiently interacts with the endocytic pathway, event after which the bacterium is able to rapidly escape to the cytosol [152]. Escaped bacteria are afterward targeted by the host autophagy pathway, through the recruitment to the bacterial vicinity of the ubiquitin conjugation system, the autophagy adaptors p62 and NDP52, and the autophagosome membrane-associated protein LC3B. However, apparently, this host cell control through autophagy ultimately fails in a high proportion of infected cells, being *B. cenocepacia* able to block the autophagosome completion and replicate in the cytosol of the host cell [152].

To better understand the intracellular behavior of *B. cenocepacia* in CF infected patients, studies have also been performed in Cystic fibrosis transmembrane conductance regulator (CFTR)-defective macrophages. Remarkably, the delayed maturation arresting of BcCV's is more exaggerated in CFTR-defective macrophages than in normal macrophages and is specific to live *B. cenocepacia* [153]. Although it is not clear how the CFTR defect enhances the *B. cenocepacia* intracellular survival, there is evidence of a link between the defective CFTR with autophagy deficiency and decreased clearance of protein aggregates and inflammation [154]. The elucidation of these survival details, especially the ability of *B. cenocepacia* to synergize with the CFTR defect and its consequences on the mechanism of autophagy will provide new avenues to explore novel therapeutic approaches for CF patients [155].

4. Toward a vaccine to prevent Bcc infections

No objective guidelines for eradication strategies are available for Bcc infections, as these pathogens are intrinsically resistant to the majority of the clinical available antimicrobials [156]. Currently, no immunotherapeutic strategy to protect CF patients from Bcc infections is available. Several studies on the immune response elicited by Bcc species in CF patients have been performed; however, they are challenging due to the ability of this bacteria to modulate and overcome the host immune responses and the ability to survive intracellularly in phagocytes and epithelial cells [157, 158].

An important aspect to consider during vaccine design is the optimal balance of Th1 and Th2 responses required for effective pathogen clearance. For example, a Th1 bias elicits a cell-mediated response, while Th2 induces a humoral immune response [159]. In the case of CF, their immune phenotype appears to be skewed toward Th2 responses [160]. In the case of Bcc, the type of host response necessary to clear the pathogen is still not fully understood, making it difficult to develop a protective vaccine (**Table 3**). Recently, BALB/c mice immunized intraperitoneally with the proteins Linocin and OmpW showed a significant reduction of *B. cenocepacia* and *B. multivorans* cells in the lung and lower dissemination of bacteria to the spleen [161]. While Linocin led to a robust Th1 response, the OmpW led to a mixed Th1/Th2 response [161]. The protection achieved with these proteins was greater against *B. cenocepacia* infection, and OmpW immunization was more efficient in reducing the lung bacterial load [161].

Nonpurified outer membrane proteins (OMP) from *B. multivorans*, supplemented with the mucosal adjuvant adamantylamide dipeptide (AdDP) that promotes a robust Th2 response, were tested for immunization of BALB/c mice [162]. A statistically significant increase in IgG and in mucosal IgA OMP-specific antibodies was observed, together with a reduction of *B. multivorans* burden and lung pathology, but only a moderate cross protection to *B. cenocepacia* was reported. The specificity of the immune response was found to be against

90, 72, 66, and 60 kDa proteins. Elicitation of specific IgA antibodies by mucosal immunization was also reported to be important to prevent the colonization of the respiratory tract by Bcc bacteria. In another study, the intranasal immunization of CD-1 mice with outer membrane proteins (OMP) from *B. cenocepacia* was described to originate a Th2-biased response with the maintenance of the bacterial burden, while mice immunized with OMP and the noninflammatory mucosal adjuvant nanoemulsion (NE) elicited a Th1/Th2-balanced response that led to a significant reduction of the *B. cenocepacia* cell burden [163]. The serum derived from mice vaccinated with OMP-NE could also inhibit *B. multivorans* growth by 80.1%, showing that induction of cross-reactive antibodies occurred after mice immunization. Additionally, a highly conserved 17-kDa OmpA-like protein was recently identified as a new immunedominant epitope in mucosal immunization [163].

Metalloproteases are also considered as potential effective candidates for vaccine development [90]. It was demonstrated that immunizations of rats using a conserved zinc metalloprotease peptide 15 (PSCP) decreased the severity of *B. cenocepacia* infection and the lung damage was reduced by 50% upon challenge with a *B. cenocepacia* strain after immunization [90].

In 2012, it was shown that the bacterial surface polysaccharide poly-β-(1-6)-N-acetyl-glucosamine (PNAG) confers protective immunity against Bcc infection in a lethal peritonitis mice model [164]. In this study by Skurnik and colleagues using opsophagocytic assays, it was observed that goat-raised antibodies against PNAG could kill Bcc strains (>80%) of the *B. ceno-*

Antigen	**Immune response**	**Bcc animal model**	***In vitro* models**	**References**
OmpW	Mixed Th1/Th2	BALB/c mice immunosuppressed with cyclophosphamide	Spleen cells from mice	[161]
Linocin	Th1	BALB/c mice immunosuppressed with cyclophosphamide	Spleen cells from mice	[162]
OMP plus NE	Mixed Th1/Th2	CD-1 mice	Murine splenocytes	[163]
OMP plus AdDP	Higher IgG and IgA titers	BALB/c mice immunosuppressed with cyclophosphamide	ND	[162]
PNAG	ND	FVB/N mice	Opsonophagocytic assay	[164]
Zinc metalloprotease peptide 15 (PSCP)	Higher IgG and IgA titers	Sprague-Dawley rat agar bead model	ND	[90]
FliC	ND	ND	T cell hybridoma assays	[165]
BCAL2958	High IgG titers in human CF serum samples	ND	Human neutrophils	[166]

ND—Not determined.

Table 3. Summary of vaccine development against Bcc infections.

cepacia, *Burkholderia dolosa* and *B. multivorans* species. Furthermore, bacterial killing was found to depend of the presence of the complement [164].

Other proteins of putative immunogenic activity have been reported as potential vaccine candidates. However, studies in a Bcc infection animal model are still lacking (**Table 3**). One of these promising antigens is the OmpA-like BCAL2958 protein that was shown to be highly conserved in Bcc, to elicit IgG antibodies in CF patients and to elicit an increase of TNFα, elastase, NO, and MPO in neutrophils [166].

Musson and colleagues have shown that T-cell hybridomas against the *Burkholderia pseudomallei* flagellar protein FliC epitope cross-reacted with orthologous FliC sequences from *B. multivorans* and *B. cenocepacia* [165]. FliC epitopes were accessible for processing and presentation from live or heat-killed *B. cenocepacia* bacteria, demonstrating that flagellin enters the HLA class II Ag presentation pathway during infection of macrophages with *B. cenocepacia*.

Studies referred above revealed that subunit vaccines that only produce an antibody response cannot fully prevent an infection caused by Bcc bacteria [157, 161, 164]. Therefore, Bcc vaccines containing multiple antigens that elicit a balanced Th1 and Th2 response are expected to be effective in preventing Bcc infections. With this aim, immunoproteomics approaches have been performed. For instance, Mariappan and colleagues identified 18 immunogenic proteins from culture supernatants of *B. cepacia* that reacted with mice antibodies raised against inactivated *B. cepacia* whole cells [167]. More recently, the analysis of the imunoproteome of two clinical relevant strains of *B. cenocepacia* and *B. multivorans* revealed 15 common immunoreactive proteins that reacted with CF human serum samples [168].

5. Concluding remarks

An overview of Bcc infections in CF from early 1980s until the more recent available data was presented. The prevalence of Bcc species in CF patients worldwide is still evolving, most probably as a result of infection control measures and segregation policies. Many virulence factors have been identified, and the resulting wealth of information prompted the establishment of new research lines envisaging the development of novel protective strategies and products, namely vaccines and vaccine components.

Acknowledgements

Funding received by iBB-Institute for Bioengineering and Biosciences from FCT-Portuguese Foundation for Science and Technology (UID/BIO/04565/2013) and from Programa Operacional Regional de Lisboa 2020 (Project N. 007317) is acknowledged. This work was also partially funded by FCT through contract PTDC/BIA-MIC/1615/2014 and grants to SAS (SFRH/BPD/102006/2014), JRF (BL184), and TP (BL183).

Author details

Jorge H. Leitão*, Joana R. Feliciano, Sílvia A. Sousa, Tiago Pita and Soraia I. Guerreiro

*Address all correspondence to: jorgeleitao@tecnico.ulisboa.pt

Departamento de Bioengenharia, Instituto Superior Técnico (IST), Universidade de Lisboa, iBB – Institute for Bioengineering and Biosciences, Lisboa, Portugal

References

[1] Govan JR, Deretic V. Microbial pathogenesis in cystic fibrosis: mucoid *Pseudomonas aeruginosa* and *Burkholderia cepacia*. Microbiol Rev. 1996; 60:539-574.

[2] Isles A, Maclusky I, Corey M, Gold R, Prober C, Fleming P, Levison H. *Pseudomonas cepacia* infection in cystic fibrosis: an emerging problem. J Pediatr. 1984; 104:206-210. DOI:10.1016/S0022-3476(84)80993-2.

[3] Burkholder WH. Sour skin, a bacterial rot of onion bulbs. Phytopathology. 1950; 40: 115-117.

[4] Yabuuchi E, Kosako Y, Oyaizu H, Yano I, Hotta H, Hashimoto Y, Ezaki T, Arakawa M. Proposal of *Burkholderia* gen. nov. and transfer of seven species of the genus *Pseudomonas* homology group II to the new genus, with the type species *Burkholderia cepacia* (Palleroni and Holmes 1981) comb. nov. Microbiol Immunol. 1992; 36:1251-1275. DOI:10.1111/j.1348-0421.1992.tb02129.x.

[5] Vandamme P, Holmes B, Vancanneyt M, Coenye T, Hoste B, Coopman R, Revets H, Lauwers S, Gillis M, Kersters K, Govan JR. Occurrence of multiple genomovars of *Burkholderia cepacia* in cystic fibrosis patients and proposal of *Burkholderia multivorans* sp. nov. Int J Syst Bacteriol. 1997; 47:1188-1200. DOI:10.1099/00207713-47-4-1188.

[6] Burkholderia Genome DB. Available from: http://www.burkholderia.com/ [Accessed 2016-07-31].

[7] Integrated Microbial Genomes & Microbiomes. Available from: https://img.jgi.doe.gov/. [Accessed 2016-07-31].

[8] Coenye T, Mahenthiralingam E, Henry D, LiPuma JJ, Laevens S, Gillis M, Speert DP,Vandamme P. *Burkholderia ambifaria* sp. nov., a novel member of the *Burkholderia cepacia* complex including biocontrol and cystic fibrosis-related isolates. Int J Syst Evol Microbiol. 2001; 51:1481-1490. DOI:10.1099/00207713-51-4-1481.

[9] Vandamme P, Henry D, Coenye T, Nzula S, Vancanneyt M, LiPuma JJ, Speert DP, Govan JR, Mahenthiralingam E. *Burkholderia anthina* sp. nov. and *Burkholderia pyrrocinia*, two additional *Burkholderia cepacia* complex bacteria, may confound results of new molecular

diagnostic tools. FEMS Immunol Med Microbiol. 2002; 33:143-149. DOI:10.1111/j.1574-695X.2002.tb00584.x.

[10] Vanlaere E, Lipuma JJ, Baldwin A, Henry D, De Brandt E, Mahenthiralingam E, Speert D, Dowson C, Vandamme P. *Burkholderia latens* sp. nov., *Burkholderia diffusa* sp. nov., *Burkholderia arboris* sp. nov., *Burkholderia seminalis* sp. nov. and *Burkholderia metallica* sp. nov., novel species within the *Burkholderia cepacia* complex. Int J Syst Evol Microbiol. 2008; 58:1580-1590. DOI:10.1099/ijs.0.65634-0.

[11] Vandamme P, Holmes B, Coenye T, Goris J, Mahenthiralingam E, LiPuma JJ, Govan JR. *Burkholderia cenocepacia* sp. nov.--a new twist to an old story. Res Microbiol. 2003; 154:91-96. DOI:10.1016/S0923-2508(03)00026-3.

[12] Vanlaere E, Baldwin A, Gevers D, Henry D, De Brandt E, LiPuma JJ, Mahenthiralingam E, Speert DP, Dowson C, Vandamme P. Taxon K, a complex within the *Burkholderia cepacia* complex, comprises at least two novel species, *Burkholderia contaminans* sp. nov. and *Burkholderia lata* sp. nov. Int J Syst Evol Microbiol. 2009; 59:102-111. DOI:10.1099/ijs.0.001123-0.

[13] Vermis K, Coenye T, LiPuma JJ, Mahenthiralingam E, Nelis HJ, Vandamme P. Proposal to accommodate *Burkholderia cepacia* genomovar VI as *Burkholderia dolosa* sp. nov. Int J Syst Evol Microbiol. 2004; 54:689-691. DOI:10.1099/ijs.0.02888-0.

[14] Peeters C, Zlosnik JE, Spilker T, Hird TJ, LiPuma JJ, Vandamme P. *Burkholderia pseudo-multivorans* sp. nov., a novel *Burkholderia cepacia* complex species from human respiratory samples and the rhizosphere. Syst Appl Microbiol. 2013; 36:483-489. DOI:10.1016/j.syapm.2013.06.003.

[15] Vandamme P, Mahenthiralingam E, Holmes B, Coenye T, Hoste B, De Vos P, Henry D, Speert DP. Identification and population structure of *Burkholderia stabilis* sp. nov. (formerly *Burkholderia cepacia* genomovar IV). J Clin Microbiol. 2000; 38:1042-1047.

[16] De Smet B, Mayo M, Peeters C, Zlosnik JE, Spilker T, Hird TJ, LiPuma JJ, Kidd TJ, Kaestli M, Ginther JL, Wagner DM, Keim P, Bell SC, Jacobs JA, Currie BJ, Vandamme P. *Burkholderia stagnalis* sp. nov. and *Burkholderia territorii* sp. nov., two novel *Burkholderia cepacia* complex species from environmental and human sources. Int J Syst Evol Microbiol. 2015; 65:2265-2271. DOI:10.1099/ijs.0.000251.

[17] Yabuuchi E, Kawamura Y, Ezaki T, Ikedo M, Dejsirilert S, Fujiwara N, Naka T. and Kobayashi K. *Burkholderia ubonensis* sp. nov., L-arabinose-assimilating but different from *Burkholderia thailandensis* and *Burkholderia vietnamiensis*. Microbiol Immunol. 2000; 44:307-317. DOI:10.1111/j.1348-0421.2000.tb02500.x.

[18] Gillis M, Van TV, Bardin R, Goor M, Hebbar P, Willems A, Segers P, Kersters K, Heulin T, Fernandez MP. Polyphasic taxonomy in the genus *Burkholderia* leading to an amended description of the genus and proposition of *Burkholderia vietnamiensis* sp. nov. for N_2-fixing isolates from rice in Vietnam. Int J Syst Bacteriol. 1995; 45:274-289. DOI:10.1099/00207713-45-2-274.

[19] Johnson WM, Tyler SD, Rozee KR. Linkage analysis of geographic and clinical clusters in *Pseudomonas cepacia* infections by multilocus enzyme electrophoresis and ribotyping. J Clin Microbiol. 1994; 32:924-930.

[20] Mahenthiralingam E, Urban TA, Goldberg JB. The multifarious, multireplicon *Burkholderia cepacia* complex. Nat Rev Microbiol. 2005; 3:144-156. DOI:10.1038/nrmicro1085.

[21] Chen JS, Witzmann KA, Spilker T, Fink RJ, LiPuma JJ. Endemicity and inter-city spread of *Burkholderia cepacia* genomovar III in cystic fibrosis. J Pediatr. 2001; 139 :643-649. DOI:10.1067/mpd.2001.118430.

[22] Coenye T, Spilker T, Van Schoor A, LiPuma JJ, Vandamme P. Recovery of *Burkholderia cenocepacia* strain PHDC from cystic fibrosis patients in Europe. Thorax. 2004; 59:952-954. DOI:10.1136/thx.2003.019810.

[23] Coenye T, LiPuma JJ. Multilocus restriction typing: a novel tool for studying global epidemiology of *Burkholderia cepacia* complex infection in cystic fibrosis. J Infect Dis. 2002; 185:1454-1462. DOI:10.1086/340279.

[24] Drevinek P, Mahenthiralingam E. *Burkholderia cenocepacia* in cystic fibrosis: epidemiology and molecular mechanisms of virulence. Clin Microbiol Infect. 2010; 16:821-830. DOI:10.1111/j.1469-0691.2010.03237.x.

[25] Thomassen MJ, Demko CA, Klinger JD, Stern RC. *Pseudomonas cepacia* colonization among patients with cystic fibrosis. A new opportunist. Am Rev Respir Dis. 1985; 131:791-796. DOI:10.1164/arrd.1985.131.5.791.

[26] Whiteford ML, Wilkinson JD, McColl JH, et al. Outcome of *Burkholderia* (*Pseudomonas*) *cepacia* colonisation in children with cystic fibrosis following a hospital outbreak. Thorax. 1995:50; 1194-1198. DOI:10.1136/thx.50.11.1194.

[27] Muhdi K, Edenborough FP, Gumery L, et al. Outcome for patients colonised with *Burkholderia cepacia* in a Birmingham adult cystic fibrosis clinic and the end of an epidemic. Thorax. 1996; 51:374-377. DOI:10.1136/thx.51.4.374.

[28] Lynch JP 3rd. *Burkholderia cepacia* complex: impact on the cystic fibrosis lung lesion. Semin Respir Crit Care Med. 2009; 30:596-610. DOI:10.1055/s-0029-1238918.

[29] Cystic Fibrosis Foundation 2014 report. Available from: (https://www.cff.org/2014-Annual-Data-Report.pdf) [Accessed 2016-09-8].

[30] European Cystic Fibrosis Society Patient Registry Annual Data report 2013. Available from: (https://www.ecfs.eu/sites/default/files/images/ECFSPR_Report2013_02.2016.pdf). [Accessed 2016-09-8].

[31] Brisse S, Cordevant C, Vandamme P, Bidet P, Loukil C, Chabanon G, Lange M, Bingen E. Species distribution and ribotype diversity of *Burkholderia cepacia* complex isolates from French patients with cystic fibrosis. J Clin Microbiol. 2004; 42:4824-4827. DOI:10.1128/JCM.42.10.4824-4827.2004.

[32] Reik R, Spilker T, Lipuma JJ. Distribution of *Burkholderia cepaci*a complex species among isolates recovered from persons with or without cystic fibrosis. J Clin Microbiol. 2005; 43:2926-2928. DOI:10.1128/JCM.43.6.2926-2928.2005.

[33] Cunha MV, Leitão JH, Mahenthiralingam E, Vandamme P, Lito L, Barreto C, et al. Molecular analysis of *Burkholderia cepacia* complex isolates from a Portuguese cystic fibrosis center: a 7-year study. J Clin Microbiol. 2003; 41(9):4113-4120. DOI:10.1128/JCM.41.9.4113-4120.2003.

[34] Jordá-Vargas L, Degrossi J, Castañeda NC, D'Aquino M, Valvano MA, Procopio A, Galanternik L, Centrón D. Prevalence of indeterminate genetic species of B*urkholderia cepacia* complex in a cystic fibrosis center in Argentina. J Clin Microbiol. 2008; 46:1151-1152. DOI:10.1128/JCM.01595-07.

[35] Martina P, Bettiol M, Vescina C, Montanaro P, Mannino MC, Prieto CI, Vay C, Naumann D, Schmitt J, Yantorno O, Lagares O, Bosch A. Genetic diversity of *Burkholderia contaminans* isolates from cystic fibrosis patients in Argentina. J Clin Microbiol. 2013; 51:339-344. DOI:10.1128/JCM.02500-12.

[36] Cunha MV, Pinto-de-Oliveira A, Meirinhos-Soares L, Salgado MJ, Melo-Cristino J, Correia S, Barreto C, Sá-Correia I. Exceptionally high representation of *Burkholderia cepacia* among *B. cepacia* complex isolates recovered from the major Portuguese cystic fibrosis center. J Clin Microbiol. 2007; 45:1628-1633. DOI:10.1128/JCM.00234-07.

[37] Medina-Pascual MJ, Valdezate S, Carrasco G, Villalón P, Garrido N, Saéz-Nieto JA. Increase in isolation of *Burkholderia contaminans* from Spanish patients with cystic fibrosis. Clin Microbiol Infect. 2015; 21:150-156. DOI:10.1016/j.cmi.2014.07.014.

[38] Lupo A, Isis E, Tinguely R, Endimiani A. Clonality and antimicrobial susceptibility of *Burkholderia cepacia* complex isolates collected from cystic fibrosis patients during 1998-2013 in Bern, Switzerland. New Microbiol. 2015; 38:281-288. DOI:10.7892/boris.81553.

[39] Zlosnik JEA, Zhou G, Brant R, Henry DA, Hird TJ, Mahenthiralingam E, Chilvers MA, Wilcox P, Speert DP. *Burkholderia* species infections in patients with cystic fibrosis in British Columbia, Canada. 30 Years' Experience. Ann Am Thorac Soc. 2015; 12:70-78. DOI:10.1513/AnnalsATS.201408-395OC.

[40] Sajjan US, Forstner JF. Role of a 22-kilodalton pilin protein in binding of *Pseudomonas cepacia* to buccal epithelial cells. Infect Immun. 1993; 61:3157-3163.

[41] Tomich M, Herfst CA, Golden JW, Mohr CD. Role of flagella in host cell invasion by *Burkholderia cepacia*. Infect Immun. 2002; 70(4):1799-1806. DOI:10.1128/IAI.70.4.1799-1806.2002.

[42] Lefebre M, Valvano M. In vitro resistance of *Burkholderia cepacia* complex isolates to reactive oxygen species in relation to catalase and superoxide dismutase production. Microbiology. 2001; 147:97-109. DOI:10.1099/00221287-147-1-97.

[43] Miethke M, Marahiel MA. Siderophore-based ion acquisition and pathogen control. Microbiol Mol Biol Rev. 2007; 71:413-451. DOI:10.1128/MMBR.00012-07.

[44] Flannagan RS, Valvano MA. *Burkholderia cenocepacia* requires RpoE for growth under stress conditions and delay of phagolysosomal fusion in macrophages. Microbiology. 2008; 154:643-653. DOI:10.1099/mic.0.2007/013714-0.

[45] Saldías MS, Lamothe J, Wu R, Valvano MA. *Burkholderia cenocepacia* requires the RpoN sigma factor for biofilm formation and intracellular trafficking within macrophages. Infect Immun. 2008; 76:1059-1067. DOI:10.1128/IAI.01167-07.

[46] Lardi M, Aguilar C, Pedrioli A, et al. σ(54)-dependent response to nitrogen limitation and virulence in *Burkholderia cenocepacia* strain H111. Appl Environ Microbiol. 2015; 81:4077-4089. DOI:10.1128/AEM.00694-15.

[47] Hunt TA, Kooi C, Sokol PA, Valvano MA. Identification of *Burkholderia cenocepacia* genes required for bacterial survival in vivo. Infect Immun. 2004; 72(7):4010-4022. DOI:10.1128/IAI.72.7.4010-4022.2004.

[48] Vinion-Dubiel AD, Goldberg JB. Lipopolysaccharide of *Burkholderia cepacia* complex. J Endotoxin Res. 2003; 9:201-213. DOI:10.1177/09680519030090040101.

[49] Holden MTG, Seth-Smith HMB, Crossman LC, et al. The genome of *Burkholderia cenocepacia* J2315, an epidemic pathogen of cystic fibrosis patients. J Bacteriol. 2009; 191(1):261-277. DOI:10.1128/JB.01230-08.

[50] Loutet SA, Flannagan RS, Kooi C, Sokol PA, Valvano MA. A complete lipopolysaccharide inner core oligosaccharide is required for resistance of *Burkholderia cenocepacia* to antimicrobial peptides and bacterial survival in vivo. J Bacteriol. 2006; 188:2073-2080. DOI:10.1128/JB.188.6.2073-2080.2006.

[51] De Soyza A, Silipo A, Lanzetta R, Govan JR, Molinaro A. Review: chemical and biological features of *Burkholderia cepacia* complex lipopolysaccharides. Innate Immun. 2008; 14(3):127-144. DOI:10.1177/1753425908093984.

[52] Khodai-Kalaki M, Andrade A, Fathy Mohamed Y, Valvano MA. *Burkholderia cenocepacia* lipopolysaccharide modification and flagellin glycosylation affect virulence but not innate immune recognition in plants. MBio. 2015; 6(3):e00679-e00615. DOI:10.1128/mBio.00679-15.

[53] Hughes JE, Stewart J, Barclay GR, Govan JR. Priming of neutrophil respiratory burst activity by lipopolysaccharide from *Burkholderia cepacia*. Infect Immun. 1997; 65:4281-4287.

[54] Hutchison ML, Bonell EC, Poxton IR, Govan JRW. Endotoxic activity of lipopolysaccharides isolated from emergent potential cystic fibrosis pathogens. FEMS Immunol Med Microbiol. 2000; 27(1):73-77. DOI:10.1111/j.1574-695X.2000.tb01414.x.

[55] Shimomura H, Matsuura M, Saito S, Hirai Y, Isshiki Y, Kawahara K. Lipopolysaccharide of *Burkholderia cepacia* and its unique character to stimulate murine macrophages with relative lack of interleukin-1β-inducing ability. Infect Immun. 2001; 69:3663-3669. DOI:10.1128/IAI.69.6.3663-3669.2001.

[56] Saldías MS, Ortega X, Valvano MA. *Burkholderia cenocepacia* O antigen lipopolysaccharide prevents phagocytosis by macrophages and adhesion to epithelial cells. J Med Microbiol. 2009; 58:1542-1548. DOI:10.1099/jmm.0.013235-0.

[57] Richau JA, Leitão JH, Correia M, Lito L, Salgado MJ, Barreto C, Cescutti P, Sá-Correia I. Molecular typing and exopolysaccharide biosynthesis of *Burkholderia cepacia* isolates from a Portuguese cystic fibrosis center. J Clin Microbiol. 2000; 38:1651-1655.

[58] Cunha M V, Sousa SA, Leitão JH, Moreira LM, Videira PA, Sá-Correia I. Studies on the involvement of the exopolysaccharide produced by cystic fibrosis-associated isolates of the *Burkholderia cepacia* complex in biofilm formation and in persistence of respiratory infections. J Clin Microbiol. 2004; 42(7):3052-3058. DOI:10.1128/JCM.42.7.3052-3058.2004.

[59] Ferreira AS, Leitão JH, Silva IN, et al. Distribution of cepacian biosynthesis genes among environmental and clinical *Burkholderia* strains and role of Cepacian exopolysaccharide in resistance to stress conditions. Appl Environ Microbiol. 2010; 76(2):441-450. DOI:10.1128/AEM.01828-09.

[60] Goldberg JB. Polysaccharides of *Burkholderia* spp. In: Coenye T, Peter V, eds. *Burkholderia* Molecular Microbiology and Genomics. Wymondham: Horizon Bioscience; 2007:93-110.

[61] Herasimenka Y, Cescutti P, Impallomeni G, et al. Exopolysaccharides produced by clinical strains belonging to the *Burkholderia cepacia* complex. J Cyst Fibros. 2007; 6(2):145-152. DOI:10.1016/j.jcf.2006.06.004.

[62] Moreira LM, Videira PA, Sousa SA, Leitão JH, Cunha M V, Sá-Correia I. Identification and physical organization of the gene cluster involved in the biosynthesis of *Burkholderia cepacia* complex exopolysaccharide. Biochem Biophys Res Commun. 2003; 312(2):323-333. DOI:10.1016/j.bbrc.2003.10.118.

[63] Chiarini L, Cescutti P, Drigo L, et al. Exopolysaccharides produced by *Burkholderia cenocepacia* recA lineages IIIA and IIIB. J Cyst Fibros. 2004; 3(3):165-172. DOI:10.1016/j.jcf.2004.04.004.

[64] Bylund J, Burgess LA, Cescutti P, Ernst RK, Speert DP. Exopolysaccharides from *Burkholderia cenocepacia* inhibit neutrophil chemotaxis and scavenge reactive oxygen species. J Biol Chem. 2006; 281:2526-2532. DOI:10.1074/jbc.M510692200.

[65] Conway BAD, Chu KK, Bylund J, Altman E, Speert DP. Production of exopolysaccharide by *Burkholderia cenocepacia* results in altered cell-surface interactions and altered bacterial clearance in mice. J Infect Dis. 2004; 190:957-966. DOI:10.1086/423141.

[66] Cuzzi B, Cescutti P, Furlanis L, et al. Investigation of bacterial resistance to the immune system response: Cepacian depolymerisation by reactive oxygen species. Innate Immun. 2012; 18(4):661-671. DOI:10.1177/1753425911435954.

[67] Zlosnik JEA, Hird TJ, Fraenkel MC, Moreira LM, Henry DA, Speert DP. Differential mucoid exopolysaccharide production by members of the *Burkholderia cepacia* complex. J Clin Microbiol. 2008; 46:1470-1473. DOI:10.1128/JCM.02273-07.

[68] Messiaen A-S, Nelis H, Coenye T. Investigating the role of matrix components in protection of *Burkholderia cepacia* complex biofilms against tobramycin. J Cyst Fibros. 2014; 13:56-62. DOI:10.1016/j.jcf.2013.07.004.

[69] Huber B, Riedel K, Köthe M, Givskov M, Molin S, Eberl L. Genetic analysis of functions involved in the late stages of biofilm development in *Burkholderia cepacia* H111. Mol Microbiol. 2002; 46(2):411-426. DOI:10.1046/j.1365-2958.2002.03182.x.

[70] Berlutti F, Morea C, Battistoni A, et al. Iron availability influences aggregation, biofilm, adhesion and invasion of *Pseudomonas aeruginosa* and *Burkholderia cenocepacia*. Int J Immunopathol Pharmacol. 2005; 18:661-670. DOI:10.1177/039463200501800407.

[71] Tomlin KL, Malott RJ, Ramage G, Storey DG, Sokol PA, Ceri H. Quorum-sensing mutations affect attachment and stability of *Burkholderia cenocepacia* biofilms. Appl Environ Microbiol. 2005; 71:5208-5218. DOI:10.1128/AEM.71.9.5208-5218.2005.

[72] Bernier SP, Nguyen DT, Sokol PA. A LysR-type transcriptional regulator in *Burkholderia cenocepacia* influences colony morphology and virulence. Infect Immun. 2008; 76:38-47. DOI:10.1128/IAI.00874-07.

[73] Aubert DF, Flannagan RS, Valvano MA. A novel sensor kinase-response regulator hybrid controls biofilm formation and type VI secretion system activity in *Burkholderia cenocepacia*. Infect Immun. 2008; 76(5):1979-1991. DOI:10.1128/IAI.01338-07.

[74] Häussler S, Lehmann C, Breselge C, et al. Fatal outcome of lung transplantation in cystic fibrosis patients due to small-colony variants of the *Burkholderia cepacia* complex. Eur J Clin Microbiol Infect Dis. 2003; 22(4):249-253. DOI:10.1007/s10096-003-0901-y.

[75] Peeters E, Nelis HJ, Coenye T. In vitro activity of ceftazidime, ciprofloxacin, meropenem, minocycline, tobramycin and trimethoprim/sulfamethoxazole against planktonic and sessile *Burkholderia cepac*ia complex bacteria. J Antimicrob Chemother. 2009; 64:801-809. DOI:10.1093/jac/dkp253.

[76] Caraher E, Reynolds G, Murphy P, McClean S, Callaghan M. Comparison of antibiotic susceptibility of *Burkholderia cepacia* complex organisms when grown planktonically or as biofilm in vitro. Eur J Clin Microbiol Infect Dis. 2007; 26:213-216. DOI:10.1007/s10096-007-0256-x.

[77] Van Acker H, Sass A, Bazzini S, et al. Biofilm-grown *Burkholderia cepacia* complex cells survive antibiotic treatment by avoiding production of reactive oxygen species. PLoS One. 2013; 8:e58943. DOI:10.1371/journal.pone.0058943.

[78] Murphy MP, Caraher E. Residence in biofilms allows *Burkholderia cepacia* complex (Bcc) bacteria to evade the antimicrobial activities of neutrophil-like dHL60 cells. Pathog Dis. 2015; 73(8):ftv069. DOI: 10.1093/femspd/ftv069.

[79] Venturi V, Friscina A, Bertani I, Devescovi G, Aguilar C. Quorum sensing in the *Burkholderia cepacia* complex. Res Microbiol. 2004; 155(4):238-244. DOI:10.1016/j.resmic.2004.01.006.

[80] Kooi C, Subsin B, Chen R, Pohorelic B, Sokol PA. *Burkholderia cenocepacia* ZmpB is a broad-specificity zinc metalloprotease involved in virulence. Infect Immun. 2006; 74(7):4083-4093. DOI:10.1128/IAI.00297-06.

[81] Sokol PA, Sajjan U, Visser MB, Gingues S, Forstner J, Kooi C. The CepIR quorum-sensing system contributes to the virulence of *Burkholderia cenocepacia* respiratory infections. Microbiology. 2003; 149(Pt 12):3649-3658. DOI:10.1099/mic.0.26540-0.

[82] Uehlinger S, Schwager S, Bernier SP, et al. Identification of specific and universal virulence factors in *Burkholderia cenocepacia* strains by using multiple infection hosts. Infect Immun. 2009; 77:4102-4110. DOI:10.1128/IAI.00398-09.

[83] Vergunst AC, Meijer AH, Renshaw SA, O'Callaghan D. *Burkholderia cenocepacia* creates an intramacrophage replication niche in Zebrafish embryos, followed by bacterial dssemination and establishment of systemic infection. Infect Immun. 2010; 78:1495-1508. DOI:10.1128/IAI.00743-09.

[84] Baldwin A, Sokol PA, Parkhill J, Mahenthiralingam E. The *Burkholderia cepacia* epidemic strain marker is part of a novel genomic island encoding both virulence and metabolism-associated genes in *Burkholderia cenocepacia*. Infect Immun. 2004; 72(3):1537-1547. DOI:10.1128/IAI.72.3.1537-1547.2004.

[85] Subramoni S, Sokol PA. Quorum sensing systems influence *Burkholderia cenocepacia* virulence. Future Microbiol. 2012; 7(12):1373-1387. DOI:10.2217/fmb.12.118.

[86] Huber B, Riedel K, Hentzer M, et al. The cep quorum-sensing system of *Burkholderia cepacia* H111 controls biofilm formation and swarming motility. Microbiology. 2001; 147(Pt 9):2517-2528. DOI:10.1099/00221287-147-9-2517.

[87] Lewenza S, Conway B, Greenberg EP, Sokol PA. Quorum sensing in *Burkholderia cepacia*: identification of the LuxRI homologs CepRI. J Bacteriol. 1999; 181:748-756.

[88] Fehlner-Gardiner CC, Hopkins TMH, Valvano MA. Identification of a general secretory pathway in a human isolate of *Burkholderia vietnamiensis* (formerly *B. cepacia* complex genomovar V) that is required for the secretion of hemolysin and phospholipase C activities. Microb Pathog. 2002; 32(5):249-254. DOI:10.1006/mpat.2002.0503.

[89] Whitby PW, Vanwagoner TM, Springer JM, Morton DJ, Seale TW, Stull TL. *Burkholderia cenocepacia* utilizes ferritin as an iron source. J Med Microbiol. 2006; 55:661-668. DOI:10.1099/jmm.0.46199-0.

[90] Corbett CR, Burtnick MN, Kooi C, Woods DE, Sokol PA. An extracellular zinc metalloprotease gene of *Burkholderia cepacia*. Microbiology. 2003; 149:2263-2271. DOI:10.1099/mic.0.26243-0.

[91] Zhang R, LiPuma JJ, Gonzalez CF. Two type IV secretion systems with different functions in *Burkholderia cenocepacia* K56-2. Microbiology. 2009; 155(Pt 12):4005-4013. DOI:10.1099/mic.0.033043-0.

[92] Sajjan SU, Carmody LA, Gonzalez CF, LiPuma JJ. A type IV secretion system contributes to intracellular survival and replication of *Burkholderia cenocepacia*. Infect Immun. 2008; 76:5447-5455. DOI:10.1128/IAI.00451-08.

[93] Tomich M, Griffith A, Herfst CA, Burns JL, Mohr CD. Attenuated virulence of a *Burkholderia cepacia* type III secretion mutant in a murine model of infection. Infect Immun. 2003; 71:1405-1415. DOI:10.1128/IAI.71.3.1405-1415.2003.

[94] Lamothe J, Huynh KK, Grinstein S, Valvano MA. Intracellular survival of *Burkholderia cenocepacia* in macrophages is associated with a delay in the maturation of bacteria-containing vacuoles. Cell Microbiol. 2007; 9(1):40-53. DOI:10.1111/j.1462-5822.2006.00766.x.

[95] Flannagan RS, Jaumouillé V, Huynh KK, et al. *Burkholderia cenocepacia* disrupts host cell actin cytoskeleton by inactivating Rac and Cdc42. Cell Microbiol. 2012; 14:239-254. DOI:10.1111/j.1462-5822.2011.01715.x.

[96] Rosales-Reyes R, Skeldon AM, Aubert DF, Valvano MA. The Type VI secretion system of *Burkholderia cenocepacia* affects multiple Rho family GTPases disrupting the actin cytoskeleton and the assembly of NADPH oxidase complex in macrophages. Cell Microbiol. 2012; 14:255-273. DOI:10.1111/j.1462-5822.2011.01716.x.

[97] Gavrilin MA, Abdelaziz DHA, Mostafa M, et al. Activation of the pyrin inflammasome by intracellular *Burkholderia cenocepacia*. J Immunol. 2012; 188:3469-3477. DOI:10.4049/jimmunol.1102272.

[98] Allan ND, Kooi C, Sokol PA, Beveridge TJ. Putative virulence factors are released in association with membrane vesicles from *Burkholderia cepacia*. Can J Microbiol. 2003; 49(10):613-624. DOI:10.1139/w03-078.

[99] Letoffe S, Redeker V, Wandersman C. Isolation and characterization of an extracellular haem-binding protein from *Pseudomonas aeruginosa* that shares function and sequence similarities with the *Serratia marcescens* HasA haemophore. Mol Microbiol. 1998; 28(6):1223-1234. DOI:10.1046/j.1365-2958.1998.00885.x.

[100] Guzzo J, Pages JM, Duong F, Lazdunski A, Murgier M. *Pseudomonas aeruginosa* alkaline protease: evidence for secretion genes and study of secretion mechanism. J Bacteriol. 1991; 173(17):5290-5297. http://www.ncbi.nlm.nih.gov/pmc/articles/PMC208238/.

[101] Duong F, Bonnet E, Géli V, Lazdunski A, Murgier M, Filloux A. The AprX protein of *Pseudomonas aeruginosa*: a new substrate for the Apr type I secretion system. Gene. 2001; 262(1-2):147-153. DOI:10.1016/S0378-1119(00)00541-2.

[102] Olson JC, Ohman DE. Efficient production and processing of elastase and LasA by *Pseudomonas aeruginosa* require zinc and calcium ions. J Bacteriol. 1992; 174(12):4140-4147. http://www.ncbi.nlm.nih.gov/pmc/articles/PMC206126/.

[103] Cahan R, Axelrad I, Safrin M, Ohman DE, Kessler E. A secreted aminopeptidase of *Pseudomonas aeruginosa*: identification, primary structure, and relationship to other aminopeptidases. J Biol Chem. 2001; 276(47):43645-43652. DOI:10.1074/jbc.M106950200.

[104] Engel LS, Hill JM, Caballero AR, Green LC, O'Callaghan RJ. Protease IV, a unique extracellular protease and virulence factor from *Pseudomonas aeruginosa*. J Biol Chem. 1998; 273(27):16792-16797. DOI:10.1074/jbc.273.27.16792.

[105] Diaz-Laviada I, Larrodera P, Diaz-Meco MT, et al. Evidence for a role of phosphatidylcholine-hydrolysing phospholipase C in the regulation of protein kinase C by *ras* and *src* oncogenes. EMBO J. 1990; 9(12):3907-3912. http://www.ncbi.nlm.nih.gov/pmc/articles/PMC552161/.

[106] Ostroff RM, Vasil AI, Vasil ML. Molecular comparison of a nonhemolytic and a hemolytic phospholipase C from *Pseudomonas aeruginosa*. J Bacteriol. 1990; 172(10):5915-5923. http://www.ncbi.nlm.nih.gov/pmc/articles/PMC526912/.

[107] Folders J, Tommassen J, van Loon LC, Bitter W. Identification of a chitin-binding protein secreted by *Pseudomonas aeruginosa*. J Bacteriol. 2000; 182(5):1257-1263. http://www.ncbi.nlm.nih.gov/pmc/articles/PMC94410/.

[108] Allured VS, Collier RJ, Carroll SF, McKay DB. Structure of exotoxin A of *Pseudomonas aeruginosa* at 3.0-Angstrom resolution. Proc Natl Acad Sci U S A. 1986; 83(5):1320-1324. http://www.ncbi.nlm.nih.gov/pmc/articles/PMC323067/.

[109] Barbieri JT, Sun J. *Pseudomonas aeruginosa* ExoS and ExoT. In: Reviews of Physiology, Biochemistry and Pharmacology. Berlin, Heidelberg: Springer Berlin Heidelberg; 2005:79-92. DOI:10.1007/s10254-004-0031-7.

[110] Yahr TL, Vallis AJ, Hancock MK, Barbieri JT, Frank DW. ExoY, an adenylate cyclase secreted by the *Pseudomonas aeruginosa* type III system. Proc Natl Acad Sci U S A. 1998; 95(23):13899-13904. http://www.ncbi.nlm.nih.gov/pmc/articles/PMC24955/.

[111] Sato H, Frank DW. ExoU is a potent intracellular phospholipase. Mol Microbiol. 2004; 53(5):1279-1290. DOI:10.1111/j.1365-2958.2004.04194.x.

[112] Juhas M, Crook DW, Dimopoulou ID, et al. Novel type IV secretion system involved in propagation of genomic islands. J Bacteriol. 2007; 189(3):761-771. DOI:10.1128/JB.01327-06.

[113] Klockgether J, Würdemann D, Reva O, Wiehlmann L, Tümmler B. Diversity of the abundant pKLC102/PAGI-2 family of genomicislands in *Pseudomonas aeruginosa*. J Bacteriol. 2007; 189(6):2443-2459. DOI:10.1128/JB.01688-06.

[114] Mikkelsen H, Hui K, Barraud N, Filloux A. The pathogenicity island encoded PvrSR/RcsCB regulatory network controls biofilm formation and dispersal in *Pseudomonas aeruginosa*. Mol Microbiol. 2013; 89(3):450-463. DOI:10.1111/mmi.12287.

[115] Wilhelm S, Gdynia A, Tielen P, Rosenau F, Jaeger K-E. The autotransporter esterase EstA of *Pseudomonas aeruginosa* is required for rhamnolipid production, cell motility, and biofilm formation. J Bacteriol. 2007; 189(18):6695-6703. DOI:10.1128/JB.00023-07.

[116] Kida Y, Higashimoto Y, Inoue H, Shimizu T, Kuwano K. A novel secreted protease from *Pseudomonas aeruginosa* activates NF-kappaB through protease-activated receptors. Cell Microbiol. 2008; 10(7):1491-1504. DOI:10.1111/j.1462-5822.2008.01142.x.

[117] Ruer S, Ball G, Filloux A, de Bentzmann S. The "P-usher", a novel protein transporter involved in fimbrial assembly and TpsA secretion. EMBO J. 2008; 27(20):2669-2680. DOI:10.1038/emboj.2008.197.

[118] Faure LM, Garvis S, de Bentzmann S, Bigot S. Characterization of a novel two-partner secretion system implicated in the virulence of *Pseudomonas aeruginosa*. Microbiology. 2014; 160:1940-1952. DOI:10.1099/mic.0.079616-0.

[119] Ballister ER, Lai AH, Zuckermann RN, Cheng Y, Mougous JD. In vitro self-assembly of tailorable nanotubes from a simple protein building block. Proc Natl Acad Sci U S A. 2008; 105(10):3733-3738. DOI:10.1073/pnas.0712247105.

[120] Leiman PG, Basler M, Ramagopal UA, et al. Type VI secretion apparatus and phage tail-associated protein complexes share a common evolutionary origin. Proc Natl Acad Sci U S A. 2009; 106(11):4154-4159. DOI:10.1073/pnas.0813360106.

[121] Bomberger JM, MacEachran DP, Coutermarsh BA, Ye S, O'Toole GA, Stanton BA. Long-distance delivery of bacterial virulence factors by *Pseudomonas aeruginosa* outer membrane vsicles. Ausubel FM, ed. PLoS Pathog. 2009; 5(4):e1000382. DOI:10.1371/journal.ppat.1000382.

[122] Thomas MS. Iron acquisition mechanisms of the *Burkholderia cepacia* complex. BioMetals. 2007; 20:431-452. DOI:10.1007/s10534-006-9065-4.

[123] Darling P, Chan M, Cox AD, Sokol PA. Siderophore production by cystic fibrosis isolates of *Burkholderia cepacia*. Infect Immun. 1998; 66:874-877.

[124] Agnoli K, Lowe CA, Farmer KL, Husnain SI, Thomas MS. The ornibactin biosynthesis and transport genes *of Burkholderia cenocepacia* are regulated by an extracytoplasmic function σ factor which is a part of the Fur regulon. J Bacteriol. 2006; 188(10):3631-3644. DOI:10.1128/JB.188.10.3631-3644.2006.

[125] Sokol PA, Darling P, Woods DE, Mahenthiralingam E, Kooi C. Role of Ornibactin biosynthesis in the virulence of *Burkholderia cepacia*: characterization of *pvdA*, the gene encoding l-ornithine N(5)-oxygenase. Infect Immun. 1999; 67(9):4443-4455.

[126] Sokol PA, Darling P, Lewenza S, Corbett CR, Kooi CD. Identification of a siderophore receptor required for ferric ornibactin uptake in *Burkholderia cepacia*. Infect Immun. 2000; 68(12):6554-6560.

[127] Visser MB, Majumdar S, Hani E, Sokol PA. Importance of the ornibactin and pyochelin siderophore transport systems in *Burkholderia cenocepacia* lung infections. Infect Immun. 2004; 72:2850-2857. DOI:10.1128/IAI.72.5.2850-2857.2004.

[128] Høiby N, Ciofu O, Bjarnsholt T. *Pseudomonas aeruginosa* biofilms in cystic fibrosis. Future Microbiol. 2010; 5(11):1663-1674. DOI:10.2217/fmb.10.125.

[129] Imperi F, Tiburzi F, Visca P. Molecular basis of pyoverdine siderophore recycling in *Pseudomonas aeruginosa*. Proc Natl Acad Sci. 2009; 106(48):20440-20445. DOI:10.1073/pnas.0908760106.

[130] Nikaido H, Pagès J-M. Broad-specificity efflux pumps and their role in multidrug resistance of Gram-negative bacteria. FEMS Microbiol Rev. 2012; 36(2):340-363. DOI:10.1111/j.1574-6976.2011.00290.x.

[131] Rushton L, Sass A, Baldwin A, Dowson CG, Donoghue D, Mahenthiralingam E. Key role for efflux in the preservative susceptibility and adaptive resistance of *Burkholderia cepacia* complex bacteria. Antimicrob Agents Chemother. 2013; 57:2972-2980. DOI:10.1128/AAC.00140-13.

[132] Leitão JH, Sousa SA, Cunha MV, Salgado MJ, Melo-Cristino J, Barreto MC, Sá-Correia I. Variation of the antimicrobial susceptibility profiles of *Burkholderia cepacia* complex clonal isolates obtained from chronically infected cystic fibrosis patients: a five-year survey in the major Portuguese treatment center. Eur J Clin Microbiol Infect Dis. 2008; 27:1101-1111. DOI:10.1007/s10096-008-0552-0.

[133] Pope CF, Gillespie SH, Pratten JR, McHugh TD. Fluoroquinolone-resistant mutants of *Burkholderia cepacia*. Antimicrob Agents Chemother. 2008; 52(3):1201-1203. DOI:10.1128/AAC.00799-07.

[134] Crowley D, Daly M, Lucey B, et al. Molecular epidemiology of cystic fibrosis-linked *Burkholderia cepacia* complex isolates from three national referral centres in Ireland. J Appl Microbiol. 2002; 92(5):992-1004. DOI:10.1046/j.1365-2672.2002.01612.x.

[135] Ramírez MS, Vargas LJ, Cagnoni V, Tokumoto M, Centrón D. Class 2 Integron with a novel cassette array in a *Burkholderia cenocepacia* isolate. Antimicrob Agents Chemother. 2005; 49(10):4418-4420. DOI:10.1128/AAC.49.10.4418-4420.2005.

[136] Aronoff SC. Outer membrane permeability in *Pseudomonas cepacia*: diminished porin content in a beta-lactam-resistant mutant and in resistant cystic fibrosis isolates. Antimicrob Agents Chemother. 1988; 32:1636-1639. DOI:10.1128/AAC.32.11.1636.

[137] Moore RA, Hancock RE. Involvement of outer membrane of *Pseudomonas cepacia* in aminoglycoside and polymyxin resistance. Antimicrob Agents Chemother. 1986; 30(6):923-926. DOI:10.1128/AAC.30.6.923.

[138] Bazzini S, Udine C, Sass A, et al. Deciphering the role of RND efflux transporters in *Burkholderia cenocepacia*. PLoS One. 2011; 6:e18902. DOI:10.1371/journal.pone.0018902.

[139] Buroni S, Pasca MR, Flannagan RS, et al. Assessment of three resistance-nodulation-cell division drug efflux transporters of *Burkholderia cenocepacia* in intrinsic antibiotic resistance. BMC Microbiol. 2009; 9:1-11. DOI:10.1186/1471-2180-9-200.

[140] Nair BM, Cheung KJ, Griffith A, Burns JL. Salicylate induces an antibiotic efflux pump in *Burkholderia cepacia* complex genomovar III (*B. cenocepacia*). J Clin Invest. 2004; 113:464-473. DOI:10.1172/JCI19710.

[141] Podnecky NL, Rhodes KA, Schweizer HP. Efflux pump-mediated drug resistance in *Burkholderia*. Front Microbiol. 2015; 6:305. DOI:10.3389/fmicb.2015.00305.

[142] Coenye T, Van Acker H, Peeters E, et al. Molecular mechanisms of chlorhexidine tolerance in *Burkholderia cenocepacia* biofilms. Antimicrob Agents Chemother. 2011; 55:1912-1919. DOI:10.1128/AAC.01571-10.

[143] Buroni S, Matthijs N, Spadaro F, et al. Differential roles of RND efflux pumps in antimicrobial drug resistance of sessile and planktonic *Burkholderia cenocepacia* cells. Antimicrob Agents Chemother. 2014; 58:7424-7429. DOI:10.1128/AAC.03800-14.

[144] Tseng SP, Tsai WC, Liang CY, et al. The contribution of antibiotic resistance mechanisms in clinical *Burkholderia cepacia* complex isolates: an emphasis on efflux pump activity. PLoS One. 2014; 9(8):e104986. DOI:10.1371/journal.pone.0104986.

[145] Drevinek P, Holden MTG, Ge Z, et al. Gene expression changes linked to antimicrobial resistance, oxidative stress, iron depletion and retained motility are observed when *Burkholderia cenocepacia* grows in cystic fibrosis sputum. BMC Infect Dis. 2008; 8:121. DOI:10.1186/1471-2334-8-121.

[146] Urban TA, Griffith A, Torok AM, Smolkin ME, Burns JL, Goldberg JB. Contribution of *Burkholderia cenocepacia* flagella to infectivity and inflammation. Infect Immun. 2004; 72:5126-5134. DOI:10.1128/IAI.72.9.5126-5134.2004.

[147] Kumar B, Cardona ST. Synthetic cystic fibrosis sputum medium regulates flagellar biosynthesis through the *flhF* gene in *Burkholderia cenocepacia*. Front Cell Infect Microbiol. 2016; 6:65. DOI:10.3389/fcimb.2016.00065.

[148] Kalferstova L, Kolar M, Fila L, Vavrova J, Drevinek P. Gene expression profiling of *Burkholderia cenocepacia* at the time of cepacia syndrome: loss of motility as a marker of poor prognosis? J Clin Microbiol. 2015; 53:1515-1522. DOI:10.1128/JCM.03605-14.

[149] Lamothe J, Thyssen S, Valvano MA. *Burkholderia cepacia* complex isolates survive intracellularly without replication within acidic vacuoles of *Acanthamoeba polyphaga*. Cell Microbiol. 2004; 6(12):1127-1138. DOI:10.1111/j.1462-5822.2004.00424.x.

[150] Keith KE, Hynes DW, Sholdice JE, Valvano MA. Delayed association of the NADPH oxidase complex with macrophage vacuoles containing the opportunistic pathogen *Burkholderia cenocepacia*. Microbiology. 2009; 155(Pt 4):1004-1015. DOI:10.1099/mic.0.026781-0.

[151] Rosales-Reyes R, Aubert DF, Tolman JS, Amer AO, Valvano MA. *Burkholderia cenocepacia* type VI secretion system mediates escape of type II secreted proteins into the cytoplasm of infected macrophages. PLoS One. 2012; 7(7):e41726. DOI:10.1371/journal.pone.0041726.

[152] Al-Khodor S, Marshall-Batty K, Nair V, Ding L, Greenberg DE, Fraser IDC. *Burkholderia cenocepacia* J2315 escapes to the cytosol and actively subverts autophagy in human macrophages. Cell Microbiol. 2014; 16:378-395. DOI:10.1111/cmi.12223.

[153] Lamothe J, Valvano MA. *Burkholderia cenocepacia*-induced delay of acidification and phagolysosomal fusion in cystic fibrosis transmembrane conductance regulator (CFTR)-defective macrophages. Microbiology. 2008; 154(Pt 12):3825-3834. DOI:10.1099/mic.0.2008/023200-0.

[154] Luciani A, Villella VR, Esposito S, et al. Defective CFTR induces aggresome formation and lung inflammation in cystic fibrosis through ROS-mediated autophagy inhibition. Nat Cell Biol. 2010; 12:863-875. DOI:10.1038/ncb2090.

[155] Valvano MA. Intracellular survival of *Burkholderia cepacia* complex in phagocytic cells. Can J Microbiol. 2015; 61:607-615. DOI:10.1139/cjm-2015-0316.

[156] Regan KH, Bhatt J. Eradication therapy for *Burkholderia cepacia* complex in people with cystic fibrosis. Cochrane Database Syst Rev. 2014; 10:1-21. CD009876. DOI:10.1002/14651858.CD009876.pub2.

[157] Pradenas, GA, Ross BN, Torres AG. *Burkholderia cepacia* Complex Vaccines: Where Do We Go from here? Vaccines. 2016; 4, 10:1-14. doi:10.3390/vaccines4020010.

[158] Schwab U, Abdullah LH, Perlmutt OS, et al. Localization of *Burkholderia cepacia* complex bacteria in cystic fibrosis lungs and interactions with *Pseudomonas aeruginosa* in hypoxic mucus. Infect Immun. 2014; 82:4729-4745. DOI:10.1128/IAI.01876-14.

[159] Kaiko GE, Horvat JC, Beagley KW, Hansbro PM. Immunological decision-making: how does the immune system decide to mount a helper T-cell response? Immunology. 2008; 123:326-338. DOI:10.1111/j.1365-2567.2007.02719.x.

[160] Moser C, Kjaergaard S, Pressler T, Kharazmi A, Koch C, Høiby N. The immune response to chronic *Pseudomonas aeruginosa* lung infection in cystic fibrosis patients is predominantly of the Th2 type. APMIS. 2000; 108:329-335. DOI:10.1034/j.1600-0463.2000.d01-64.x.

[161] McClean S, Healy ME, Collins C, Carberry S, O'Shaughnessy L, Dennehy R, Adams Á, Kennelly H, Corbett JM, Carty F, et al. Linocin and OmpW are involved in attachment of the cystic fibrosis associated pathogen *Burkholderia cepacia* complex to lung epithelial cells and protect mice against infection. Infect Immun. 2016; 84:1424-1437. DOI:10.1128/IAI.01248-15.

[162] Bertot GM, Restelli MA, Galanternik L, Aranibar Urey RC, Valvano MA, Grinstein S. Nasal immunization with *Burkholderia multivorans* outer membrane proteins and the mucosal adjuvant adamantylamide dipeptide confers efficient protection against experimental lung infections with *B. multivorans* and *B. cenocepacia*. Infect Immun. 2007; 75:2740-2752. DOI:10.1128/IAI.01668-06.

[163] Makidon PE, Knowlton J, Groom JV, Blanco LP, LiPuma JJ, Bielinska AU, Baker JR, Jr. Induction of immune response to the 17 kDa OMPA *Burkholderia cenocepacia* polypeptide and protection against pulmonary infection in mice after nasal vaccination with an OMP nanoemulsion-based vaccine. Med Microbiol Immunol. 2010; 199:81-92. DOI:10.1007/s00430-009-0137-2.

[164] Skurnik D, Davis MR Jr, Benedetti D, Moravec KL, Cywes-Bentley C, Roux D, Traficante DC, Walsh RL, Maira-Litràn T, Cassidy SK, Hermos CR, Martin TR, Thakkallapalli EL, Vargas SO, McAdam AJ, Lieberman TD, Kishony R, Lipuma JJ, Pier GB, Goldberg JB, Priebe GP. Targeting pan-resistant bacteria with antibodies to a broadly conserved surface polysaccharide expressed during infection. J Infect Dis. 2012; 205:1709-1718. DOI:10.1093/infdis/jis254.

[165] Musson JA, Reynolds CJ, Rinchai D, et al. CD4+ T cell epitopes of FliC conserved between strains of *Burkholderia* - implications for vaccines against melioidosis and cepacia complex in Cystic Fibrosis. J Immunol (Baltimore, Md : 1950). 2014; 193(12):6041-6049. DOI:10.4049/jimmunol.1402273.

[166] Sousa SA, Morad M, Feliciano JR, Pita T, Nady S, El-Hennamy RE, Abdel-Rahman M, Cavaco J, Pereira L, Barreto C, Leitão JH. The *Burkholderia cenocepacia* OmpA-like protein BCAL2958: identification, characterization, and detection of anti-BCAL2958 antibodies in serum from *B. cepacia* complex-infected Cystic Fibrosis patients. AMB Express. 2016; 6(1):41. DOI:10.1186/s13568-016-0212-1.

[167] Mariappan V, Vellasamy KM, Thimma JS, Hashim OH, and Vadivelu J. Identification of immunogenic proteins from *Burkholderia cepacia* secretome using proteomic analysis. Vaccine. 2010; 28:1318-1324. DOI:10.1016/j.vaccine.2009.11.027.

[168] Shinoy M, Dennehy R, Coleman L, Carberry S, Schaffer K, Callaghan M, Doyle S, McClean S. Immunoproteomic analysis of proteins expressed by two related pathogens, *Burkholderia multivorans* and *Burkholderia cenocepacia,* during human infection. PLoS One. 2013; 8(11):e80796. DOI:10.1371/journal.pone.0080796.

Chapter 5

Pseudomonas aeruginosa Extracellular Secreted Molecules Have a Dominant Role in Biofilm Development and Bacterial Virulence in Cystic Fibrosis Lung Infections

Theerthankar Das and Jim Manos

Additional information is available at the end of the chapter

http://dx.doi.org/10.5772/66308

Abstract

Cystic fibrosis (CF) is a genetic disorder that predominantly affects Caucasian populations. *Pseudomonas aeruginosa* is the most important Gram-negative pathogen that persists in CF patients' lungs. By evading host defence mechanisms and persisting, it is ultimately responsible for the morbidity and mortality of about 80% of CF patients worldwide. *P. aeruginosa* is also responsible for infections in burns, wounds, eyes, nosocomial patients and HIV patients. Prevalence and progression of infection by *P. aeruginosa* in the host is dependent on secretion of numerous extracellular molecules such as polysaccharides, proteases, eDNA, pyocyanin and pyoverdine. These molecules have multiple roles in facilitating *P. aeruginosa* colonisation and virulence. Pyocyanin is one of the major factors dictating progression of infection and biofilm formation. Pyocyanin is a potent virulence factor causing host cell death in CF patients. In this chapter, we have outlined the roles of various extracellular molecules secreted by *P. aeruginosa* and specifically focused on the role of pyocyanin in inducing eDNA production, binding to eDNA via intercalation and facilitating biofilm promoting factors, whilst inducing oxidative stress to host cells via production of reactive oxygen species. In line with this, we have described the current challenges in treatment of CF infections and the development of new strategies to control *P. aeruginosa* infections.

Keywords: *Pseudomonas aeruginosa*, polysaccharides, protease, pyoverdine, pyocyanin, eDNA, glutathione, biofilm

1. Introduction

Cystic fibrosis (CF) is a genetic disorder whose effects are felt from birth. It predominantly affects Caucasian populations; however, it is also present in non-Caucasians [1]. The prevalence of CF varies around the globe; however, extensive evidence suggests that in the USA, Canada, Australia, New Zealand and European countries the ratio of newborns with CF is 1:2000–3000 [2]. CF is induced by mutations (amino acid deletions/substitutions) in the cystic fibrosis transmembrane conductance regulator (CFTR), with a loss of the phenylalanine at position 508 (ΔF508) leading to the most severe outcome. The dysfunctional CFTR leads to greatly reduced transport of ions across epithelial cells and membranes, resulting in dehydration of the mucus in the host respiratory tract/lungs and the digestive pathway, reduced mucus clearance and severe breathing problems [1, 2]. The slow-moving mucous facilitates the growth of microbes, including potentially life-threatening bacteria such as *Pseudomonas aeruginosa, Staphylococcus aureus, Haemophilus influenzae* and *Burkholderia cenocepacia*, as well as fungal species such as *Candida, Aspergillus* and *Malassezia* spp. and viruses [3]. Chronic microbial infections and concomitant airway inflammation induced by the bacterial are primarily responsible for respiratory failure in about 95% of CF patients [1]. In spite of intensive antibiotic therapy and other associated therapy (chest physical therapy, pure oxygen therapy) and finally lung transplantation to combat the effects of CF, the mean life expectancy of CF sufferers is still shorter than that of non-CF people, ranging between 35 and 50 years [2].

P. aeruginosa is the most important Gram-negative pathogen that persists in CF patients' lungs, and this persistence is achieved primarily by evading host defence mechanisms through a shutdown of potential trigger genes. *P. aeruginosa* is ultimately responsible for the morbidity and mortality of about 80% of CF patients worldwide [2]. Clinical research has shown that during a CF patient's infancy and childhood more infections are caused by *S. aureus* and *H. influenzae*, whereas in adulthood, the severity of infection is accelerated by *P. aeruginosa* colonisation [4]. *P. aeruginosa* is the most prevalent Gram-negative pathogen in CF patients' lungs by adolescence, by which time the strains isolated from patients are usually multidrug resistant. Evidence suggests that *P. aeruginosa* and its associated infections are more persistent and dominant in CF patients aged over 18 years (91%) than in patients less than 18 years (39%) [5]. In addition to CF-related infections, *P. aeruginosa* is also primarily responsible for airway infections in bronchiectasis, infection of burns and wounds, surgery-associated infections, eye infections due to contact lens contamination and nosocomial infections such as pneumonia and urinary tract infections in the immunocompromised [6]. In CF and bronchiectasis patients, *P. aeruginosa* infection results in chronic airway inflammation, lung tissue damage, declining lung function, respiratory failure and premature death [1, 6].

Persistence of bacterial infections in the host is due to the bacterium's ability to form biofilms via secretion of numerous extracellular biopolymers, collectively known as extracellular polymeric substances (EPS) and small molecules [7, 8]. Different extracellular biopolymers and small molecules conjugate with each other through physico-chemical interactions to form a highly complexed and structurally integrated matrix [7]. This matrix represents a critical interface between bacterial cells and the host or its environment. Extracellular biopolymers

(EPSs) play a primary role in immobilising planktonic cells (cell adhesion) and cell-cell communication (aggregation), leading to colonisation and biofilm formation on both biotic and abiotic surfaces. It also provides bacterial cells/biofilms with inherent protection against physical stress, traditional antibiotic therapy and host immune defences, thus making eradication extremely difficult [7, 9]. Potentially all biopolymers (e.g. proteins, polysaccharides, eDNA) in EPS serve as an excellent source of nutrients and specifically eDNA promotes horizontal gene transfer between cells within the biofilm [7].

P. aeruginosa EPS plays multiple roles in bacterial adhesion, colonisation, biofilm formation and pathogenesis of *P. aeruginosa* infections [7]. EPS primarily consists of bio-polymers such as polysaccharides (alginate, lipopolysaccharides), proteins (protease, elastase), nucleic acids such as extracellular DNA (eDNA) and RNA, and small molecules such as siderophores and metabolites (phenazines/pyocyanin) [8, 9]. Secretion of EPS and metabolites (phenazines) by *P. aeruginosa* is regulated by the quorum sensing (QS) system. With QS, bacterial cells communicate with each other via small molecules comprising N-acyl homoserine lactones (AHL) and the *Pseudomonas* quinolone signal (PQS). These AHL and PQS promote *P. aeruginosa* biofilm formation through activation of numerous genes expressing extracellular molecules at different stages of the bacterial growth phase [7, 8], with roles in virulence and biofilm development (**Figure 1**).

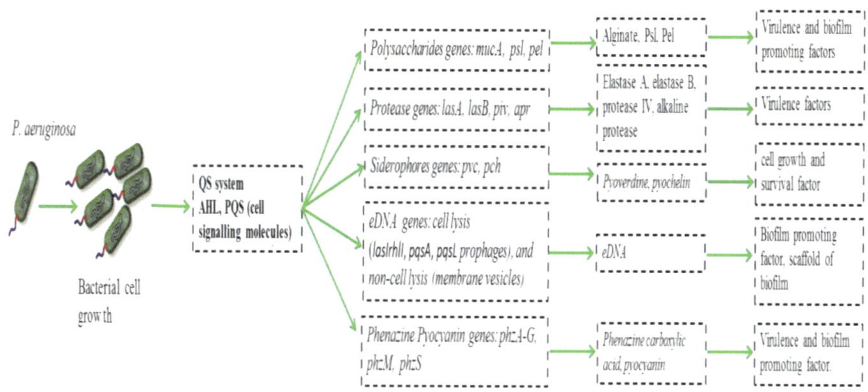

Figure 1. Schematic diagram showing quorum-sensing-mediated production of various extracellular molecules (polysaccharides, protease, pyoverdine, eDNA, pyocyanin) by *P. aeruginosa* and their potential roles in biofilm development and virulence.

Of the many extracellular molecules secreted by *P. aeruginosa*, phenazine-pyocyanin stands out as a molecule that has numerous functions including assistance in growth and multiplication of the cell population, biofilm promotion and virulence. Pyocyanin is a small metabolite with oxidant properties that act as a virulence factor by producing reactive oxygen species (ROS) and generating oxidative stress in the host [10]. Pyocyanin is also a key metabolite in strengthening the e-DNA backbone of the *P. aeruginosa* biofilm [10]. The major focus of this chapter will be on pyocyanin in its role as a *P. aeruginosa* virulence factor. This will involve a review of the literature in the field as well as our work in understanding pyocyanin's role in strengthening the *P. aeruginosa* biofilm and inducing virulence in the host. In addition, we will briefly review the role of other essential molecules such as polysaccharides, protease, e-DNA and pyoverdine, secreted by *P. aeruginosa* in establishment of the biofilm and progression of infection. This chapter will also address various developments in therapeutic treatment that involves these extracellular metabolites and biopolymers, and our development of new approach disrupts *P. aeruginosa* biofilms in vivo using a combined antioxidant/DNase-I/antibiotic approach.

2. Role of *P. aeruginosa* secreted extracellular molecules in development of biofilm and pathogenesis

2.1. Polysaccharides

Alginate (capsular polysaccharide) is acknowledged as a virulence factor responsible for mucoidal *P. aeruginosa* infection in CF lung [11]. Transformation from initial non-mucoid *P. aeruginosa* colonies occurs after a mutation in the negative regulator of mucoidy, *mucA*, leads to expression of the alginate biosynthesis operon [12] and extracellular secretion of alginate, the basis of the robust mucoid phenotype. Alginate is also partly responsible for the pathogenicity of *P. aeruginosa* infection and has been shown to enhance the resistance of biofilms against antibiotics and the host immune response, by scavenging reactive oxygen species (ROS) released by host immune cells [13, 14]. In line with this, studies have shown that mucoid *P. aeruginosa* biofilms treated with alginate lyase demonstrated enhanced efficacy to antibiotic treatment [15]. However, evidence suggests that alginate is not essential for *P. aeruginosa* biofilm development since *P. aeruginosa* wild-type alginate-producing and alginate deficient strains form morphologically and structurally similar biofilms [16].

Other polysaccharides that are essential and partly associated with biofilm formation include Psl and Pel (coded by the *psl* and *pel* gene clusters, respectively) [16]. Interestingly, studies show that *P. aeruginosa* laboratory strains that do not produce detectable amounts of alginate (UCBPP-PA14 (PA14) and PAO1), still form robust biofilms through expression of Psl, indicating that biofilm formation is independent of alginate production [16]. Psl and Pel polysaccharides are distinct biochemically and play different roles in the establishment of *P. aeruginosa* biofilms. Psl is a mannose and galactose-rich polysaccharide and is essential for initiation of *P. aeruginosa* cell surface adhesion and aggregation (cell-cell interactions) and maintenance of the structural integrity of established biofilms [17]. In respect to the host, Psl plays a significant role in initiating *P. aeruginosa* adhesion to mucin-coated surfaces, airway epithelial cells and biotic surfaces, thus triggering colonisation of CF lung [18]. Pel is a glucose-rich matrix polysaccharide that is essential for pellicle formation and biofilm structure in *P. aeruginosa* [11]. Studies with Pel-deficient mutants concluded that Pel only influences morphological changes in *P. aeruginosa* colonies and does not influence biofilm initiation [19].

2.2. Proteases

P. aeruginosa secretes several protease enzymes identified as important virulence factors, such as alkaline protease (AP), elastase (Ela) B, elastase A (LasA protease), toxin A, phospholipase

C and protease IV [20, 21]. Through their activity, these proteases contribute to the pulmonary damage seen in CF patients [21]. Interestingly, studies have shown that both environmental (soil and water) and clinical *P. aeruginosa* isolates produce similar concentrations of toxin A, phospholipase C, AP and Ela and have similar levels of elastolytic activity [22]. Protease production in *P. aeruginosa* is triggered through the QS system and numerous genes including *lasA* (elastase A/LasA protease), *lasB* (elastase B), *piv* (protease IV) and the *apr* (alkaline protease) operon are involved [23]. A significant amount of AP, Ela and protease IV has been detected in bronchial secretions from the lungs of CF patients [23]. These bacterial proteases can significantly influence a broad range of biological functions including the infection process, by hydrolysing peptide bonds and degrading proteins essential for basic biological functions in the host. They are also active against the host's humoral immunity system [23]. For example, AP and Ela cleave the major human immunoglobulins IgA and IgG in the respiratory tract [24]. In infected CF lung, protease has been shown to induce a severe inflammatory response, with increased interleukin-8 (IL-8) and interleukin-6 (IL-6) cytokine levels in the airways [25]. *P. aeruginosa* protease secretions in infected burn and wounds patients have been shown to induce sepsis, leading to an increased mortality rate [26]. However, the effectiveness of proteases is limited, as studies have shown that chronically infected CF patients produce specific antibodies against proteases and that these antibodies provide a defensive mechanism for the host by inhibiting protease-mediated cleavage of secretory immunoglobulins [27].

P. aeruginosa-secreted elastase B degrades human elastin, and over time, the decreased levels of elastin and increased levels of collagen in lung tissue result in lung fibrosis [25]. Elastase A cleaves glycine-containing proteins and interestingly influences the activity of several other host elastolytic proteases, including human leukocyte elastase, human neutrophil elastase [28]. *P. aeruginosa* protease IV potentially cleaves IgG and fibrinogen (required for blood clotting). Low levels of fibrinogen lead to haemorrhaging, which is a characteristic of *P. aeruginosa* CF infection [29, 30]. In vitro studies demonstrated that secretion of *P. aeruginosa* proteases is significantly affected by antibiotic (ciprofloxacin) treatment [31]. Biofilms of *P. aeruginosa* PA1159 and PA1230 when treated with 64 μg/ml ciprofloxacin(twice the minimum inhibitory concentration (MIC)) showed up to a 65% decrease in total proteolytic activity [31]. However, the remaining *P. aeruginosa* population displayed increased resistance to ciprofloxacin compared to their planktonic counterparts when grown in fresh medium [31].

2.3. Pyoverdine

Iron is an important cofactor required for bacterial metabolism, growth and survival and also essential for induction of infection in host by various pathogenic bacteria including *P. aeruginosa* [32]. Various iron-binding proteins (a class of ferritin) secreted by mammalian systems reduce the bioavailability of free iron essential for progress of infection and growth by pathogens, thus ferritin acts as an innate immunity molecule against bacterial infection [32]. Under iron limitation conditions, bacteria secrete siderophores (iron-chelating molecules) to acquire iron from the host [32]. *P. aeruginosa* secretes two types of siderophores: pyoverdine (the predominant siderophore) and pyochelin, with high and low affinity for Fe^{3+} ions, respectively [33, 34]. Pyoverdine production is encoded mainly bythe *pvc* gene cluster and pyochelin production by the *pch* gene cluster [35]. Pyoverdine is more efficient in releasing iron from human ferritin and also has high affinity for Fe^{2+} ions [33, 34]. Studies have demonstrated that pyoverdine is more important than its counterpart pyochelin for the development of *P. aeruginosa* biofilm and infection, whereas mutants that produce pyochelin but are deficient in pyoverdine production are significantly hampered in their biofilm-forming ability [34]. In line with this, a study using an animal model (immunosuppressed mice) showed that pyoverdine predominantly contributes to *P. aeruginosa* virulence and infection [36].

Various factors influence the bioavailability of iron for *P. aeruginosa* and other pathogens in the host; in vitro studies show mutations in the CFTR gene trigger increased release of extracellular iron from lung epithelial cells in comparison to healthy epithelial cells, while elevated iron levels in CF patients directly correlated with an increase in the *P. aeruginosa* population [34]. The proteolytic activity of *P. aeruginosa* protease degrades human ferritin so that it cannot bind iron, thus allowing pyoverdine to scavenge iron and triggering *P. aeruginosa* pathogenicity [34]. Tate et al. showed that iron acquisition by *P. aeruginosa* in CF also occurs through the heme uptake (FeoABC and EfeU) pathways, which are independent of regular siderophore uptake pathways [37]. The presence of an elevated concentration of haem in CF sputum due to haemolysis resulting from pulmonary exacerbations provides bacteria in general with an excellent source of iron. Studies have also demonstrated that under oxygen-deficient conditions in *P. aeruginosa* biofilms or in CF airways,iron exists as Fe^{2+} ions and *P. aeruginosa* takes up Fe^{2+} via the FeoABC and EfeU pathways [37].

Interestingly, mammalian biological systems have an innate defence strategy against siderophores, a neutrophil-gelatinase-associated lipocalin (NGAL). NGAL functions as a scavenger by directly binding with siderophores, blocking *P. aeruginosa's* ability to sequester iron and thereby inhibiting bacterial growth and infection [32]. However, studies have reported that pyoverdine does not bind to NGAL and consequently is able to assist *P. aeruginosa* growth, as demonstrated by biofilm formation and chronic infection in CF lung in spite of elevated amounts of NGAL in lung secretions and bronchoalveolar lavage fluid [32].

2.4. Role of eDNA

eDNA is currently recognised as an essential constituent of EPS and plays a pivotal role in the various processes of biofilm formation in numerous medicallyrelevant Gram-negative and Gram-positive bacteria [8, 9]. In *P. aeruginosa*, eDNA is recognised as an essential molecule in facilitating biofilm formation, including assisting initial bacterial adhesion to surfaces, cell-to-cell interaction (aggregation), microcolony formation and enhancement of biofilm strength and stability [38–41]. eDNA, which is similar to chromosomal DNA in its primary structure [42], is not only released by many bacterial species, predominantly through cell-lytic, but also partly through non-lytic mechanisms [9, 43, 44]. In cell-lytic release, various cell lysing agents such as prophages, autolysin proteins, enzymes and phenazines lyse bacterial cells and trigger eDNA release [8, 38]. Non-lytic eDNA release occurs through the lysis of bacterial outer membrane blebs/vesicles that contain large amounts of DNA [44, 45]. In *P. aeruginosa*, both lytic and non-lytic eDNA releases have been recorded [38, 43, 44]. Studies show that mutants deficient in eDNA production are significantly hampered in biofilm formation. In the same vein, biofilm treatment with DNase I, an enzyme that non-specifically cleaves DNA via hydrolysis of phosphodiester bonds in DNA, significantly inhibits biofilm formation and dispersal of mature biofilms [39, 40, 43].

eDNA also serves as a nutrient source (an excellent source of carbon,phosphate and nitrogen), facilitates horizontal gene transfer through Type IV pili and competence stimulating peptides and helps maintain the structural integrity of the biofilm by binding to various extracellular molecules (proteins, polysaccharides, metabolites) in the biofilm matrix [7, 8]. Recent investigations have revealed that eDNA protects bacterial cells in biofilm from physical challenges such as shear stress by increasing biofilm viscosity, and from chemical challenges by antibiotics and detergents. For example, eDNA binds to various positively charged antibiotics (aminoglycosides) thus shielding *P. aeruginosa* in biofilms against their action [46]. eDNA at sub-MIC concentrations creates a cation-limited atmosphere by chelating divalent cations such as Ca^{2+}. This results in the induction of genes involved in resistance to cationic antimicrobial peptides [47]. Swartjeset al. demonstrated that continuous exposure of bacterial cells (*P. aeruginosa* and *S. aureus*) to a DNase I-coated surface inhibits biofilm formation [40]. Treating biofilms with DNase I alters the biofilm architecture leading to penetration by antibiotics, thus promoting the efficacy of antibiotics in killing mature biofilms [48]. It is important to note that *P. aeruginosa*-infected CF lung secretions and bronchitis sputum contain a significant amount of eDNA (3–14 mg/ml), compared to none in non-CF patients [49]. eDNA aids bacterial viability by inducing antibiotic resistance [48] and it also contributes tothe high viscosity of CF sputum [49].

While eDNA is well-recognised as one of the prime factors in the establishment of *P. aeruginosa* biofilms [39, 43], it has also been demonstrated to have such a role in other biofilm-forming bacteria [50, 51]. eDNA initiates biofilm formation by binding with bacterial extracellular biomolecules such as polysaccharides, peptides/enzymes/proteins and other bacterial cell surface structures. In *Listeria monocytogenes* (a food-borne pathogen), Harmsen et al. demonstrated that eDNA binds with peptidoglycan (*N*-acetyl glucosamine), and this molecular interaction initiates adhesion by *L. monocytogenes* to surfaces [50]. In *Caulobacter crescentus* (environmental freshwater bacterium) biofilms, eDNA binds to polar adhesive structure called 'hold-fast' that is present on the tip of the stalk cell (a part of the cell wall that is essential for *C. crescentus* adherence to surfaces), while eDNA from lysed cells masking the adhesive properties of hold-fast, inhibit swarmer cell adherence to the same surface [52]. Rather than acting as an essential structural element of the biofilm, this unusual role for eDNA means that it functions as a regulatory component assisting in the escape of cells from the biofilm and thus promoting development of new, independent colonies [52]. Peptide-eDNA interactions have also been found to be an essential factor promoting biofilm growth of *Streptococcus mutans* (an oral pathogen responsible for dental plaque). In *S. mutans*, uptake of eDNA is triggered through a competence-stimulating peptide, whereas bacterial cell-to-cell interaction and biofilm formation are initiated through the DNA-binding protein ComGB [51]. In *P. aeruginosa*, Das et al. were the first to discover that the phenazine metabolite (pyocyanin) binds with DNA to facilitate *P. aeruginosa* biofilm formation [53].

2.5. Role of pyocyanin

2.5.1. Pyocyanin production in P. aeruginosa

Pyocyanin, a member of the phenazine class, is a molecule only known to be expressed by *P. aeruginosa*, and thus distinguishes it from other pathogens. Up to 95% of *P. aeruginosa* isolates synthesise pyocyanin [54]. It is a bluish-green-coloured extracellular metabolite that is secreted in copious quantities both in vitro and in vivo. In *P. aeruginosa*, phenazine production is regulated through the bacterium's complex QS mechanism. The primary QS molecules, AHL and PQS, trigger the induction of the phenazine operon (*phz A-G*) to produce phenazine-1-carboxylic acid (PCA). Seven genes have been identified as having a role in pyocyanin synthesis, namely *phzCDEFGMS*. Amongst these, *phzM* and *phzS* are central to the conversion of PCA to pyocyanin in a two-step reaction. First, PCA is converted to 5-methylphenazine-1-carboxylic acid betaine (encoded by *phzM*) and then to pyocyanin (encoded by *phzS*) [54, 55]. PCA is also converted in much lower ratios to other types of phenazines, including phenazine-1-carboxamide (PCN, encoded by *phzH*) and 1-hydroxyphenazine (1-OHPHZ, encoded by *phzS*) [54].

In chronic CF lung infection, up to 85 μM of pyocyanin has been recorded in *P. aeruginosa*-infected CF lung secretions and up to 130 μM in bronchitis sputum [56]. In vitro measurement of pyocyanin production by *P. aeruginosa* in both clinical CF and laboratory reference strains showed, in most cases, the expression of large amounts of pyocyanin within 24 h of growth in Luria-Bertani (LB) medium. Amongst CF isolates, the Liverpool Epidemic Strain LESB58 and the Australian Epidemic Strain-2 (AES-2) produced close to 100 μM pyocyanin, as did the laboratory reference strain DKN-370 (a pyocyanin overproducing strain), while the laboratory reference strain PA14 and the Australian epidemic strain-1 isolate AES-1R produced 70–80 μM pyocyanin. Conversely, the chronic infection isogen of AES-1R (AES-1M) produced less than 5 μM pyocyanin indicating expression is reduced as the strain adapts to the CF lung [11]. Evidence suggests that many factors activate pyocyanin production, including low iron [57] and phosphate depletion [58].

2.5.2. Pyocyanin facilitates eDNA release

Pyocyanin is a redox molecule and electrochemically active (has potential to accept and donate electrons as a shuttle) with a multitude of biological activities [59]. Recent investigations have demonstrated that pyocyanin facilitates eDNA release in *P. aeruginosa*. Comparison of eDNA release by *P. aeruginosa* PA14 wild-type and a phenazine/pyocyanin-deficient PA14 mutant (Δ*phzA-G*) showed up to 50% increase in eDNA release by the wild-type under laboratory growth conditions in LB. In line with this, the Δ*phzA-G* mutant showed a significant increase in eDNA release when grown in the presence of exogenous pyocyanin, with the rate of eDNA release directly correlated to the concentration of pyocyanin [38]. Pyocyanin-mediated eDNA release is induced through cell lysis due to hydrogen peroxide (H_2O_2) expression. In PAO1 and PA14 planktonic growth cultures, pyocyanin has been shown to donate electrons to molecular oxygen to form H_2O_2 and initiate an increase of up to 14% in cell lysis under laboratory growth conditions [38]. Interestingly, the surviving *P. aeruginosa* population is protected from H_2O_2 by catalase, whose expression is upregulated by *P. aeruginosa* as a self-defence mechanism against its own and host-released H_2O_2 molecules [60]. H_2O_2-mediated eDNA release has also been documented in other bacterial species including *Streptococccus sanguinis,* an oral bacterium responsible for dental disease. In this species, pyruvate oxidase activity by *S. sanguinis* induces a ca. 10% increase in cell death in its own population and consequently facilitates eDNA release [61].

2.5.3. *Pyocyanin and eDNA intercalate in biofilms*

Pyocyanin's intercalation with DNA has been demonstrated using various bio-physical techniques (circular dichroism, Fourier transform infrared spectroscopy, fluorescence and UV-Vis spectroscopy) [53]. In a preliminary study using fluorescence emission spectroscopy, it was shown that pyocyanin displaces ethidium bromide bound to dsDNA, indicating pyocyanin is an intercalating agent. Fluorescence emission spectroscopy data were further complemented using the UV-Vis spectra of the DNA-pyocyanin complex. Results indicated a significant shift (from 259 to 253 nm) and increase in absorbance intensity in the DNA peak. This marked change in the DNA peak from 259 nm indicates effective intercalation of pyocyanin molecules between the nitrogenous base-pairs of DNA [53]. Meanwhile, the circular dichroism spectra of the DNA-pyocyanin mixtures confirmed that pyocyanin binds to the sugar-phosphate backbone of DNA and strongly intercalates with the nitrogenous bases of DNA, consequently creating local perturbations in the DNA double helix structure [53]. This type of interaction is a typical characteristic feature of all intercalating molecules. In the same study, Das et al. also discovered that pyocyanin significantly increased the viscosity of DNA solutions, and that by intercalating with DNA pyocyanin-facilitated electron transfer [53]. These results are in line with previous studies concluding that in order to remain viable in biofilms, *P. aeruginosa* exploits redox-active metabolites such as pyocyanin, where direct access to electron acceptors such as oxygen or nitrate is diffusion-limited [59].

2.5.4. *Pyocyanin-eDNA binding influences biofilm formation via physico-chemical interactions*

Molecules that bind to both biological and non-biological surfaces are known to influence hydrophobicity, charge and the physico-chemical properties that assist or resist interactions. Previous studies have demonstrated that in both bacteria and fungi, the presence of such bio-molecules (eDNA or proteins) plays a significant role in dictating cell surface hydrophobicity and physico-chemical interactions [41]. In *P. aeruginosa*, the presence of eDNA has been shown to increase cell surface hydrophobicity. Water contact angle measurements on DNase I-treated *P. aeruginosa* PA14 and PAO1 reduced the angle from 50 to 34° and 46 to 31°, respectively. Interestingly, the PA14 phenazine deficient mutant (Δ*phzA-G*) had a water contact angle similar to DNase I-treated PA14, and DNase I treatment of Δ*phnzA-G* did not show any further reduction in cell surface hydrophobicity [41], indicating that pyocyanin-DNA binding is an essential factor influencing *P. aeruginosa* cell surface hydrophobicity. eDNA-mediated modulation in cell surface hydrophobicity has also been reported in other pathogenic strains, including *Staphylococcus epidermidis* and *S. aureus* [62].

Analysis of bacteria-to-bacteria and bacteria-to-substratum physico-chemical interactions (Lifshitz-Van der Waals interactions forces, acid-base interactions forces) has revealed that the presence of pyocyanin and eDNA facilitates attractive physico-chemical interactions [41]. Removal of eDNA from the *P. aeruginosa* wild-type cell surface or absence of pyocyanin in the *ΔphzA-G* strain showed significant impact, that is, resulted in non-attractive interaction, especially on the short-range acid-base interactions, which include electron donating and electron accepting parameters. However, the long-range Lifshitz-Van der Waals interactions remained unaffected between wild-type and *Δphz*A-G regardless of DNase I treatment [42]. Similarly, the effect of eDNA on physico-chemical forces between *S. epidermidis* cells has been reported, and results suggest that eDNA triggers *S. epidermidis* cell-to-cell interactions [62]. Similarly, adhesion force analysis in *S. mutans* using atomic force microscopy and phase-contrast microscopy imaging and quantification indicates that in the presence of eDNA, *S. mutans* has a stronger adhesion force and adheres to surfaces in significantly higher cell numbers [63].

It should be noted, however, that physico-chemical interactions do not explain bacterial interaction in all cases, since bacterial cell structures (pili, fimbriae) and bio-polymers (poly-saccharides, proteins, eDNA) extend up to hundreds of nanometres from the bacterial cell surface and can affect other interaction types [64]. These cell structures and bio-polymers initiate hydrogen bonding and ionic interactions by colliding with bio-molecules anchored on the bacterial cell surface to stabilise the biofilm matrix and also to its adjacent cells and thereby help bacterial cells to overcome the physico-chemical energy barrier and promote bacterial cell-to-cell interactions and biofilm formation [7, 64]. Confocal laser scanning microscopy (CLSM) analysis revealed that the intercalation of pyocyanin with eDNA facilitates *P. aeruginosa* PA14 wild-type biofilm formation while the absence of pyocyanin significantly inhibits biofilm formation [65]. To investigate this further, Klare et al. grew the CF *P. aeruginosa*AES-1 isolate R (isolated at the acute stage of infection)in an artificial sputum media (ASMDM+) that mimics CF sputum, and found it formed robust biofilms in comparison to its isogenic counterpart AES-1M (isolated at chronic infection). AES-1M which produces about 15 times less pyocyanin than AES-1R, and the exogenous addition of pyocyanin to AES-1M cultures facilitated enhanced biofilm formation [65] (**Figure 2**).

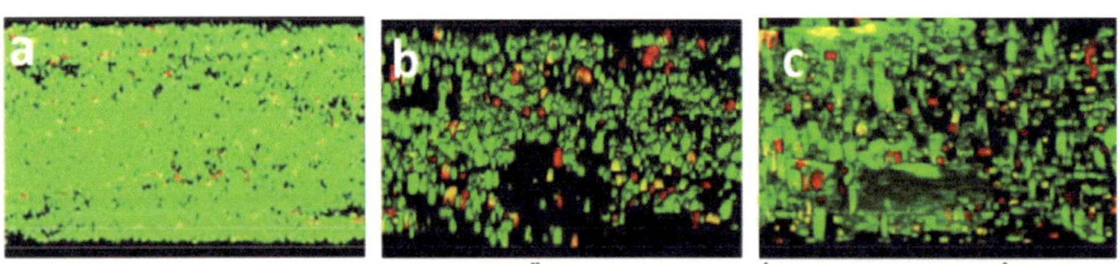

Figure 2. Biofilm formation by *P. aeruginosa* CF isogens in ASMDM+ medium (a) AES-1R, (b) AES-1M and (c) AES-1M grown in the presence of exogenous pyocyanin. The biofilm architecture of (c) indicates pyocyanin facilitates/enhances biofilm formation. Images taken with permission from Ref. [65].

2.5.5. *Pyocyanin as a virulence factor*

Pyocyanin was formerly recognised only as a bacterial secondary metabolite, but has recently gained significant attention for its involvement in a variety of crucial roles in microbial ecology, specifically correlated with the severity of *P. aeruginosa* pathogenicity in plants and humans [66]. **Figure 3** is a schematic representation of pyocyanin-induced H_2O_2 production and toxicity on bacterial, fungal and human cells. Pyocyanin also has antibacterial and antifungal activity that is toxic to other pathogenic bacteria and fungi. Pyocyanin-mediated bactericidal activity occurs through production of H_2O_2, which consequently depletes oxygen supply to cells and disables electron flow and metabolic transport processes [67]. Studies suggest that pyocyanin potentially kills *Staphylococcus* sp. and other species in the CF lung environment; and that it also has anti-*Escherichia coli* activity [67, 68] (**Figure 3**). The inhibitory effect of pyocyanin on the growth of fungi such as *Aspergillus fumigatus* and *Candida albicans* isolated from the sputum of CF patients has also been reported earlier [69] (**Figure 3**). These results could be interpreted as a pyocyanin-mediated modulation of the microbial community in the CF lung by *P. aeruginosa*, resulting in its predominance [70].

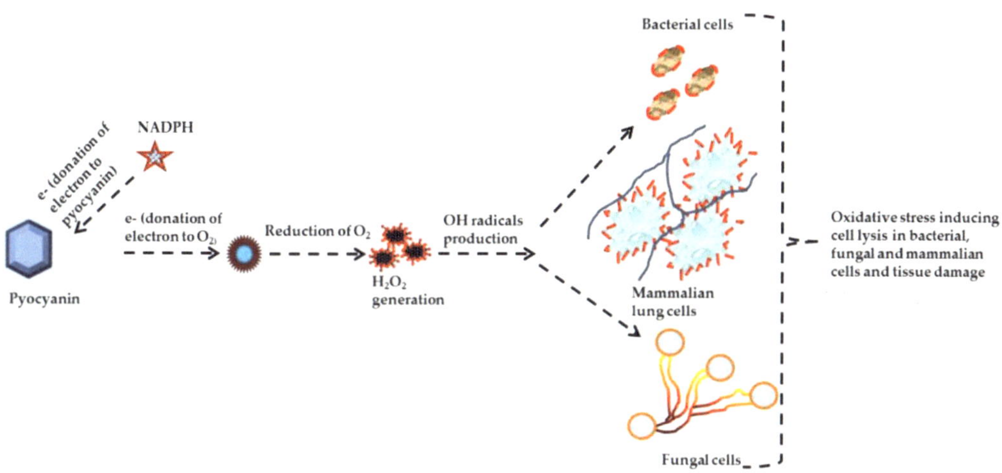

Figure 3. Schematic diagram of pyocyanin induced H_2O_2 production and toxicity on bacterial, fungal and human cells.

In the host, pyocyanin appears to participate in a reduction mechanism, which is capable of reducing and releasing the iron from transferrin in host cells to stimulate the growth of *P. aeruginosa* [71]. Previous research concluded that a direct correlation exists between pyocyanin concentration in CF sputum and severity of infection [71]. Studies using *P. aeruginosa*-infected bronchiectasis airways in a mouse model of lung infection demonstrated that pyocyanin rapidly inhibited lung function and caused cell hyperplasia and metaplasia (abnormal changes in cell or tissue morphology), airway fibrosis and alveolar airspace destruction [71]. Harmer et al. analysed the difference between *P. aeruginosa* epidemic and non-epidemic isogenic strains that were collected 5–8 years apart from five chronically infected adult CF patients, this study suggested that epidemic (FCC) strains are more virulent and more efficient in killing *Caenorhabditis elegans* than their non-epidemic counterparts [72]. The isogens collected early in the infection produced more virulence factors including elastase, pyoverdine and pyocyanin. Over the course of chronic infection, the isogens undergo a significant downregulation in virulence factors *lasB*, *rsaL*, *lecB* and *oprG*, with a significant decrease in elastase and pyoverdine production, however, pyocyanin production increased in three out of five strains and so did biofilm production [72]. Fluctuations in pyocyanin concentration observed among different CF strains are probably due to adaptation of a particular strain to the host and time of acquisition of sample, for example, at exacerbation (when the patient is seriously ill and hospitalised). At exacerbation, the pyocyanin levels may be switched on by the *P. aeruginosa* strain as a protective mechanism against host defences, and this leads to the increased lung damage seen at that time [72]. If the sample was taken when the patient was not in exacerbation, the pyocyanin expression may be very low or negligible [72]. Other phenazine-like PCA molecules secreted by *P. aeruginosa* were also shown to be highly toxic, killed *C. elegans* and caused serious cell damage in a mouse model of lung infection [73].

Pyocyanin has also been extensively studied due to its electrochemical and redox activity. The diffusible nature and small size of pyocyanin means it can easily pass through the host cell membrane and undergo redox reactions with other molecules [74]. For example, it accepts electrons from NADH and subsequently donates electrons to molecular oxygen to form reactive oxygen species (ROS) such as H_2O_2 [74] (**Figure 3**). Pyocyanin-mediated ROS cause oxidative stress and affect calcium homeostasis while also obstructing cellular respiration and depleting intracellular cAMP and ATP levels [75]. Pyocyanin significantly alters human protease activity, inhibits nitric oxide production and consequently influences blood flow, blood pressure and immune functions. It also modulates the host immune response to support evasion of the host immune system and establish chronic infection [75]. In CF, pyocyanin-mediated ROS oxidise host intracellular and extracellular reduced glutathione (GSH) to form glutathione disulphide or oxidised glutathione (GSSG) [76]. Depleted GSH levels during the chronic stage of CF infection lead to widespread epithelial cell death and consequent lung damage and leading to respiratory failure and death [75, 76]. Pyocyanin also inhibits catalase activity in airway epithelial cells, thus increasing oxidative stress in these cells and initiating pulmonary tissue damage [77]. In a recent study, Rada et al. showed that pyocyanin promotes neutrophil extracellular trap (NET) formation [78]. NET formation is an important innate immune mechanism initiated by neutrophils to trap and kill pathogens, however, the aberrant NET release triggered by pyocyanin-mediated intracellular ROS production directly damages host tissues and has been linked to the severity of many diseases including CF [78].

3. Treating *P. aeruginosa* infections

Substantial research over many decades has led to a good degree of understanding of the mechanisms *P. aeruginosa* utilises to cause infection and colonisation. In brief, *P. aeruginosa* has been shown to evade the host's innate defence system through production of various extracellular molecules and render antibiotics ineffective through several efflux pump mechanisms [6, 8, 79]. This research has particular implications for CF, burns and wounds patients, particularly as *P. aeruginosa* antibiotic resistance is a serious concern. This in turn has given impetus to the development of new therapeutic methods. Prominent amongst the extracellular molecules available to *P. aeruginosa* are the previously discussed eDNA, protease, pyocyanin and pyoverdine.

3.1. Current antibiotic treatment and challenges against *P. aeruginosa* infections in CF patients

Many antibiotics developed in recent decades such as aminoglycosides, ticarcillin, ureidopenicillins, ceftazidime, cefepime, aztreonam, the carbapenems, ciprofloxacin and levofloxacin display anti-pseudomonal activity. However, the choice of best antibiotic to use in a particular case remains a major challenge as *P. aeruginosa* can readily adapt by mutation or horizontal gene transfer to acquire resistance in a portion of remaining cells, leading to consequent treatment failure.

Antibiotics commonly used to treat *P. aeruginosa* infection in CF patients include tobramycin, colistin, aztreonam, ciprofloxacin and azithromycin. Administration methods include nebulised, dry powder inhalation, oral or intravenous, or a combination of different strategies [2, 80]. Studies have shown the size of inhaled antibiotic particles is very important in determining whether they will reach deep infection sites. Particles of 1–5 μm diameters are more effective in reaching deep lung tissue efficiently [81]. However, one of the major concerns in inhalation therapy is that most antibiotics are trapped in the thick viscous mucus that covers both the large respiratory zone (respiratory bronchioles, alveolar ducts and alveolar sacs) and the conductive zone (trachea, bronchi and terminal bronchioles) [81, 82]. With intravenous or oral therapy, antibiotics are readily transported through the bloodstream mainly reaching the respiratory zone but not effectively reaching the conductive zone. A combination of both strategies has been shown to enhance the access of antibiotics to infection sites at both the conductive zone and respiratory zones [82].

Other serious challenges with nebuliser treatment (in comparison to dry powder inhalation) strategies are that the antibiotic particles do not reach infection sites at a faster rate, but even with dry powder inhalation does not provide immediate relief to CF patients [83]. For example, studies with CF patients demonstrated that inhaled tobramycin is effective in reducing *P. aeruginosa* density from the lower airways but has no effect in reducing lung inflammation, and consequently certain infection loci and disease symptoms remain [84]. Azithromycin has been shown to improve lung function (lung inflammation, exacerbations and cough) in CF patients compared to other antibiotics and lead to a reduction in *P. aeruginosa* colonisation [85]. However, azithromycin or the macrolide class of antibiotics has significant side effects, including a significant increase in macrolide resistant *S. aureus* and *H. influenzae* strains in CF sputum [85]. In general, many antibiotics are known to cause adverse side-effects in patients, targeting the central nervous system, gastrointestinal tract and urinary tract leading to kidney failure [86, 87]. With the increase in antibiotic resistance, there is an urgent need to develop novel therapeutic approaches to disrupt bacterial biofilms and eradicate the causative bacteria in the host.

3.2. Current non-antibiotic strategies against CF lung infection

Non-antibiotic treatment strategies that have shown potential to reduce the severity of respiratory symptoms in CF patients and bacterial associated infections have largely centred on the use of aerosolised recombinant human DNase I (rhDNase I (Pulmozyme)) in a nebuliser [88]. Earlier studies showed DNase I reduced the viscosity of CF sputum by cleaving DNA present in sputum and thus leading to increased pulmonary function [49]. As noted above, eDNA is an essential biofilm promoting factor in many pathogenic bacterial species, is the backbone of the *P. aeruginosa* biofilm matrix, which by its impenetrable structure constitutes a defence strategy against antibiotics [46–48]. In line with this studies have shown that DNase I inhalation reduces the prevalence of bacterial strains in CF patients [88].

3.3. New non-antibiotic treatments

A new potential treatment strategy involves the use of reduced GSH to bind to pyocyanin and prevent its intercalation with eDNA. Intracellular GSH levels in mammalian cells are in the millimolar (mM) range, and lower concentrations are found in some bacterial cells. However, in CF patients, GSH levels in whole blood, blood neutrophils lymphocytes and epithelial lung fluid are markedly decreased [89]. Replenishment of GSH levels in CF has thus been investigated in a number of human studies using either inhaled GSH [90, 91] or oral N-acetylcysteine, a GSH precursor [92]. These studies demonstrated the feasibility of successfully delivering GSH to human lung, with a significant improvement in lung function (FEV1), especially in patients with moderate lung disease. The GSH therapy was well tolerated by CF patients with no noticeable side effects [91].

GSH, being a thiol antioxidant, will donate electrons/protons to pyocyanin directly through the –SH group from cysteine [53, 76], thereby interfering in the pyocyanin oxidation process by inhibiting H_2O_2 generation [76]. The antioxidant properties of GSH make it a potential inhibitor of pyocyanin toxicity. GSH binding to pyocyanin tends to modulate pyocyanin's structure, and this has been confirmed using nuclear magnetic resonance (NMR) spectroscopyand mass spectrometry [53, 93]. This structural change consequently inhibits the intercalation of pyocyanin with DNA, confirmed using circular dichroism [53]. In line with this, Muller and Merrett concluded that GSH forms a cell-impermanent conjugate with pyocyanin and consequently inhibits pyocyanin entry into host cells, thus preventing pyocyanin-mediated lung epithelial cell lysis [93].

Recent studies in the Manos laboratory by Klare et al. have demonstrated the excellent utility of GSH in disrupting *P. aeruginosa* biofilms. It was demonstratedusing CLSM that GSH-mediated inhibition of pyocyanin-DNA binding modulates *P. aeruginosa* biofilm architecture, significantly decreases biofilm biomass, surface coverage and leads to a significant increase in the percentage of dead bacterial cells [65]. GSH alone was shown to have a significant effect on disruption of mature 72-h-old biofilms of the epidemic isolate AES-1R grown in ASMDM+, while the combined treatment with GSH and DNase I of biofilms from a range of CF isolates showed greater disruption and significantly increased susceptibility to ciprofloxacin killing. GSH-treated biofilms were also shown by RNA-sequencing to display a transcriptomic profile that was distinctly different from those of both mature biofilms and dispersed cells, including those resulting from dispersal agents such as NO [65]. In contrast to dispersed cells, GSH-disrupted biofilm cells significantly upregulated cyclic-di-GMP synthesis genes (*siaA* and *siaB*), and there was no concomitant induction of flagellar biosynthesis genes. Cyclic-di-GMP gates the transition from sessile to motile lifestyle, and its expression prevents this transition [94]. GSH-disrupted cells also significantly upregulated the pyoverdine biosynthesis operon, in contrast to the downregulation of pyoverdine shown by dispersed cells. The active expression of pyoverdine is essential for biofilm structure formation [95]. CF sputum and ASMDM+ both have low levels of iron, and this may have triggered increased pyoverdine expression to sequester iron for processes required to re-form the disrupted biofilm.

In comparison to other techniques, GSH treatment has a distinct advantage, being an intrinsic and essential antioxidant for host cells that not only has antibiofilm properties but has also been proven to enhance lung epithelial growth and increase pulmonary function in CF patients [91].

3.4. Development of new antibacterial agents

Several new antibacterial agents are being developed and undergoing stringent testing both in vitro and in vivo (animal models) against *P. aeruginosa* and other CF pathogens. QS-inhibiting molecules against *P. aeruginosa* biofilms, such as furanone-based compounds (naturally secreted by the alga *Delisea Pulchra*) and synthetic furanone compounds have high affinity and compete with the cognate AHL signal for the LuxR receptor site in *P. aeruginosa* [96]. Thus by binding with and controlling the LuxR mechanism, these furanone molecules significantly alter biofilm architecture and enhance the efficiency of the antibiotic tobramycin against planktonic cells and biofilms [96]. Most interestingly, furanones have been shown to repress numerous QS-regulated virulence genes and production of concomitant virulence factors, including LasA protease and elastase B (encoded by *lasA* and *lasB*, respectively), rhamnolipid (encoded by the *rhlAB* operon) and phenazine biosynthesis (encoded by the *phzA-G* operon) [96].

Other antibiofilm agents under investigation include nitric oxide (NO) which has recently been discovered to induce dispersal of *P. aeruginosa* biofilms by mediating an increase in bacterial phosphodiesterase activity and a decrease in intracellular levels of the secondary messenger cyclic di-GMP, thereby inhibiting signal transduction in bacteria [97]. NO was shown to disperse released cells, and the remaining biofilms displayed enhanced sensitivity towards antibiotics [97]. A recent study by Kimyon et al. showed that prodigiosin (a heterocyclic bacterial secondary metabolite secreted by *Serratia sp.*) induces biofilm disruption and exhibits bactericidal activity against *P. aeruginosa* [98]. Prodigiosin-mediated *P. aeruginosa* biofilm disruption occurs by the release of H_2O_2 and generation of hydroxyl radicals in the presence of copper ions that consequently cleaves/damages eDNA and alters *P. aeruginosa* cell surface hydrophobicity. Prodigiosin also induces bacterial cell lysis as a consequence of the oxidative stress generated by H_2O_2 [98].

4. Conclusions

Extracellular molecules released by bacteria form a scaffold for biofilm formation. In *P. aeruginosa,* polysaccharides, eDNA and pyocyanin are major factors that integrate the biofilm matrix and provide defence against cationic antibiotics by binding to it [8]. On the other hand, molecules such as pyoverdine help promote bacterial growth and prevalence in the host by chelating iron [34]. Increased resistance to antibiotic therapies and the persistence of bacterial colonisation within the CF lung is associated with bacteria-secreted extracellular molecules. Novel treatment strategies seek to act on molecules that are essential for bacterial persistence such as biofilm constituents. Biofilm matrix disruption is associated with increased antibiotic susceptibility and clearance of bacteria. Current antibiotics strategies target growth inhibition without cleaving the biofilm matrix, whereas other strategies including DNase I and GSH cleave or disrupt biofilm matrix constituents, but have no bactericidal activity. In CF patients, the severity of disease due to *P. aeruginosa* infection is the leading cause of death, so there is an urgent need to develop new strategies that could disrupt bacterial biofilm matrix and facilitate bactericidal activity, ultimately allowing for repair and re-growth of lung epithelial tissue. The combination of biofilm-disrupting agents with traditional antibiotics could serve as a new line of therapy for CF patients in the near future.

Author details

Theerthankar Das[1,2*] and Jim Manos[1]

*Address all correspondence to: theerthankar_das11@rediffmail.com

1 Department of Infectious Diseases and Immunology, Sydney Medical School, University of Sydney, Sydney, Australia

2 School of Biotechnology and Biomolecular Sciences, University of New South Wales, Sydney, Australia

References

[1] Jeffrey BL, Carolyn LC, Gerald BP. Lung infections associated with cystic fibrosis. Clinical Microbiology Reviews. 2002;15:194–222. DOI: 10.1128/CMR.15.2.194–222.2002.

[2] Hoiby N. Recent advances in the treatment of *Pseudomonas aeruginosa* infections in cystic fibrosis. BioMed Central Medicine. 2011;9:1–7. DOI: 10.1186/1741-7015-9-32

[3] Filkins LM, O'Toole GA. Cystic fibrosis lung infections: polymicrobial, complex, and hard to treat. PLoS Pathogens. 2015;11:e1005258. DOI: 10.1371/journal.ppat.1005258

[4] Laura MF, Jyoti A G, Daniel GO, Emily LD, Lee RL, Sabin B, O'Toole GA. Coculture of *Staphylococcus aureus* with *Pseudomonas aeruginosa* drives *S. aureus* towards fermentative metabolism and reduced viability in a cystic fibrosis model. Journal of Bacteriology. 2015;197:2252–2264. DOI: 10.1128/JB.00059-15

[5] Cox MJ, Allgaier M, Taylor B, Marshall SB, Yvonne JH, Rebecca AD, Ulas K, Gary LA, Ronald B, Kei EF, Brain W, Diem T, Jonathan K, Susan VL. Airway microbiota and pathogen abundance in age-stratified cystic fibrosis patients. PLoS One. 2010;5:e11044. DOI: 10.1371/journal.pone.00111044

[6] Shaan LG, Hancock REW. *Pseudomonas aeruginosa*: new insights into pathogenesis and host defenses. Pathogens and Disease. 2013;67:159–173. DOI: 10.1111/2049-632X.12033

[7] Felming HC, Wingender J. The biofilm matrix. Nature Reviews Microbiology. 2010;8:623–633. DOI: 10.1038/nrmicro2415

[8] Das T, Sehar S, Manefield M. The roles of extracellular DNA in the structural integrity of EPS and bacterial biofilm. Environmental Microbiology Reports. 2013;5:778–786. DOI: 10.1111/1758-2229.12085

[9] Stewart PS, Costerton JW. Antibiotics resistance of bacteria in biofilms. Lancet. 2001;358:135–138. DOI: 10.1016/140-6736

[10] Das T, Ibugo A, Manefield M. Role of pyocyanin and extracellular DNA in facilitating *Pseudomonas aeruginosa* biofilm formation. Intech: Rijeka, Croatia. Microbial Applications, 2016, Chapter 2. DOI.org/10.5772/63497.

[11] Ryder C, Matthew B, Daniel JW. Role of polysaccharides in *Pseudomonas aeruginosa* biofilm development. Current Opinion Microbiology. 2007;10:644–648. DOI: 10.1016/j.mib.2007.09.010.

[12] Martin DW, Schurr MJ, Mudd MH, Govan JRW, Holloway BW, Deretic V. Mechanism of conversion to mucoidy in *Pseudomonas aeruginosa* infecting cystic fibrosis patients. Proceedings of the National Academy of Sciences of United States of America. 1993;90:8377–8381.

[13] Govan JRW, Deretic V. Microbial pathogenesis in cystic fibrosis: mucoid *Pseudomonas aeruginosa* and *Burkholderia cepacia*. Microbiological Reviews. 1996;60:539–574.

[14] Pier GB. *Pseudomonas aeruginosa*: a key problem in cystic fibrosis. ASM News. 1998;6:339–347.

[15] Alkawash MA, Soothill JS, Schiller NL. Alginate lyase enhances antibiotic killing of mucoid *Pseudomonas aeruginosa* in biofilms. APMIS. 2006;114:131–138. DOI: 10.1111/j.1600-0463.2006.apm_356.x

[16] Stapper AP, Narasimhan G, Ohman DE, Barakat J, Hentzer M, Molin S, Kharazmi A, Hoiby N, Mathee K. Alginate production affects *Pseudomonas aeruginosa* biofilm development and architecture, but is not essential for biofilm formation. Journal of Medical Microbiology. 2004;53:679–690. DOI: 10.1099/jmm.0.45539-0

[17] Friedman L, Kolter R. Two genetic loci produce distinct carbohydrate-rich structural components of the *Pseudomonas aerguinosa* biofilm matrix. Journal of Bacteriology. 2004;186:4457–4465. DOI: 10.1128/JB.186.14.4457-4465.2004

[18] Jackson KD, Starkey M, Kremer S, Parsek MR, Wozniak DJ. Identification of psl, a locus encoding a potential exopolysaccharide that is essential for *Pseudomonas aeruginosa* PAO1 biofilm formation. Journal of Bacteriology. 2004;186:4466–4475. DOI: 10.1128/JB.186.14.4466-4475.2004

[19] Matsukawa M, Greenberg EP. Putative exopolysaccharide synthesis genes influence *Pseudomonas aeruginosa* biofilm development. Journal of Bacteriology. 2004;186:4449–4456. DOI: 10.1128/JB.186.14.4449-4456.2004

[20] Suter S, Schaad UB, Roux L, Nydegger UE, Waldvogel FA. Granulocyte neutral proteases and *Pseudomonas elastase* as possible causes of airway damage in patients with cystic fibrosis. Journal of Infectious Diseases. 1984;149:523–531.

[21] Upritchard HG, Cordwell SJ, Lamont IL. Immunoproteomics to examine cystic fibrosis host interactions with extracellular *Pseudomonas aeruginosa* proteins. Infection and Immunity. 2008;76:4624–4632. DOI: 10.1128/IAI.01707-07

[22] Thalia IN, Barbara HI. Production of elastase and other exoproducts by environmental isolates of *Pseudomonas aeruginosa*. Journal of Clinical Microbiology. 1986;23:967–969.

[23] Hoge R, Pelzer A, Rosenau F, Wilhelm S. Weapons of a pathogen: proteases and their role in virulence of *Pseudomonas aeruginosa*. Current Research, Technology and Education, Topics in Applied Microbiology and Microbial Biotechnology. Formatex Research Center 2010, pp. 383–395.

[24] Doring, G., Obernesser, H.-J., Botzenhart, K. Extracellular toxins of *Pseudomonas aeruginosa*. II. Effect of two proteases on human immunoglobulins IgG, IgA and sec retory IgA. Zentralblatt für Bakteriologie, Mikrobiologie und Hygiene [A]. 1981;249:89–98.

[25] Voynow JA, Fischer BM, Zheng S. Proteases and cystic fibrosis. International Journal of Biochemistry & Cell Biology. 2008;40:1238–1245. DOI: 10.1016/j.biocel.2008.03.003

[26] Murray PR, Baron EJ, Pfaller MA, Tenover FC, Yolken RH. Manual of Clinical Microbiology. 2nd ed. Washington, MD: American Society Microbiology; 1999.

[27] Doring G, Obernesser HJ, Botzenhart K, Flehmig B, Hoilby N, Hofmann A. Proteases of *Pseudomonas aeruginosa* in patients with cystic fibrosis. The Journal of Infectious Diseases. 1983;147:744–750.

[28] Peters JE, Park SJ, Darzins A, Freck LC, Saulnier JM, Wallach JM, Galloway DR. Further studies on *Pseudomonas aeruginosa* LasA: analysis of specificity. Molecular Microbiology. 1992;6:1155–1162.

[29] Elliott BW, Cohen C. Isolation and characterization of a lysine-specific protease from *Pseudomonas aeruginosa*. Journal of Biological Chemistry. 1986;261:11259–11265.

[30] Engel LS, Hill JM, Caballero AR, Green LC, O'Callaghan RJ. Protease IV: a unique extracellular protease and virulence factor from *Pseudomonas aeruginosa*. Journal of Biological Chemistry. 1998;273:16792–16797.

[31] Ewa Ołdak and Elz˙bieta A. Trafny. Secretion of proteases by *Pseudomonas aeruginosa* biofilms exposed to Ciprofloxacin. Antimicrobial Agents and Chemotherapy. 2005;49:3281–3288. DOI: 10.1128/AAC.49.8.3281-3288.2005.

[32] Peek ME, Bhatnagar A, McCarty NA, Zughaier SM. Pyoverdine, the major siderophore in *Pseudomonas aeruginosa*, Evades NGAL Recognition. 2012; Article ID 843509. DOI: 10.1155/2012/843509

[33] Visca P, Imperi F, Lamont IL. Pyoverdine siderophores: from biogenesis to biosignificance. Trends in Microbiology. 2007;15:22–30. DOI: 10.1016/j.tim.2006.11.004

[34] Lamont IL, Konings AF, Reid DW. Iron acquisition by *Pseudomonas aeruginosa* in the lungs of patients with cystic fibrosis. BioMetals. 2009;22:53–60. DOI: 10.1007/s10534-008-9197-9

[35] Takase H, Nitanai H, Hoshino K, Otani T. Impact of siderophore production on *Pseudomonas aeruginosa* infections in immunosuppressed mice. Infection and Immunity. 2000;68:1834–1839. DOI: 10.1128/IAI.68.4.1834-1839.2000

[36] Meyer JM, Neely A, Stintzi A, Georges C, Holder IA. Pyoverdin is essential for virulence of *Pseudomonas aeruginosa*. Infection and Immunity. 1996:64:518–523.

[37] Tate S, MacGregor G, Davis M, Innes JA, Greening AP. Airways in cystic fibrosis are acidified: detection by exhaled breath condensate. Thorax. 2002;57:926–929. DOI: 10.1136/thorax.57.11.926

[38] Das T, Manefield M. Pyocyanin promotes extracellular DNA release in *Pseudomonas aeruginosa*. PLoS One. 2012;7:e46718. DOI: 10.1371/journal.pone.0046718

[39] Whitchurch CB, Tolker-Nielsen T, Ragas PC, Mattick JS. Extracellular DNA required for bacterial biofilm formation. Science. 2002;295:1487. DOI: 10.1126/science.295.5559.1487

[40] Swartjes JJTM, Das T, Sharifi S, Subbiahdoss G, Sharma PK, Krom BP, Busscher HJ, Van der Mei HC. A functional DNase I coating to prevent adhesion of bacteria and the

formation of biofilm. Advance Functional Materials. 2012;23:2843–2849. DOI: 10.1002/adfm.201202927.

[41] Das T, Kutty SK, Kumar N, Manefield M. Pyocyanin factilitates extracellular DNA binding to *Pseudomonas aeruginosa* influencing cell surface properties and aggregation. PLoS One. 2013;8:e58299. DOI: 10.1371/journal.pone.0058299

[42] Böckelmann U, Janke A, Kuhn R, Neu TR, Wecke J, Lawrence JR, Szewzyk U. Bacterial extracellular DNA forming a defined network-like structure. FEMS Microbiology Letters. 2006;262:31–38. DOI: 10.1111/j.1574-6968.2006.00361.x

[43] Allesen-Holm M, Barken KB, Yang L, Klausen M, Webb JS, Staffan K, Soren M, Michael G, Tim T-N. A characterization of DNA release in *Pseudomonas aeruginosa* cultures and biofilms. Molecular Microbiology. 2005;59:1114–1128. DOI: 10.1111/j.1365-2958

[44] Kadurugamuwa JL, Beveridge TJ. Virulence factors are released from *Pseudomonas aeruginosa* in association with membrane vesicles during normal growth and exposure to gentamicin: a novel mechanism of enzyme secretion. Journal of Bacteriology. 1995;177:3998–4008. DOI: 10.1016/j.ijppharm.09.043

[45] Barnes, AM, Ballering KS, Leibman, RS, Wells CL, Dunny GM. *Enterococcus faecalis* produces abundant extracellular structures containing DNA in the absence of cell lysis during early biofilm formation. MBio. 2012;3:e00193–00112. DOI: 10.1128//IAI.01162-10

[46] Chiang WC, Nilsson M, Jensen PO, Hoiby N, Givskov, M, Toler-Nielsen T. Extracellular DNA shields against aminoglycosides in *Pseudomonas aeruginosa* biofilms. Antimicrobial Agents and Chemotherapy. 2013;57:2352–2361. DOI: 10.1128/AAC.00001-13

[47] Mulcahy H, Mazenod LC, Lewenza S. Extracellular DNA chelates cations and induces antibiotic resistance in *Pseudomonas aeruginosa* biofilms. PLoS Pathogens. 2008;4:e1000213. DOI: 10.1371/1000213

[48] Tetz, GV, Artemenko NK, Tetz VV. Effect of DNase and antibiotics on biofilm characteristics. Antimicrobial Agents and Chemotherapy. 2009;53:1204–1209. DOI: 10.1128/AAC.00471-08

[49] Shak S, Capon DJ, Hellmiss R, Scot AM, Carrie LB. Recombinant human DNase I reduces the viscosity of cystic fibrosis sputum. Proceedings of the North American Academy of Science. 1990;87:9188–9192. DOI: 10.1073/9188

[50] Harmsen M, Lappann M, Knøchel S, Molin S. Role of extracellular DNA during biofilm formation by *Listeria monocytogenes*. Applied and Environmental Microbiology. 2010;76:2271–2279. DOI: 10.1128/AEM.02361-09

[51] Petersen FC, Tao L, Scheie AA. DNA binding-uptake system: a link between cell-to-cell communication and biofilm formation. Journal of Bacteriology. 2005;187:4392–4400. DOI: 10.1128/JB.187.13

[52] Berne C, Kysela DT, Brun YV. A bacterial extracellular DNA inhibits settling of motile progeny cells within a biofilm. Molecular Microbiology. 2010:77:815–829. DOI: 10.1111/j.1365-2958.2010.07267.x

[53] Das T, Kutty SK, Tavallaie R, Amaye I I, Janjira P, Shama S, Leigh A, Amanda WSY, Shane RT, Naresh K, Justin, JG, Mike M. Phenazine virulence factor binding to extracellular DNA is important for *Pseudomonas aeruginosa* biofilm formation. Nature Scientific Reports. 2015;5:8398. DOI: 10.1038/08398

[54] Mavrodi DV, Bonsall RF, Delaney SM, Soule MJ, Philipps G, Thomashow, LS. Functional analysis of genes for biosynthesis of pyocyanin and Phenazine-1-Carboxamide from *Pseudomonas aeruginosa* PAO1. Journal of Bacteriology. 2001;183:6454–6465. DOI: 10.1128/JB 183.21.64546465

[55] Parsons JF, Greenhagen BT, Shi K, Calabrese K, Robinson H, Ladner JE. Structural and functional analysis of the pyocyanin biosynthetic protein Phz M from *Pseudomonas aeruginosa*. Biochemistry. 2007;46:1821–1828. DOI: 10.1021/bi6024403

[56] Wilson R, Sykes DA, Watson D, Rutman, A, Taylor G.W, Cole PJ. Measurement of *Pseudomonas aeruginosa* phenazine pigments in sputum and assessment of their contribution to sputum sol toxicity for respiratory epithelium. Infection and Immunity. 1988;56:2515–2517. DOI: 10.1111/1751

[57] Cox CD. Role of pyocyanin in the acquisition of iron from transferring. Infection and Immunity. 1986;52:263–270.

[58] Porter RC. Studies in pigment production by *Pseudomonas aeruginosa*. MS thesis, Texas Tech University, TX, 59 p.

[59] Price-Whelan A, Dietrich LEP, Newman DK. Rethinking secondary metabolism: physiological roles for phenazine antibiotics. Nature Chemical Biology. 2006;2:71–78. DOI: 10.1038/764

[60] Elkins JG, Hassett DJ, Stewart PS, Schweizer HP, McDermott TR. Protective role of catalase in*Pseudomonas aeruginosa*biofilm resistance to hydrogen peroxide. Applied and Environmental Microbiology. 1999;65:4594–4600.

[61] Zheng L, Chen Z, Itzek A, Ashby M, Kreth J. Catabolite control protein A controls hydrogen peroxide production and cell death in *Streptococccus sanguinis*. Journal of Bacteriology. 2011;193:516–526. DOI: 10.1128/JB.01131-10

[62] Das T, Krom BP, van der Mei HC,Busscher HJ, Sharma PK. DNA-mediated bacterial aggregation is dictated by acid-base interactions. Soft Matters. 2011;7:2927–2935. DOI: 10.1039/C0SM01142H

[63] Das T, Sharma PK, Krom BP, van der Mei HC, Busscher HJ. Role of eDNA on the adhesion forces between *Streptococcus mutans* and substratum surfaces: influence of ionic strength and substratum hydrophobicity. Langmuir. 2011;27:10113–10118. DOI: 10.1021/la202013m.

[64] Boks NP, Norde W, Van der Mei, HC, Busscher HJ. Forces involved in bacterial adhesion to hydrophilic and hydrophobic surfaces. Microbiology. 2008;154:3122–3133. DOI: 10.1099/mic.018622-0

[65] Klare W, Das T, Ibugo A, Buckle E, Manefield M, Manos J. The glutathione-disrupted biofilm of clinical *Pseudomonas aeruginosa* strains: enhanced antibiotic effect and a novel biofilm transcriptome. Antimicrobial Agents and Chemotherapy. 2016;60:4539–4551. DOI: 10.1128/AAC.02919-15

[66] Ran H, Hassett DJ, Lau GW. Human targets of *Pseudomonas aeruginosa* pyocyanin. Proceedings of the North American Academy of Science. 2003;100:14315–14320. DOI: 10.1073/pnas.2332354100.

[67] Sweden EG. Study the effect of antibiotics on pyocyanin production from *Pseudomonas aeruginosa* and pyocyanin as antibiotic against different pathogenic bacteria. Journal of University Anbar Pure Science. 2010;4:15–18.

[68] Hassan HM, Fridorich I. Mechanism of the antibiotic action of pyocyanine. Journal of Bacteriology. 1980;141:156–163.

[69] Kerr JR, Taylor GW, Rutman A, Hoiby N, Cole PJ, Wilson R. *Pseudomonas aeruginosa* pyocyanin and 1-hydroxyphenazine inhibit fungal growth. Journal of Clinical Pathology. 1999;52:385–387

[70] Hunter RC, Vanja K, Magen ML, Hannah G, Thomas RM, Dianne KN. Phenazine content in the cystic fibrosis respiratory tract negatively correlates with lung function and microbial complexity. American Journal of Respiratory Cell and Molecular Biology. 2012;47:738–745. DOI: 10.1165/rcmb.2012-0088OC

[71] Charles CC, Yi C, Goetzmann HS, Hao Y, Borchers MT, Hassett DJ, Young LR, Mavrodi D, Thomashow L, Lau GW. *Pseudomonas aeruginosa* exotoxin pyocyanin causes cystic fibrosis airway pathogenesis. The American Journal of Pathology. 2009;175:2473–2488. DOI: 10.2353/ajpath.2009.090166

[72] Harmer C, Alnassafi K, Hu H, Elkins M, Bye P, Rose B, Cordwell S, Triccas JA, Harbour C, Manos J. Modulation of gene expression by *Pseudomonas aeruginosa* during chronic infection in the adult cystic fibrosis lung. Microbiology. 2013;159:2354–2363. DOI: 10.1099/mic.0.066985-0

[73] Brent C, Vinayavekhin N, Grenfell-Lee D, Yuen GJ, Saghatelian A, Ausubel FM. Identification of *Pseudomonas aeruginosa* phenazines that kill Caenorhabditis elegans. PLoS Pathogens. 2013;9:e1003101. DOI: 10.1371/journal.ppat.1003101

[74] Schwarzer C, Fischer H, Kim EJ, Baba KJ, Mills AD, Kurtt MJ, Gruenert DC, Suh JH, Machen TE, Illek B. Oxidative stress by pyocyanin impairs CFTR Cl^- transport in human bronchial epithelial cells. Free Radical Biology & Medicine. 2008;45:1653–1662. DOI: 10.1016/freeradbiomed.09.011

[75] Winstanley C, Fothergill JL. The role of quorum sensing in chronic cystic fibrosis *Pseudomonas aeruginosa* infections. FEMS Microbiology Letters. 2008;290:1–9. DOI: 10.1111/j.1574-6968.2008.01394.x.

[76] O'Malley YQ, Reszka KJ, Spitz DR, Denning GM, Britigan BE. *Pseudomonas aeruginosa* pyocyanin directly oxidizes glutathione and decreases its levels in airway epithelial cells. American Journal of Physiology Lung Cellular and Molecular Physiology. 2004;287:94–103. DOI: 10.1152/apjplung.00025

[77] O'Malley YXQ, Krzysztof JR, George TR, Maher YA, Gerene MD, Bradley EB. The Pseudomonas secretory product pyocyanin inhibits catalase activity in human lung epithelial cells. American Journal of Physiology Lung Cellular and Molecular Physiology. 2003;285:L1077–L1086. DOI: 10.1152/ajplung.00198.

[78] Rada B, Jendrysik MA, Pang L, Craig PH, Dae-goon Y, Jonathan JP, Samuel MM, Harry LM, Thomas LL. Pyocyanin-enhanced neutrophil extracellular trap formation requires the NADPH oxidase. PLoS One. 2013;8:e54205. DOI: 101371/0054205.

[79] Aeschlimann JR. The role of multidrug efflux pumps in the antibiotic resistance of *Pseudomonas aeruginosa* and other gram-negative bacteria. Pharmacotherapy. 2003;23: 916–923.

[80] Heijerman H, Westerman E, Conway S, Touw D, Döring G, Consensus working group. Inhaled medication and inhalation devices for lung diseases in patients with cystic fibrosis: a European consensus. Journal of Cystic Fibros. 2009;8:295–315. DOI: 10.1016/ j.jcf.2009.04.005

[81] Ratjen F, Rietschel E, Kasel D, Schwiertz R, Starke K, Beier H, van Koningsbruggen S, Grasemann H. Pharmacokinetics of inhaled colistin in patients with cystic fibrosis. Journal of Antimicrobial and Chemotherapy. 2006;57:306–311. DOI: 10.1093/jac/dki461

[82] Permin H, Koch C, Høiby N, Christensen HO, Møller AF, Møller S. Ceftazidime treatment of chronic *Pseudomonas aeruginosa* respiratory tract infection in cystic fibrosis. Journal of Antimicrobial and Chemotherapy. 1983;12:313–323.

[83] Duff AJ, Latchford GJ. Inhaled medication and inhalation devices for lung disease in patients with cystic fibrosis: poor adherence and the need to address it. Journal of Cystic Fibrosis. 2010;9:455–456. DOI: 10.1016/j.jcf.2010.08.012

[84] Noah TL, Ivins SS, Abode KA, Stewart PW, Michelson PH, Harris WT, Henry MM, Leigh MW. Inhaled versus systemic antibiotics and airway inflammation in children with cystic fibrosis and Pseudomonas. Pediatric Pulmonology. 2010;45:281–290. DOI: 10.1002/ppul.21176

[85] Saiman L, Anstead M, Mayer-Hamblett N, Lands LC, Kloster M, Hocevar- Trnka J, Goss CH, Rose LM, Burns JL, Marshall BC, Ratjen F, AZ0004 Azithromycin Study Group. Effect of azithromycin on pulmonary function in patients with cystic fibrosis uninfected with *Pseudomonas aeruginosa*: a randomized controlled trial. Journal of the American Medical Association. 2010;303:1707 1715. DOI: 10.1001/jama.2010.563

[86] De Sarro A, De Sarro G. Adverse reactions to fluoroquinolones. An overview on mechanistic aspects. Current Medicinal Chemistry. 2001;8:371–384.

[87] De Broe ME, Paulus GJ, Verpooten GA, Roels F, Buyssens N, Wedeen R, Van Hoof F, Tulkens PM. Early effects of gentamicin, tobramycin, and amikacin on the human kidney. Kidney International. 1984;25:643–652.

[88] Frederiksen B, Pressler T, Hansen A, Koch C, Høiby N. Effect of aerosolized rhDNase (Pulmozyme) on pulmonary colonization in patients with cystic fibrosis. Acta Paediatrica 2006;95:1070–1074. DOI: 10.1080/08035250600752466

[89] Lands LC, Grey V, Smountas AA, Kramer VG, McKenna D. Lymphocyte glutathione levels in children with cystic fibrosis. Chest. 1999;116:201–205.

[90] Calabrese C, Tosco A, Abete P, Carnovale V, Basile C, Magliocca A, Quattrucci S, De Sanctis S, Alatri F, Mazzarella G, De Pietro L, Turino C, Melillo E, Buonpensiero P, Di Pasqua A, Raia V. Randomized, single blind, controlled trial of inhaled glutathione vs placebo in patients with cystic fibrosis. Journal of Cystic Fibros. 2015;14:203–210. DOI: 10.1016/j.jcf.2014.09.014

[91] Griese M, Kappler M, Eismann C, Ballmann M, Junge S, Rietschel E, van Koningsbruggen-Rietschel S, Staab D, Rolinck-Werninghaus C, Mellies U, Köhnlein T, Wagner T, König S, Teschler H, Heuer HE, Kopp M, Heyder S, Hammermann J, Küster P, Honer M, Mansmann U, Beck-Speier I, Hartl D, Fuchs C; Glutathione Study Group, Hector A. Inhalation treatment with glutathione in patients with cystic fibrosis: a randomized clinical trial. American Journal of Respiratory Critical Care Medicine. 2013;188:83–89. DOI: 10.1164/rccm.201303-0427OC

[92] Conrad C, Lymp J, Thompson V, Dunn C, Davies Z, Chatfield B, Nichols D, Clancy J, Vender R, Egan ME, Quittell L, Michelson P, Antony V, Spahr J, Rubenstein RC, Moss RB, Herzenberg LA, Goss CH, Tirouvanziam R. Long-term treatment with oral N-acetylcysteine: affects lung function but not sputum inflammation in cystic fibrosis subjects. A phase II randomized placebo-controlled trial. Journal of Cystic Fibrosis. 2015;14:219–27. DOI: 10.1016/j.jcf.2014.08.008

[93] Muller M, Merrett ND. Mechanism for glutathione-mediated protection against the *Pseudomonas aeruginosa* redox toxin, pyocyanin. Chemico-Biological Interactions. 2015;5:232:30–7. DOI: 10.1016/j.cbi.2015.03.011.

[94] Chua SL, Liu Y, Yam JK, Chen Y, Vejborg RM, Tan BG, Kjelleberg S, Tolker-Nielsen T, Givskov M, Yang L. Dispersed cells represent a distinct stage in the transition from bacterial biofilm to planktonic lifestyles. Nature Communications. 2014;5:Article No: 4462. DOI: 10.1038/ncomms5462

[95] Banin E, Vasil ML, Greenberg EP. Iron and *Pseudomonas aeruginosa* biofilm formation. Proceedings of the National Academy of Sciences of United States of America. 2005;102:11076–11081. DOI: 10.1073/pnas.0504266102

[96] Hentzer M, Givskov M. Pharmacological inhibition of quorum sensing for the treatment of chronic bacterial infections. Journal of Clinical Investigation. 2003;112:1300–1307. DOI: 10.1172/JCI200320074.

[97] Nguyen T-K, Selvanayagam R, Ho KKK, Chen R, Kutty SK, Rice SA, Kumar N, Barraud N, Duong HTT, Boyer C. Co-delivery of nitric oxide and antibiotic using polymeric nanoparticles. Chemical Science. 2016;7:1016. DOI: 10.1039/c5sc02769a

[98] Kimyon Ö, Das T, Ibugo AI, Kutty SK, Ho KK, Tebben J, Kumar N, Manefield M. Serratia secondary metabolite prodigiosin inhibits *Pseudomonas aeruginosa* biofilm development by producing reactive oxygen species that damage biological molecules. Frontiers in Microbiology. 2016;7:Article 972 DOI: 10.3389/fmicb.2016.00972.

Chapter 6

Structure-Function Relationships of Rhamnolipid and Exopolysacharide Biosurfactants of *Pseudomonas aeruginosa* as Therapeutic Targets in Cystic Fibrosis Lung Infections

Milena G. Rikalovic, Natasa S. Avramovic and Ivanka M. Karadzic

Additional information is available at the end of the chapter

http://dx.doi.org/10.5772/66687

Abstract

Chronic *Pseudomonas aeruginosa* lung infection is the cause of much morbidity and most of the mortality in cystic fibrosis (CF) patients. The high prevalence of *P. aeruginosa* infections in CF is related to the microbe's large genome and mechanisms of adaptation to the CF lung environment, the host immune system and antibiotic resistance. Among a wide range of *P. aeruginosa* metabolites involved in infection development in CF, the biosurfactant compounds, rhamnolipids (RLs) and exopolysaccharides (EPSs), have important roles in the early stages of *P. aeruginosa* infection in CF. RLs and EPSs are involved in bacterial adhesion, biofilm formation, antibiotic resistance, and impairment of host immune system pathways, as well as in processes such as biofilm maintenance and the mucoid phenotype of *P. aeruginosa,* which lead to development of chronic infection. Due to the proposed roles of RLs and EPSs and the importance of prevention and treatment of *P. aeruginosa* respiratory infections in CF, these compounds are promising targets for patient therapy. In the future, impairment of *P. aeruginosa* quorum sensing (QS) pathways and modification of host respiratory mucus epithelial membranes should be considered as potential approaches in preventing respiratory infections caused by this microbe in CF patients.

Keywords: cystic fibrosis, *Pseudomonas aeruginosa,* biosurfactant, rhamnolipid, exopolysaccharide, biofilm

1. Introduction

Cystic fibrosis is a congenital, recessively inherited disorder. The genetic background of CF development is >1500 mutations in the cystic fibrosis transmembrane conductance regulator gene (CFTR) on chromosome 7, which lead to malfunction of the chloride channel in CF patients. CF affects a large number of organs and tissues (airways, pancreas, the small intestine, liver, the reproductive tract and sweat glands), resulting in numerous clinical symptoms (viscid mucus, respiratory infections, intestinal malabsorption of fat, diabetes mellitus, meconium ileus, impaired liver function, male infertility and salt loss) [1].

The malfunction of the chloride channel in CF patients leads to impairment of the non-inflammatory defense mechanism of the lower respiratory tract. Therefore, CF patients, from early childhood, suffer recurrent and chronic respiratory tract infections caused by *P. aeruginosa*, *Burkholderia cepaci*, *Achromobacter xylosoxidans*, *Staphylococcus aureus*, *Haemophilus influenzae*, *Stenotrophomonas maltophilia*, nontuberculous *Mycobacteria* and *Aspergillus fumigatus*. In spite of the host inflammatory response and intensive antibiotic therapy, infections persist and lead to respiratory failure requiring lung transplantation or death [1].

Chronic *P. aeruginosa* lung infection is the cause of much of the morbidity and most of the mortality in CF patients. Chronic infection is considered as growth of *P. aeruginosa* from multiple respiratory cultures over a 6-month period [2]. About 80% of adults with CF have chronic *P. aeruginosa* infection [3]. *P. aeruginosa* is able to survive and persist for several decades in the respiratory tract of CF patients, in spite of the defense mechanisms of the host and intensive antibiotic therapy. However, the microbe has adaptive mechanisms, which explain why it can survive in the hostile CF lung for so long. These include phenotype splitting due to mutations (into nonmucoid or mucoid), their different distributions in respiratory and conductive zones in the lungs and switching to a biofilm mode of growth—mucoid phenotype [4–7].

Recent research indicates that chronic *P. aeruginosa* infections are caused by the ability of bacteria to organize themselves into microcolonies regarding to formation of biofilms. In this state, the bacteria are incorporated in a self-produced protective matrix, often with surrounding inflammatory cells, which is very well protected against antibiotics and the host defense [4]. The biosurfactant compounds (RLs and EPSs), due to their structures and physicochemical properties, as well as their interactions and correlation with other metabolites, significantly contribute to colonization, motility and biofilm formation [8–10]. Additionally, the mucoid colony morphology of *P. aeruginosa* is highly correlated with overproduction of alginate (a type of EPS) [8]. Therefore, it is important to consider these biosurfactants and their biosynthetic pathways as possible targets and approaches for CF therapy in order to impair *P. aeruginosa* mechanisms of pathogenicity. Furthermore, cell-to-cell communication and QS signaling pathways together with their genetic aspects, closely related to RL and EPS biosynthesis, are the most significant targets for new therapy approaches in CF treatment [10–13].

2. *P. aeruginosa* infection in CF

2.1. *P. aeruginosa*

Pseudomonas is ubiquitously present worldwide, being an extremely diverse bacterial genus. Pseudomonads are frequently closely associated with animals and plants; they are common and numerous in a wide range of environmental habitats. Their ability to adapt genetically, producing varying physiological advantages as a response to their pervasiveness, is the subject of much scientific speculation and study. *P. aeruginosa,* as all species that belong to the genus *Pseudomonas,* due to its metabolic diversity, has potential for adaptation, survival and growth in a wide range of environmental conditions [14, 15].

P. aeruginosa produces an arsenal of secondary metabolites, including EPSs, RLs, enzymes (elastase, alkalne protease, exoenzyme S, phospholipase C and hemolysins), pigments and toxins (exotoxin A), using these virulence factors for infecting and colonizing a wide range of hosts (animals, plats, insect and nematodes) and surfaces [12–24]. The major biosurfactant compounds produced by *P. aeruginosa,* RLs and EPSs, are involved in bacterial adherence, biofilm formation and maintenance, which all are necessary for respiratory infection establishment, development and progression in CF patients [4, 8, 12, 13, 16].

2.2. Pathogenesis of *P. aeruginosa* infection in CF

Despite constant exposure to a wide range of microorganisms, CF patients are predisposed to infection by only specific groups of microorganisms [8]. The proximal event in development of CF is mutation of the CFTR gene (see Introduction), but still, it remains unclear how this primary step causes particular infections in CF patients. However, numerous proposed mechanisms are related to CFTR gene mutation, defective CFTR channels and infection development [8]: (1) reduced ion transport; (2) modified salt content in the airway surface liquid; (3) increased levels of acylated glycolipids on the surface of CF airway epithelial cells; (4) defective CFTR exposed on airway epithelial cell membranes become receptors; (5) low levels of antimicrobial compounds (inducible nitric oxide synthase and nitric oxide); and (6) intrinsic hyperinflammation of airways (**Table 1**) [25–36].

The first step in infection of CF airways by *P. aeruginosa* is microbe acquisition [8]. Due to the abundance of *P. aeruginosa* in many natural environments, most individuals acquire *P. aeruginosa* through casual contact with natural bacterial sources, while some individuals acquire *P. aeruginosa* directly or indirectly from other CF patients. Transmission data and genotype/phenotype properties of clinical and environmental *P. aeruginosa* isolates indicate that characterizing the ecology of *P. aeruginosa* originating from natural environments would lead to a better understanding CF epidemiology [8].

Initially, infection of *P. aeruginosa* in CF is usually the result of an alternating series of acquisitions of different isolates and in the first stage of infection, most of the isolates are nonmucoid and highly antibiotic sensitive [8, 37–39]. Eventually, one or two isolates establish themselves and, due to their genetic, phenotypic and physiological changes, develop chronic infection [13, 16, 40].

Mechanism	Effect
Decreased ion transport, which results from defective CFTR channels enhances fluid absorption in the airways	Lowered airways surface liquid and impaired ciliary transport of the mucous layer, which results in defects in microbial clearance
Altered salt content in the airway surface liquid	Inactivation of immune system defenses pathways; defected neutrophils activity
Increased levels of acylated glycolipids on the surface of CF airway epithelial cells due to defective CFTR molecules	Modified glycolipids are receptors for *P. aeruginosa* adherence
Binding of *P. aeruginosa* to defective CFTR molecule exposed on airway epithelial cells membranes	Internalisation of *P. aeruginosa*
Lowered level of antimicrobial compounds	Propensity of individuals to lung infection
Istrinical hyperinflammation of airways	Damage of host cells and disruption of effective microbe clearance

Table 1. Proposed mechanisms of *P. aeruginosa* in development of respiratory infection in CF airways.

2.2.1. P. aeruginosa quorum sensing systems and biofilm

One of the most important factors which facilitate *P. aeruginosa* to colonize and persist in acute and chronic lung infection in CF patients is the ability of this microbe to grow as a biofilm, assembly of which is regulated by a QS system [13, 30, 40].

QS is the mechanism by which bacteria engage in cell-to-cell communication using diffusible molecules based on a critical cell density [41]. QS molecules manage and regulate diverse physiological processes, some of which are interrelated. In *P. aeruginosa*, expression, production and/or secretion of many virulence factors, such as EPSs, RLs, enzymes, pigments production, biofilm formation and antibiotic resistance, are controlled by QS [10, 13, 42]. *P. aeruginosa* possesses two interrelated QS systems, the *las* and *rhl* systems. The *las* system comprises the transcriptional regulatory protein, LasR and its cognate autoinducer, N-(3-oxododecanoyl) homoserine lactone (3O-C_{12}-HSL). The *rhl* system comprises the RhlR transcription regulator protein (also known as R-protein) and N-butyryl homoserine lactone (C_4-HSL), its cognate autoinducer [13]. Additionally, these two systems are not independent but are interlinked in a hierarchical manner (the *las* system directs the *rhl* system). They are linked by a third signal molecule, 2-heptyl-3-hydroxy-4-quinolone, known as the *Pseudomonas* quinolone signal (PQS). PQS is produced under the control of the *pqs* system, which is considered as the third distinct QS system [11, 42]. Interestingly, transcriptome analyses have revealed that between 6 and 10% of the *P. aeruginosa* genome is regulated by the *las* and/or *rhl* systems [13].

Biofilms are matrix-enclosed microbial accretions that adhere to biological or nonbiological surfaces [43]. *P. aeruginosa* biofilms are related to development of different acute and chronic infections, not only in CF patients [16, 44, 45]. Formation of *P. aeruginosa* biofilm occurs in stages: bacterial attachment and irreversible adhesion to surface, microcolony development, biofilm maturation and dispersion of bacterial cells from the biofilm [46]. Heterogeneous microenvironments due to oxygen and nutrient diffusion limitations occur in biofilms and they lead to physiological and phenotype diversity [47, 48]. Suggested mechanisms of *P. aeruginosa* biofilm formation involve QS signaling, which coordinates and protects biofilm assembly and maintenance [44, 49–52]. The *las I*, which encodes the biosynthetic pathway for 3O-C_{12}-HSL, is critical for biofilm maturation [50]. Heterogeneity of the bacterial population in biofilm is an important characteristic of *P. aeruginosa* pathogenicity and contributes to the microbe's resistance to antimicrobial therapy. In laboratory conditions, *P. aeruginosa* can form two types of biofilm, "flat" and "structured", and alginate-producing isolates (the mucoid phenotype) form complex structured type of biofilm which is resistant to tobramycin [53]. Additionally, the QS system is involved in regulation of several genes such as *rhlA, rpoS, sad A* and genes in the denitrification pathways. These genes are important for all stages of biofilm development, maintenance, or dispersion: (1) biosynthesis of the biofilm matrix (EPSs, extracellular DNA); (2) biosynthesis of RLs; and (3) other metabolic pathways (not discussed here) [13, 42].

2.2.2. *Adaptation mechanisms of P. aeruginosa in CF lungs*

The CF lungs are an unfriendly and varied environment for invading bacteria due to the presence of stressors such as osmotic stress of viscous mucus, oxidative and nitrosative stresses of the host responses, sublethal concentrations of antibiotics and other microbes presence. Regarding to the environment of CF lungs, it is a great challenge of *P. aeruginosa* populations to overcome these stressors and persist [54].

It is believed that mechanisms that allow *P. aeruginosa* to cause persistent chronic infection are related to its remarkable potential for adaptation to environmental changes [8, 15]. *P. aeruginosa* adaptations in CF patients' lungs are dynamic and generate subpopulations of bacteria with differing phenotypes [8]. It is thought that primary infection is related to the large *P. aeruginosa* genome, while development of persistent infection is dependent on spontaneous mutations [55, 56]. Mutations are multiple due to different factors such as the presence of hypermutable strains, development of biofilm and downregulation of antioxidant enzymes [57–59]. Environmental conditions in CF airways then further favor specific *P. aeruginosa* phenotypes. This set of adaptations finally leads to development of the subpopulations of bacteria (mentioned above) within the same respiratory tract, which are relatively similar, but which carry unique groups of genes [56, 60, 61]. Some commonly and intensively studied *P. aeruginosa* adaptation mechanisms present during respiratory infections in CF involve: transition to mucoid phenotype, antibiotic resistance, alterations in lipopolysacharride (LPS), loss of type III secretion and motility, auxotrophy, small-colony variants, defects in the QS system and hypermutability [8, 54].

3. Biosurfactants of *P. aeruginosa*—rhamnolipids and exopolysaccharides

Biosurfactants are a group of amphiphilic compounds, comprise a hydrophobic and a hydrophilic moiety and are produced by a range of microorganisms [9, 62]. *Pseudomonas* spp. are the most common producers of biosurfactants [63], with *P. aeruginosa* being the preeminent RL and EPS biosurfactant-producing species [9, 63]. Up to date, a variety of biosurfactants have been studied, but RLs (glycolipid biosurfactants) and EPSs (polymeric biosurfactants) are currently attracting the most attention, as they are relevant in medicine, environmental protection, food and the pharmaceutical industry [15, 24, 64–66].

3.1. *P. aeruginosa* rhamnolipids

Rhamnolipids comprise one or two L-rhamnose units and one or two units of 3-hydroxy fatty acid. Variations in lipid components contribute to the biodiversity of RLs [9, 67]. Due to their chemical composition, RLs are classified into four homologue groups (**Figure 1**): RL1—mono-rhamno-di-lipidic, RL2—mono-rhamno-mono-lipidic, RL3—di-rhamno-di-lipidic and RL4–di-rhamno-mono-lipidic structures. RL1 and RL3 are usually classified as principal—common RLs, while RL2 and RL4 are classed as atypical–uncommon RLs [68]. The development of sensitive, high throughput analytical techniques, such as soft ionization mass spectrometry, has led to the further discovery of a wide diversity of RL congeners and homologues (about 60) produced in different concentrations by various *Pseudomonas* spp. and other bacteria [9].

3.1.1. Diversity of rhamnolipid structures

RL biosurfactants are always produced as mixtures of different RL congeners, as observed with various *P. aeruginosa* isolates [15, 69–74]. The complexity of the RL mixtures produced depends on various factors such as bacterial isolate origin, type of carbon substrate, culture conditions and isolation procedure and age of the culture and of course, the *P. aeruginosa* isolate itself [15, 23, 63, 72, 75–80]. Despite the number of such factors reported, some particular RL congeners are predominant in all *P. aeruginosa* producer isolates. These are classified as the major RL structures (Rha-C_{10}-C_8, Rha-C_{10}-C_{10}, Rha-C_{10}-C_{12}, Rha-C_{10}-$C_{12:1}$, Rha-Rha-C_{10}-C_8, Rha-Rha-C_{10}-C_{10}, Rha-Rha-C_{10}-C_{12} and Rha-C_{10}-$C_{12:1}$) [23, 72, 81–84]. Other RLs, produced only sometimes or in low abundance, are the minor RL structures [23, 72, 81–84]. Both the major and the minor RL congeners contribute to the complete profile of RLs. In all studies of RL mixtures produced by various *P. aeruginosa* isolates, mono-rhamnolipid Rha–C_{10}–C_{10} and di-rhamnolipid Rha–Rha–C_{10}–C_{10} were the predominant congeners, in spite of the varying compositions produced [23, 72, 81–84].

The presence of different functional groups in RL molecules (the hydrophobic, lipid part and the hydrophilic and carbohydrate part) gives RLs important physicochemical properties. Due to their amphipathic structure, RLs behave as wetting agents, surface active compounds, emulsifiers and detergents. These RL functional groups are, therefore, utilized in enhancing and facilitating bacterial movement, adhesion and contact with surfaces, as well as substrate uptake, or solubilization.

3.1.2. Rhamnolipid biosynthesis and quorum sensing

Biosynthesis of RLs requires three rhamnosyltransferases. The fatty acid dimer moiety in RLs and free 3-(3-hydroxyalkanoyloxy) alkanoic acid (HAA) are both synthesized by the rhamnosyltransferase RhlA. Next, dTDP-L-rhamnose is transferred to HAA by the rhamnosyltransferase RhlB, or to a previously generated mono-RL by the rhamnosyltransferase RhlC [85]. HAA precursors are derived from the FASII cycle (bacterial fatty acid synthesis system), while activated L-rhamnose is derived from the glucose moiety of deoxythymidine

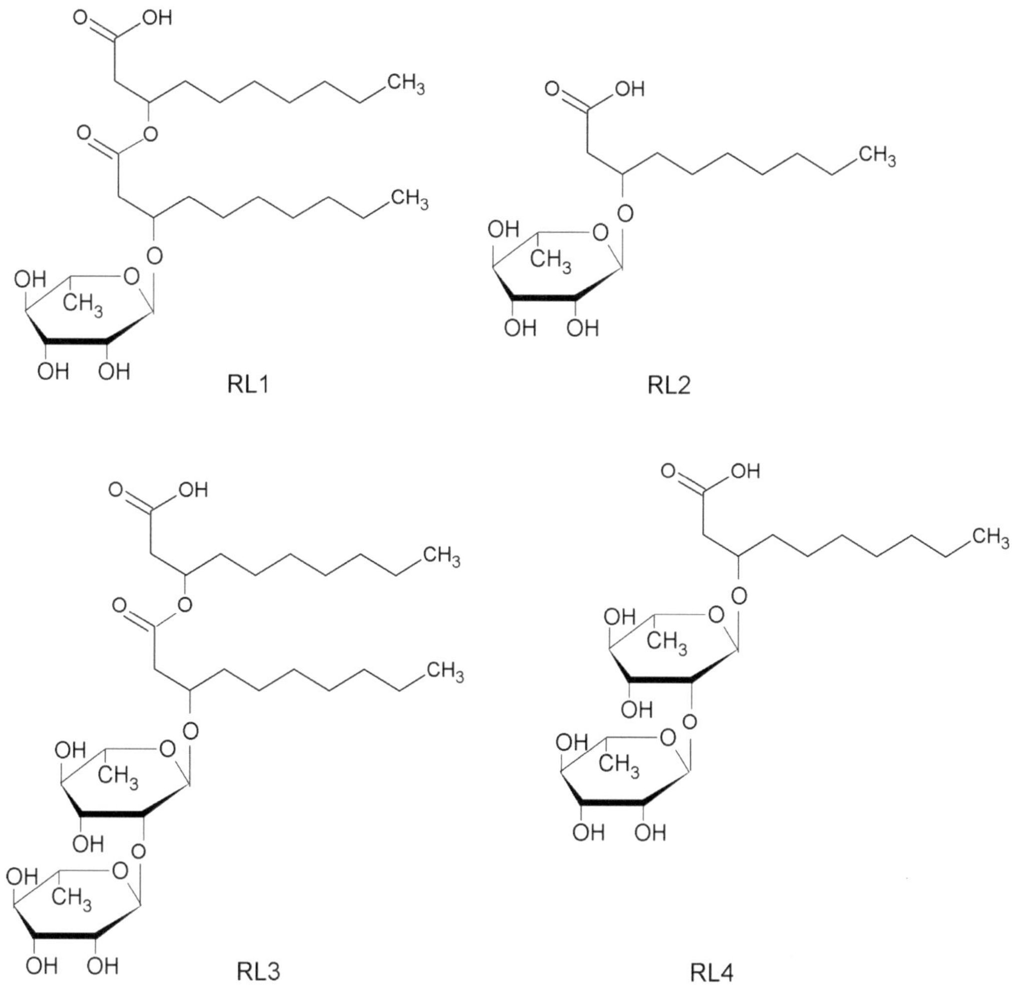

Figure 1. Structure of rhamnolipid congeners: RL1 (mono-rhamno-di-lipidic), RL2 (mono-rhamno-mono-lipidic), RL3 (di-rhamno-di-lipidic) and RL4 (di-rhamno-di-lipidic).

di-phospho (dTDP)-L-rhamnose through several reactions catalyzed by four enzymes that, in *P. aeruginosa,* belong to single operon, *rmlBDA* [11]. dTDP-L-rhamnose has an important role in the regulation of RL biosynthesis, as it is an allosteric regulator for RmlA (which catalyzes transfer of a thymidylmonophosphate nucleotide to glucose-1-phosphate and is a sensor enzyme in this metabolic pathway). Also, this molecule is a precursor for other L-rhamnose containing molecules (LPSs and EPSs). dTDP-L-rhamnose affects the production of mono-RL through coexpression of the operons *rmlBDAC* and *rhlAB,* which are responsible for expression of rhamnosyltransferases RhaA and RhaB [86, 87]. However, in *P. aeruginosa,* the QS system has an essential role in regulation of the *rhlAB* operon and, therefore, in RL biosynthesis.

In Section 2.2.1, we stated that *P. aeruginosa* QS has two interrelated systems, *las* and *rhl,* which are linked by the PQS molecule and that their relationship influences the biosynthesis of various metabolites. Production of RLs is governed by three *QS* molecules: *Pseudomonas* autoinducer 1 (PAI-1, also known as 3O-C_{12}-HSL), *Pseudomonas* autoinducer 2 (PAI-2, also known as C_4-HSL) and PQS. In *P. aeruginosa*, the *las* operon consists of two transcriptional activator proteins, LasR and LasI, which direct the synthesis of PAI-1. The production of RLs is regulated by the *rhl* system. The synthesis of RLs takes place under the coordinated guidance of the *rhlAB* genes. The *rhl* system consists of the transcriptional activator proteins, RhlR and RhlI, which regulate the synthesis of PAI-2. The transcriptional activator RhlR activates the transcription of *rhlAB* operon and gene *rhlC* (encoding RhlC) [10, 11].

The *rhlAB* operon is clustered on *P. aeruginosa* DNA together with *rhlR* and *rhlI*, which together direct the synthesis of all proteins required for RL production (the rhamnosyltransferases and the transcriptional activators, RhlR and RhlI) [10]. RL synthesis is upregulated and promoted at transcriptional level, related to the QS system, by the Vfr (global virulence regulation) and the *pqs* systems through activation of RhlR expression and *rhlRI* operon, respectively [11]. RasL (repressor of *las* system) and AlgR (biofilm formation) downregulate RL synthesis by repression of LasI and *rhlAB*/*rhlI*, respectively [11]. For instance, increasing bacterial cell density induces the *las* system, resulting in an increased concentration of PAI-1 that binds to the transcriptional activator site LasR and forms the LasR–PAI-1 complex. The LasR–PAI-1 complex induces genes controlled by the *rhl* system, including the regulator gene *rasL*, *rhlR* and *pqsH*, required for PQS production. PQS acts as a link between the *las* and *rhl* systems. The activity of these signals depends on their ability to dissolve in and freely diffuse through aqueous solution [10]. PQS induces the *rhlI* gene, which directs the production of PAI-2 that binds to and activates RhlR (RhlR–PAI-2 complex). The RhlR–PAI-2 complex induces genes for RL production, which are controlled by the *rhl QS* system (operons *rhlAB*, *rhlC*, *rhlI*, *rhlR* and *rhlG*). The RLs produced enhance the solubility of PQS in aqueous solutions and promote cell-to-cell communication. This is important because of the role PQS plays in the *P. aeruginosa* stress response, in conditions related to the CF lung environment (oxidative stress and antimicrobial agents) [88].

In conclusion, in the complex QS network, there is a hierarchy between *las* and *rhl* systems in RLs biosynthesis. Furthermore, RL biosynthesis is regulated at the transcriptional level according to nutritional and environmental conditions, as well as at the posttranscriptional level [11, 42]. However, most of the regulatory mechanisms are not completely understood [11, 42].

3.2. *P. aeruginosa* exopolysaccharides

Pseudomonads have the potential to produce various types of EPSs such as alginate, levan, marginalan and cellulose, as well as different heteropolysaccharides and protein polysaccharides complexes [89]. Nearly all *Pseudomonas* isolates, including *P. aeruginosa*, *Pseudomonas putida* and *Pseudomonas fluorescens* can produce alginate as the main acidic EPS [90–92]. Alginate is composed of β-1,4-D-mannuronic and L-guluronic acids linked via β-1,4-glycosidic bonds [93]. Alginates are also produced by *Azotobacter* isolates and some genera of brown and red algae. In comparison to algal alginates, bacterial alginates are O-acetylated at some of the C-2 and C-3 carbons of the mannuronic acid residues and acetylation occurs during transport through the periplasm. A high degree of O-acetylation increases the viscosity and flexibility of alginate, as well as its ability to bind water [94].

3.2.1. *Diversity of exopolysaccharide structures*

P. aeruginosa has the genetic ability to produce at least three polysaccharides: alginate, Psl (polysaccharide synthesis locus) and Pel (pellicle formation locus). Alginate and Psl have different chemical structures (**Figure 2a**) although they have similar biosynthetic mechanisms [89]. In comparison to alginate, a highly O-acetylated linear polymer of 1,4-linked mannuronic acid (M) and guluronic acid (G), Psl is a helicoid polysaccharide composed of a repeating pentamer containing D-mannose, L-rhamnose and D-glucose (**Figure 2b**). The structure of Pel is not completely characterized and it is supposed that it differs from alginate and Psl

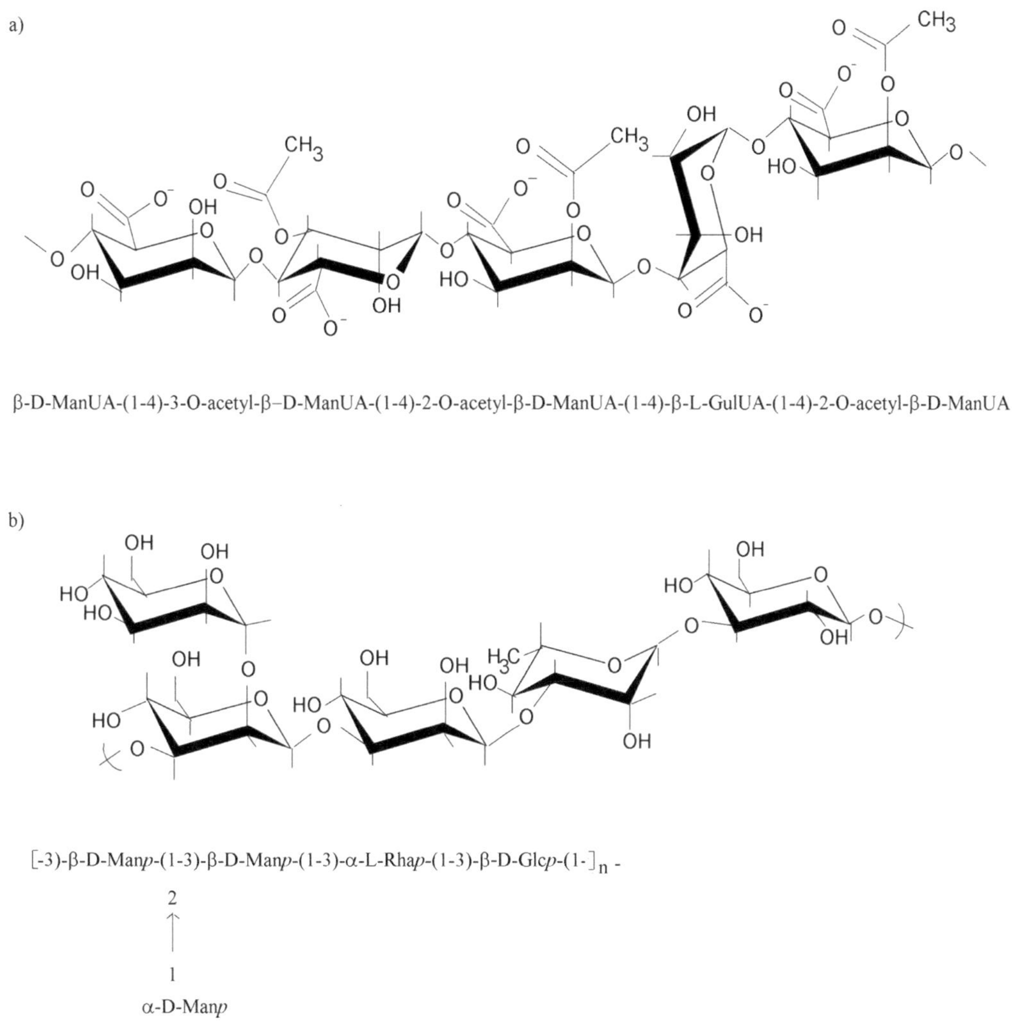

Figure 2. Structures of extracellular polysaccharides produced by *P. aeruginosa*: (a) alginate and (b) exopolysaccharide Psl.

[95]. Pel is proposed to be a glucose-rich polysaccharide, different to cellulose [96]. Each EPS has distinct physiological properties, affecting the cells and the biofilm matrix. While alginate is secreted into the surrounding medium without covalently linking to the cell surface, Psl has helical distribution around the cell surface with a key role in cell-to-cell and cell-to-surface interactions during biofilm formation. Pel forms a connecting matrix allowing it a structured assembly at the air-liquid interface connecting the cells. This matrix could also contain O-antigen-LPS and cyclic glucans [95]. The diversity of EPSs produced by bacterial biofilm subpopulations is one of the proposed *P. aeruginosa* survival strategies for adaptation to environmental changes, as related to the conditions in CF lungs.

3.2.2. Exopolysaccharide biosynthesis and quorum sensing

EPS biosynthesis requires sugar-nucleotide precursors and for alginate production, this is GDP-mannuronate. The enzymes required for GDP-mannuronate production include: (1) the bifunctional enzyme, AlgA which exhibits phosphomannose isomerase (PMI) and GDP-mannose pyrophosphorylase (GMP) activity; (2) AlgC, a phosphomannomutase; and (3) AlgD, which is a GDP mannose dehydrogenase [97–99]. AlgD catalyzes the first step in alginate biosynthesis, which is responsible for the mucoid phenotype often observed in clinical *P. aeruginosa* from chronically infected CF patients [13].

Alginate is first synthesized as a linear homopolymer of D-mannuronic acid residues. The polymer is then modified in the periplasm through selective O-acetylation by the concerted action of AlgI, AlgJ and AlgF and epimerized by AlgG [100, 101]. Alginate has a reasonably random structure (**Figure 2a**). This differentiates alginate from Psl and numerous *E. coli* capsule polysaccharides, the structures of which are more regular, with repeating subunits (**Figure 2b**). The randomness of alginate's structure occurs because during polymerization, AlgG converts D-mannuronic acid residues to L-guluronic acid and critically, either the C-2 and/or C-3 carbons can have acetylated hydroxyl functional groups, which become available for linking the residues.

AlgC appears to be crucial for general EPS biosynthesis, not just alginate, as it is also required for precursor synthesis of Psl, as well as LPSs and RLs [102, 103]. The LasR from the *las* system might, to some extent, regulate expression of *algC* and *algD*, confirming the correlation of QS systems with EPS production [13].

4. Physiological role of *P. aeruginosa* biosurfactants in CF infection

4.1. Physiological role of rhamnolipids and exopolysaccharides

Among proposed functions of RL biosurfactants, related to their physicochemical properties (surface activity, wetting ability, detergency and other amphipathic-related properties), are promotion of the uptake and biodegradation of poorly soluble substrates, immune modulators and virulence factors [9, 15]. Additionally, these molecules are involved in the process of swarming, as surface wetting agents and chemotaxis stimuli and in *P. aeruginosa* biofilm structuring, maturation (the formation of water channels in mature biofilms) and dispersion

[10]. Probably because they do not present the profile of typical or traditional virulence factors, RLs are sometimes not considered significant members of the virulence arsenal of *P. aeruginosa* [9]. However, published data strongly demonstrate their importance as virulence determinants and their significant role in infection establishment and persistence [8, 9].

Physicochemical properties of EPSs, such as surface activity, viscosity, flexibility of molecule, as well as its ability to bind water, protect the microbe from dehydration in the unique CF microenvironment following the switch from nonmucoid to mucoid phenotype [94]. In this regard, the *P. aeruginosa* mucoid phenotype is the most studied adaptation in patients with CF and it is directly proportional to overproduction of EPSs, which is widely considered to be a marker for the transition to chronic infection [8, 54]. Alginates are well studied as compounds associated with biofilm formation and invasion of pathogenic microorganisms. The alginate-containing matrix of mucoid *P. aeruginosa* is thought to allow the formation of protected microcolonies and provide increased resistance to opsonization, phagocytosis and destruction by antibiotics [104]. Alginates also have a protective role in *P. aeruginosa* infection because they scavenge free radicals released by activated macrophages *in vitro*, prevent phagocytic clearance and protect the microorganism from the host defense system [13].

4.2. Rhamnolipids and exopolysaccharides in *P. aeruginosa* biofilm formation

Swarming motility is the rapid and coordinated movement of a bacterial population across a surface, which often results in characteristic flowery, dendritic colony shapes on agar plates [105]. This type of colony movement is related to the production of an extracellular slime layer, mainly composed of EPSs and surface active compounds, which is a pivotal feature of swarming cells, acting as a wetting agent that reduces the surface tension [106]. Several studies suggest that *P. aeruginosa* expresses swarming motility and that it requires flagella and the production of wetting agents (RLs and its lipidic precursors HAAs) [85, 107–109]. Also, HAAs and di-RLs actually modulate the swarming process, as di-RLs and HAAs behave as self-produced chemotactic attractants with opposite activity, while mono-RLs seem to be act solely as wetting agents [107, 109]. Additionally, swarming motility is clearly related to biofilm formation [105].

The importance of swarming motility for biofilm formation indicates that RLs are involved in the process of biofilm formation. Indeed, it was shown that RLs enhance adhesion of planktonic cells in the early stages of biofilm development, when an initial microcolony is formed (**Figure 3**). Proposed mechanisms for RL effects on cell adhesion include regulation of cell-surface hydrophobicity and modification of adhesive interactions, especially when nutritional conditions are changed [85, 110–112]. Also, RLs are involved in later differentiation of the biofilm structure, the detachment and dispersion of *P. aeruginosa* cells, where RLs behave as mediators which disturb cell-to-cell and cell-to-substratum interactions and maintenance of open channels inside the biofilm [111, 113]. Furthermore, regulation of RL production by *P. aeruginosa* is regulated not only in temporal terms, but also in quantifiable terms, because overproduction of RLs disrupts biofilm structure or impedes biofilm formation [113].

EPSs also play an important role in biofilm formation and invasion of pathogenic microorganisms. During biofilm maturation, *P. aeruginosa* begin to excrete EPSs, such that the bacteria in the mature biofilm are encased in a matrix of EPSs that they have produced [114]. Overproduction of alginate is the main indicator of *P. aeruginosa* converting to the mucoid phenotype and is responsible for the notable microbial resistance to antibiotics as well as defense from the host immune system of CF patients (**Figure 3**). The mucoid phenotype of *P. aeruginosa* produces a great amount of alginate as a result of several genes, including *algD,* which encodes GDP-mannose dehydrogenase, responsible for synthesis of alginate precursor [8, 94]. The alginate-containing matrix of the mucoid phenotype allows the formation of protected microcolonies and provides increased resistance to opsonization, phagocytosis and antibiotics, resulting in persistent infection and a worsening prognosis for CF patients [104].

In the context of immune system pathways, polymorphonuclear leukocytes (PMNs) are considered as the central line of defense in innate immunity and they are produced as a predominant response to infection, especially in CF lungs [115]. When PMNs phagocytose bacteria, the host cells produce highly reactive oxygen species, which kill *P. aeruginosa* or induce mutations in the microbial *mucA* gene. However, the alginate produced by mucoid phenotype *P. aeruginosa* is also an oxygen radical scavenger, helping to protect this pathogen against host inflammatory defense mechanisms [116]. Airway epithelial cells play a crucial role during establishment of respiratory infection because *P. aeruginosa* attaches to and enters respiratory epithelia, producing an immune response in the lung by activating lymphocytes at the site of infection [117].

Surfactant protein A (SP-A) is involved in prevention of alginate-induced *P. aeruginosa* invasion of lung epithelial cells. SP-A plays a part in the innate immunity in the lung, with a

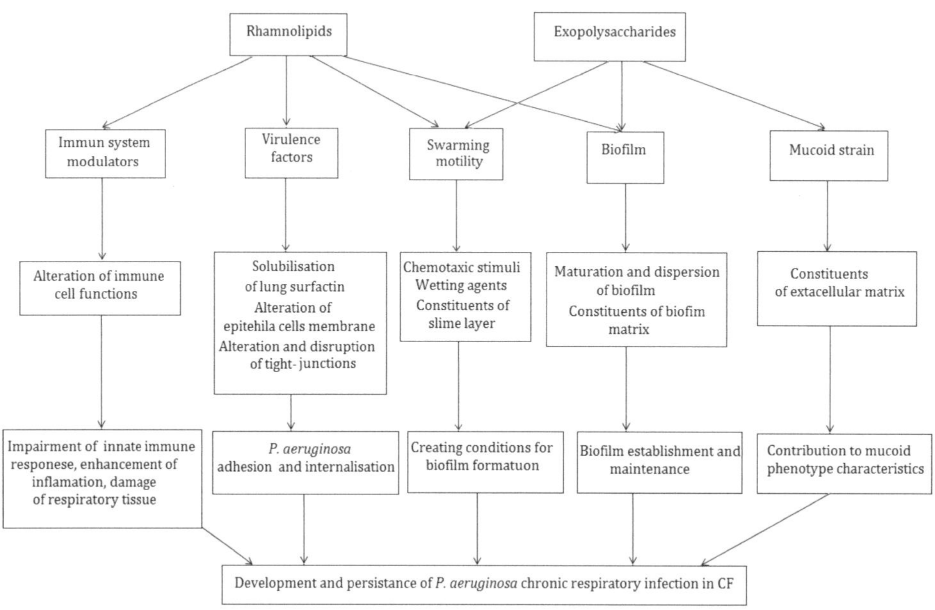

Figure 3. Proposed roles, relations and effects of *P. aeruginosa* biosurfactants RLs and EXPs in development and persistence of chronic respiratory infection in CF patients.

direct role in bacteria opsonization and killing, as well as impairment of bacterial membrane permeabilization [117]. Alginate is surface exposed and levels of SP-A could be crucial in modulating the interaction of *P. aeruginosa* with the epithelial barrier.

4.3. Effect of *P. aeruginosa* rhamnolipids and exopolysaccharides

Respiratory mucosa protects host airways from microbial infection. *P. aeruginosa* and other microbial species capable of causing lung infections have developed mechanisms to overcome this barrier, such as alteration of the apical membrane of epithelial cells or alteration and disruption of tight junctions (TJ) [118]. Proposed mechanisms involve alterations of respiratory epithelial ion transport, inhibition of transcellular ion transport and interference with the normal tracheal ciliary function. Bacterial adherence to the basolateral domain of epithelial cells and internalization are suggested as a potential mechanism of *P. aeruginosa* pathogenicity (**Figure 3**). The physiological pathways of these processes are not still completely clarified, but reports indicate involvement of virulence factors, production of which is controlled by the type III secretion (cytotoxic proteins) and the *las* and *rhl* QS (RLs, elastase) systems [119, 120].

RLs concentration of up to 8 μg/ml was found in the sputum of CF patients infected by *P. aeruginosa* [120], while secretions from a lung removed contained 65 μg/ml RLs [121]. These concentrations of RLs are likely adequate for promotion of *P. aeruginosa* epithelial cell infiltration. Furthermore, this indicates link between elevated levels of RLs and worsening of patient clinical status.

RLs produce damage to the bronchial epithelium and inhibit ciliary function [122–124]. Damage to the bronchial epithelia is related to impairment of the protective layer of lung surfactant in CF patients. Phospholipase C and RLs produced by *P. aeruginosa* can act synergistically to break down lipids and lecithin from lung surfactant [12]. It is believed that RLs, due to their detergency, solubilize the phospholipids in lung surfactant, making them more accessible to cleavage by phospholipase C [12].

The effects of *P. aeruginosa* RLs on the respiratory epithelia function were studied in several animal models [122]. RLs caused ciliostasis and cell membrane damage to rabbit tissue were a secretagogue in cats and inhibited epithelial ion transport in sheep tissue. Additionally, the authors investigated the effect of RLs on mucociliary transport in the anesthetized guinea pig and guinea pig and human respiratory epithelia *in vitro* [122]. Reduction of tracheal mucus velocity (TMV) *in vivo* occurred depending on the applied RL concentration (10 μg of RLs caused cessation of TMV without recovery; 5 μg of RLs reduced TMV by 22.6% over a period of 2 h and 2.5 μg of RLs caused no overall change in TMV). RLs (10 μg) did not disrupt the ultrastructure of guinea pig tracheal epithelium. RL (250 μg/ml) stopped ciliary beating of guinea pig tracheal. Treatment with RL concentration of 100 μg/ml caused immediate slowing of the cilliar beat frequency (CBF) of human nasal brushings, as well as CBF of human nasal turbinate organ culture. Mono- and di-RL had equivalent effects [122]. In addition, RLs stimulate the release of mucus glycoconjugates from feline trachea or human bronchial mucosa [125, 126].

In vitro reconstructed respiratory epithelium was exposed to several *P. aeruginosa* isolates with alterations in genotype: wild type, CF isolates and strains with altered QS system expression

[118]. The authors found that only RL-producing *P. aeruginosa* (those that expressed the *rhl* QS system) was able to infiltrate the epithelia by modulating the permeability of the tissue. The early stages of infection did not correlate with type III secretion and elastase activity [118], in contrast to previous reports [127, 128]. The effect of exogenously applied purified RLs on the epithelial barrier was also studied [118]. The authors used JBR 515, which is commercial mixture of 50% w/v Rha-C_{10}-C_{10} and 50% w/m Rha-Rha-C_{10}-C_{10}. RLs produced by bacteria *in situ* or purified. The applied RLs caused loss of epithelial cell polarity by: incorporation in first, the apical and later, the basolateral epithelial membranes (due to chemical structure); cilia loss; ezrin displacement; and alterations of TJ. The final result was a decrease of transepithelial resistance and higher permeability of respiratory epithelia, without affecting cell viability [118]. After disruption of TJ, paracellular invasion by some *P. aeruginosa*, involving RL deficient strains, was observed, but they were not internalized [118]. This was in contrast to previous reports [129, 130], perhaps due to the *in vitro* conditions used in the studies as difference. Altogether, the importance of RL biosurfactant and the QS system in *P. aeruginosa* invasion of respiratory epithelium is acknowledged, but the exact mechanisms of cell polarity and structure alterations remain unclear.

The effect of RLs on immune system pathways with direct impairment and modulation of immune cell activity is well known [9] (**Figure 3**). RLs are reported to have hemolytic activity on various erythrocyte species; induce direct neutrophil chemotactic activity [130]; enhance the oxidative burst response of monocytes; stimulate and release inflammatory mediators from mast cells and platelets; induce lysis of PMNs; stimulate both chemotaxis and chemokinesis of PMNs (depending on concentration); and enhance production of several interleukins produced by granulocyte-macrophage and nasal epithelial cells (at noncytoxic levels) [131–135]. Furthermore, RLs, especially di-RLs, are cytolytic for human monocyte-derived macrophages and at lower concentrations, they inhibit the phagocytic response of macrophages [136].

The response of *P. aeruginosa* mutants (PAO1 and QS, *rhlA* and *pqsA* deficient) to the presence of PMNs was studied [115]. Previously reported data showed that *in vitro*, PMNs performed their immune function and eliminated QS-deficient *P. aeruginosa* biofilms, although they were incapable of eliminating QS-proficient biofilms [51]. Additionally, purified RLs induced necrosis in PMNs [134]. In biofilm, *P. aeruginosa* (PAO1 wild type) produced increased levels of various virulence factors in response to PMNs, while *P. aeruginosa rhlA* mutant was eliminated by PMNs [115]. Additionally, 2000-fold higher levels of RLs from *P. aeruginosa* PAO1 occurred in biofilm than in surrounding fluid, indicating that RL molecules were grouped around biofilm [115]. Similarly, a *P. aeruginosa rhlA* mutant was cleared more quickly than the wild strain from two *in vivo* mouse models of lung infection [137]. Also, microscopic analysis showed that there were no intact PMNs in close contact with outer layers of biofilm. This correlated with microscopic investigations of *P. aeruginosa* infected *ex vivo* tissues samples from CF lungs, where PMNs were located peripherally [115]. The RLs isolated in this study were a mixture of mono- and di-RL congeners (Rha-C_{10}-C_{10}, Rha-C_{10}-C_{12}, Rha-C_{10}-$C_{12\Delta}$ and respective di-RL derivates) [137]. Van et al. [137] proposed that RLs have a role as a protective mechanism in biofilm resistance to phagocytosis and supported a "launch a shield" model, where

RLs surround the biofilm and on contact destroy PMNs. This study [137], in correlation with previous reports about QS regulation of bacterial response to PMNs [50, 134] showed that *P. aeruginosa pqsA* mutant was unable to respond to exposure to PMNs by increasing RL production and that there was impairment of the QS hierarchy. These studies show that RLs probably contribute to the inflammatory-related tissue damage observed in lungs of CF patients, which involves complex and tight regulation by the QS system. RL production, though, is not continued because it affects all host cells, not only immune cells and high levels of RL may create conditions (due to inflammation and host tissue damage) which are not favorable for *P. aeruginosa* persistence [137]. This study supports a model by which cross-kingdom-based communication contributes significantly to immunomodulation and evasion and which is one reason studying the infective properties of *P. aeruginosa* is so fascinating.

Modification of membrane LPSs in *P. aeruginosa* is also an important mechanism in the development of chronic infection in CF patients [138–140]. Membrane LPSs in *P. aeruginosa* are composed of three parts: highly acylated lipid A; a central core oligosaccharide bound to lipid A and O-antigen; and a variable polysaccharide composed of repeated units located out from the core [138, 140]. It is not surprising that the structure of LPSs is modified in *P. aeruginosa* isolated from CF patients because of their direct interface position with the pulmonary environment [8]. Compared to normal lipid A, that from CF patients contains more hexa- and hepta-acylated moieties as well as added aminoarabinose, a cationic amino sugar residue which is responsible for resistance to antimicrobials [140]. Acylation levels of lipid A are responsible for LPS recognition by the host and induction of the proinflammatory response, so their modification causes *P. aeruginosa* to be less visible to the host immune system [141]. Also, in CF isolates, O-antigen is lost, due to mutations in genes responsible for O-antigen production. This loss can facilitate chronic persistence in respiratory tracts of CF patients [138–140]. Modification of LPS can directly correlate with overproduction of alginate, which is typical for the mucoid phenotype. Alginate might interact via the carboxylic groups in polyguluronic acid units with modified membrane LPSs in *P. aeruginosa,* across cationic amino sugar aminoarabinose residues. This likely enhances polymerization and facilitates release of EPSs from the membrane. Thus, study of factors that influence increased production of EPSs and RLs, as well as the structure-function relationships of these compounds would likely be of great importance for improved therapy of CF patients [8].

Figure 3 summarizes the proposed roles, relationships and effects of the biosurfactant RLs and EPSs produced by *P. aeruginosa* in the development of chronic respiratory CF infection.

5. Rhamnolipids and exopolysaccharides as targets—current and future perspectives

The importance of biofilm formation and maintenance for the establishment and persistence of *P. aeruginosa* chronic respiratory infection in CF has been discussed in Section 2.2.1. The complex regulation of biofilm development includes the QS network, swarming motility and production of extracellular metabolites and involves significant roles for RLs and EPSs.

Agents	Type	Strategy	Resistance	References
Ticarcillin, Piperacillin Cefrazidime, Cefepime Imipenem, Meropenem Aztreonam	β-Lactams	Impairment of biofilm structure and *QS* inhibitors	Antibiotic cleavage by β-lactamase enzymes, antibiotic expulsion by encoded efflux mechanisms and reduced drug uptake due to loss of outer membrane porin proteins	[16, 155]
Ciprofloxacin	Fluoroquinolones	*QS* inhibitors	Mutations by DNA gyrase and topoisomerase IV enzymes and efflux systems	[155, 156]
Tobramycin, Gentamicin, Amikacin	Aminoglycosides	Impairment of biofilm structure	Aminoglycoside-modifying enzymes AMEs and rRNA methylases as well as efflux mechanisms	[16, 155, 157]
Patulin, penicillin acid, cis-2 decanoic acid	Bacterial metabolites	Impairment of biofilm structure and *QS* inhibitors	No resistance	[16, 158]
Solenopisin A	Fire ant venom	Impairment of biofilm structure and *QS* inhibitors	No resistance	[16, 154]
Salicylic acid and 4-nitro-pyridine oxide (4-NPO)	Synthetic compounds	Impairment of biofilm structure and *QS* inhibitors	No resistance	[16, 152, 154]
Garlic extract	Natural mixture	Impairment of biofilm structure and *QS* inhibitors	No resistance	[16, 152, 159]
Halogenated furanones from algae *D. pulchra*, Furanone C-30	Synthetic or modifies natural derived furanones	*QS*-inhibitor and *P. aeruginosa* elimination in combination with antibiotics	No resistance	[16, 160]

Table 2. Antibiofilm approaches in therapy of P. *auruginosa* infection of CF patients.

Therefore, a logical approach in preventing and treating chronic *P. aeruginosa* infection in CF patients is focused on antibiofilm strategies. Antibiofilm strategies can take two differing approaches, one common, related to antibiotic therapy and the other novel, related to interruption of QS (**Table 2**). Furthermore, vaccination is proposed as a modern approach to prevent *P. aeruginosa* infection in CF, where virulence factors, such as alginate, have been used as the antigen. However, most vaccines are still in the clinical research phase and have not reached the market [142].

Traditional antibiotic therapy is related to the early colonization period, the only possible phase when *P. aeruginosa* can be eradicated from CF airways [143, 144]. The effectiveness of antibiotics later is significantly reduced due to microbe adaptation mechanisms (membrane changes, efflux system changes, production of various virulence factors and EPS-containing extracellular matrix, mutation and modification of enzymes) [16] (**Table 2**). Furthermore, tobramycin (an aminoglycoside) is the most common antibiotic for *P. aeruginosa* therapy choice in CF lungs [145]. This is in spite of the fact that alginates produced by the microbe decrease, the movement of aminoglycosides, cationic antimicrobial peptides and quaternary ammonium compounds through *P. aeruginosa* biofilms [27, 146] (**Table 2**). To overcome obstacles related to antibiotic resistance and increase the antimicrobial effects, an inhaled version of tobramycin, as well as liposomal-encased current antibiotics are available. These antibiotic formulations have improved delivery times and provide higher drug concentrations at the site of infection. Additionally, the importance of biofilm formation as having a crucial role in the antibiotic resistance of *P. aeruginosa* (as well as other CF pathogens) is now being recognized. Recent research trends include analysis of biofilm formation in terms of *P. aeruginosa* antibiotic resistance/susceptibility and the potential for antibiotics as efficient therapy agents for biofilm impairment [147–150].

A more novel antibiofilm strategy, QS interruption, is a promising approach for treating CF respiratory infections. In this strategy, the QS system is targeted, due to its regulation of the biosynthesis of RLs and EPSs [151–153]. The QS impairment approach involves identification of molecules which can interrupt QS pathways. Generally, these compounds have one of following mechanisms of activity: blocking production of QS signal molecules, degradation of QS signal molecules or prevention of microbe recognition and response to QS stimuli [16]. Various natural compounds inhibited QS or directly impaired biofilm (**Table 2**) (e.g., garlic extract, metabolites from *Penicillium* spp., salicylic acid, the *P. aeruginosa* metabolite *cis*-2-decanoic acid). Furanones are QS blockers and the furanone produced by *Delisea pulchra and* synthetic furanones, enhanced *P. aeruginosa* elimination in combination with antibiotic therapy [16]. Furanone C-30 repressed 77% of *P. aeruginosa* genes induced by exposure to PMNs [50]. The great advantage of using QS inhibitors in CF therapy is that they are not expected to induce bacterial resistance, because their activity is not closely related to bacterial growth [154].

In the context of the physiological roles of RLs and EPSs discussed in Section 4, these compounds are also promising targets for future strategies in CF therapy related to specific modulation of respiratory mucus [118].

6. Conclusion

RLs and EPSs, biosurfactant molecules, play significant roles in bacterial acquisition, biofilm development and establishment of chronic *P. aeruginosa* infections in CF patients. Specifically, RLs and EPSs are, due to their amphipathic structures and physicochemical properties, involved in processes of respiratory mucus alteration, modulation of immune system defense pathways, biofilm development and maintenance and the *P. aeruginosa* mucoid phenotype. These compounds are responsible for antibiotic resistance and survival and general persistence of *P. aeruginosa* in the specific, dynamic environmental conditions in CF patients' lungs. Consequently, RLs and EPSs are the direct or indirect cause of bad outcomes and high mortality rates among these patients. Currently, therapy generally based on application of antibiotics fails to prevent and treat chronic *P. aeruginosa* infection. Therefore, RLs and EPSs are interesting novel targets for dealing with respiratory infection in CF patients. In addition, the

P. aeruginosa QS system is an important aspect of CF lung infection, as it regulates synthesis of the biosurfactants and other virulence factors, as well as biofilm formation. Future perspectives to prevent and treat *P. aeruginosa* respiratory infections in CF certainly should involve impairment of QS pathways. Finally, further study of potential approaches to modify host respiratory mucus epithelial membranes is required.

Acknowledgment

This work was supported by projects III43004 and III46010, granted by the Ministry of Education, Science and Technological Development of the Republic of Serbia.

Author details

Milena G. Rikalovic[1,*], Natasa S. Avramovic[2] and Ivanka M. Karadzic[2]

*Address all correspondence to: mrikalovic@gmail.com

1 Sport Academy Belgrade College of Higher Vocational Studies, Belgrade, Serbia

2 University School of Medicine, University of Belgrade, Belgrade, Serbia

References

[1] Høiby N: Mini review recent advances in the treatment of *Pseudomonas aeruginosa* infections in cystic fibrosis. BMC Medicine. 2011;**9**:32. DOI: 10.1186/1741-7015-9-32

[2] Jansen HK, Høiby N: Seasonal onset of initial colonisation and chronic infection with *Pseudomonas aeruginosa* in patients with cystic fibrosisi in Denmark. Thorax. 1992;**47**:109-111. DOI: 10.1136/thx.47.2.109

[3] Hansen CR, Pressler T, Høiby N: Early aggressive eradication therapy for intermittent *Pseudomonas aeruginosa* airway colonization in cystic fibrosis patients: 15 years experience. J. Cyst. Fibros. 2008;**7**:523-530. DOI: 10.1016/**j**.jcf.2008.06.009

[4] Bjarnsholt T, Jensen PØ, Fiandaca MJ, Pedersen J, Hansen CR, Andersen CB, Pressler T, Givskov M, Høiby N: *Pseudomonas aeruginosa* biofilms in the respiratory tract of cystic fibrosis patients. Pediatr. Pulmonol. 2009;**44**:547-558. DOI: 10.1002/ppul.21011

[5] Hoffmann N, Rasmussen TB, Jensen PØ, Stub C, Hentzer M, Molin S, Ciofu O, Givskov M, Johansen HK, Høiby N: Novel mouse model of chronic *Pseudomonas aeruginosa* lung infection mimicking cystic fibrosis. Infect. Immun. 2005;**73**:2504-2514. DOI: 10.1128/IAI.73.4.2504-2514.2005

[6] Høiby N, Ciofu O, Bjarnsholt T: *Pseudomonas aeruginosa* biofilms in cystic fibrosis. Future Microbiol. 2010;**5**:1663-1674. DOI: 10.2217/fmb.10.125

[7] Jelsbak L, Johansen HK, Frost AL, Thøgersen R, Thomsen LE, Ciofu O, Yang L, Haagensen JA, Høiby N, Molin S: Molecular epidemiology and dynamics of *Pseudomonas aeruginosa* populations in lungs of cystic fibrosis patients. Infect. Immun. 2007;**75**:2214-2224. DOI:10.1128/IAI.01282-06

[8] Hauser AR, Jain M, Bar-Meir M, McColley SA: Clinical significance of microbial infection and adaptation in cystic fibrosis. Clin. Microbiol. Rev. 2011;**24**:29-70. DOI: 10.1128/CMR.00036-10

[9] Abdel-Mawgoud AM, Lépine F, Déziel E: Rhamnolipids: diversity of structures, microbial origins and roles. Appl. Microbiol. Biotechnol. 2010;**86**:1323-1336. DOI: 10.1007/s00253-010-2498-2

[10] Dusane DH, Zinjarde, SS, Smita S, Venugopalan, VP, Mclean, RJC, Weber MM, Rahman PKSM, Quorum sensing: implications on rhamnolipid biosurfactant production. Biotechnol. Genet. Eng. Rev, 2010; **27**:159-184. http://hdl.handle.net/10149/113428

[11] Reis RS, Pereira AG, Neves BC, Freire DMG: Gene regulation of rhamnolipid production in *Pseudomonas aeruginosa*—A review. Bioresor. Technol. 2011;**102**:6377-6384. DOI:10.1016/j.biortech.2011.03.074

[12] Van Delden C, Iglewski BH: Cell-to-cell signaling and *Pseudomonas aeruginosa* infections. Emerg. Infect. Dis. 1998;**4**:551-560. DOI: 10.3201/eid0404.980405

[13] Wagner VE, Iglewski BH: *P. aeruginosa* biofilms in infestion. Clin. Rev. Allerg. Immunol. 2008.**35**:124-134. DOI 10.1007/s12016-008-8079-9

[14] Grbavčić S, Bezbradica D, Izrael-Živković L, Avramović N, Milosavić N, Karadžić I, Jugović-Knežević Z: Production of lipase and protease from an indigenous *Pseudomonas aeruginosa* strain and their evaluation as detergent additives: Compatibility study with detergent ingredients and washing performance. Bioresour. Technol. 2011;**102**:11226-11233. DOI:10.1016/j.biortech.2011.09.076

[15] Rikalovic M, Vrvic M, Karadzic I. Bioremediation by rhamnolipids produced by environmetal isolates of *Pseudomonas aeruginosa*. In: Velázquez-Fernández JB, Muñiz-Hernándes S, editors. Bioremediation: Processes, Challenges and Future Prospects. Nova Science Publishers, USA; 2014. pp. 299-332, ISBN: 978-1-62948-513-3

[16] Anderson GG. Pseudomonas aeruginosa biofilm formation in the CF lung and its implications for therapy. In: Sriramulu D, editor. The Cystic Fibrosis—Renewed Hopes Through Research, InTech, Croatia; 2012. pp. 154-180, DOI: 10.5772/30529

[17] Avramović NS, Nikolić-Mandić SD, Karadžić IM: Influence of rhamnolipids, produced by *Pseudomonas aeruginosa* NCAIM (P) B001380 on their Cr (VI) removal capacity in liquid medium. J. Serb. Chem. Soc. 2013;**78**:639-651. DOI: 10.2298/JSC120831115A

[18] Dimitrijevic AS, Velickovic DV, Rikalovic MG, Avramovic NS, Milosavic NB, Jankov RM, Karadzic IM: Simultaneous production of exopolysaccharide and lipase from extremophylic *Pseudomonas aeruginosa san-ai* strain: A novel approach for lipase

immobilization and purification. Carbohydr. Polym. 2011;**83**:1397-1401. DOI:10.1016/j.carbpol.2010.10.005

[19] Izrael-Zivkovic L, Gojgic-Cvijovic G, Gopcevic K, Vrvic M, Karadzic I: Enzymatic characterization of 30 kDa lipase from *Pseudomonas aeruginosa* ATCC 27853. J. Basic. Microbiol. 2009;**49**:452-462. DOI: 10.1002/jobm.200800229

[20] Jakovetić SM, Knezević-Jugović ZD, Grbavčić SŽ, Bezbradica DI, Avramović NS, Karadžić IM: Rhamnolipid and lipase production by *Pseudomonas aeruginosa san-ai*: The process comparison analysis by statistical approach. Chem. Ind. 2013;**67**:677-685. DOI: 10.2298/HEMIND121008114J

[21] Karadzic I, Masui A, Izrael-Zivkovic L, Fujiwara N: Purification and characterization of an alkaline lipase from *Pseudomonas aeruginosa* isolated from putrid mineral cutting oil as metal working fluid. J. Biosc. Bioeng. 2006;**102**:82-89. DOI: 10.1263/jbb.102.82

[22] Karadzic I, Masui A, Fujiwara N: Purification and characterization of a protease from *Pseudomonas aeruginosa* grown in cutting oil. J. Biosci. Bioeng. 2004;**98**:145-152. DOI: 10.1263/jbb.98.145

[23] Rikalovic MG, Abdel-Mawgoud AM, Déziel E, Gojgic-Cvijovic G Dj, Nestorovic Z, Vrvic MM, Karadzic IM: Comparative analysis of rhamnolipids from novel environmental isolates of *Pseudomonas aeruginosa*. J. Surfact.. Deterg. 2013;**16**:673-682. DOI: 10.1007/s11743-013-1462-4 DOI:10.1007/s11743-013-1462-4

[24] Rikalovic MG, Vrvic MM, Karadžić IM: Rhamnolipid biosurfactant from *Pseudomonas aeruginosa*—From discovery to application in contemporary technology. J. Serb. Chem. Soc. 2015;**80**:279-304. DOI: 10.2298/JSC140627096R

[25] Davies JC: *Pseudomonas aeruginosa* in cystic fibrosis: Pathogenesis and persistence. Paediatr. Respir. Rev. 2002;**3**:128-134. DOI: http://dx.doi.org/10.1016/S1526-0550(02)00003-3

[26] Doring G, Gulbins E: Cystic fibrosis and innate immunity: How chloride channel mutations provoke lung disease. Cell. Microbiol. 2009;**11**:208-216. DOI: 10.1111/j.1462-5822.2008.01271.x

[27] Gibson RL, Burns JL, Ramsey BW: Pathophysiology and management of pulmonary infections in cystic fibrosis. Am. J. Respir. Crit. Care. Med. 2003;**168**:918-951. DOI: 10.1164/rccm.200304-505SO

[28] Kelley TJ, Drumm ML: Inducible nitric oxide synthase expression is reduced in cystic fibrosis murine and human airway epithelial cells. J. Clin. Invest. 1998;102:1200-1207. DOI: 10.1172/JCI2357 DOI:10.1172%2FJCI2357#pmc_ext

[29] Konstan MW: Therapies aimed at airway inflammation in cystic fibrosis. Clin. Chest. Med. 1998;**19**:505-513. DOI: 10.1016/S0272-5231(05)70096-4

[30] Lyczak JB, Cannon CL, Pier GB: Lung infections associated with cystic fibrosis. Clin. Microbiol. Rev. 2002;**15**:194-222. DOI: 10.1128/CMR.15.2.194-222.2002

[31] Machen TE: Innate immune response in CF airway epithelia: Hyperinflammatory? Am. J. Physiol. Cell. Physiol. 2006;**291**:C218-C230. DOI: 10.1152/ajpcell.00605.2005

[32] Matsui H, Grubb BR, Taran R, Randell SH, Gatzy JT, Davis CW, Boucher RC: Evidence for pericilliary liquid layer depletion, not abnormal ion composition, in the pathogenesis of cystic fibrosis airways disease. Cell. 1998;**95**:1005-1015. DOI: http://dx.doi.org/10.1016/S0092-8674(00)81724-9

[33] Rajan S, Saiman L: Pulmonary infections in patients with cystic fibrosis. Semin. Respir. Infect. 2002;**17**:47-56. DOI: 10.1053/srin.2002.31690

[34] Saiman L, Prince A: *Pseudomonas aeruginosa* pili bind to asialoGM1 which is increased on the surface of cystic fibrosis epithelial cells. J. Clin. Invest. 1993;**92**:1875-1880. DOI: 10.1172/JCI116779 DOI:10.1172%2FJCI116779#pmc_ext

[35] Smith JJ, Travis SM, Greenberg EP, Welsh MJ: Cystic fibrosis airway epithelia fail to kill bacteria because of abnormal airway surface fluid. Cell. 1996;**85**:229-236. DOI: http://dx.doi.org/10.1016/S0092-8674(00)81099-5 DOI:10.1016/S0092-8674(00)81099-5#doilink

[36] Starner TD, McCray Jr PB: Pathogenesis of early lung disease in cystic fibrosis: A window of opportunity to eradicate bacteria. Ann. Intern. Med. 2005;**143**:816-822. http://www.the-aps.org/mm/publications/journals/pim/starner-pdf.pdf

[37] Adams C, Morris-Quinn M, McConnell F, West J, Lucey B, Shortt C, Cryan B, Watson JBG, O'Gara F: Epidemiology and clinical impact of *P. aeruginosa* infection in cystic fibrosis using AP-PCR fingerprinting. J. Infect. 1998;**37**:151-158. DOI: doi:10.1016/S0163-4453(98)80170-9

[38] Burns JL, Gibson RL, McNamara S, Yim D, Emerson J, Rosenfeld M, Hiatt P, McCoy K, Castile R, Smith AL, Ramsey BW: Longitudinal assessment of *Pseudomonas aeruginosa* in young children with cystic fibrosis. J. Infect. Dis. 2001;**183**:444-452. DOI: 10.1086/318075

[39] Speert DP, Campbell ME, Henry DA, Milner R, Taha F, Gravelle A, Davidson AG, Wong LT, Mahenthiralingam E: Epidemiology of *Pseudomonas aeruginosa* in cystic fibrosis in British Columbia, Canada. Am. J. Respir. Crit. Care. Med. 2002;**166**:988-993. DOI: 10.1164/rccm.2203011

[40] Winstanley C, Fothergill JL: The role of quorum sensing in chronic cystic fibrosis *Pseudomonas aeruginosa* infections. FEMS Microbiol. Lett. 2009:**290**:1-9. DOI:10.1111/j.1574-6968.2008.01394.x

[41] Williams P, Winzer K, Chan WC, Camara M: Look who's talking: Communication and quorum sensing in the bacterial world. Philos. Trans. R. Soc. Lond. B Biol. Sci. 2007;**362**:1119-1134. DOI:10.1098/rstb.2007.2039 DOI:10.1098%2Frstb.2007.2039#pmc_ext

[42] Lee J, Zhang L: The hierarchy quorum sensing network in *Pseudomonas aeruginosa*. Protein Cell. 2015;**6**:26-41. DOI: 10.1007/s13238-014-0100-x

[43] Hall-Stoodley L, Costerton JW, Stoodley P: Bacterial biofilms: from the natural environment to infectious diseases. Nat. Rev. Microbiol. 2004;**2**:95-108. DOI:10.1038/nrmicro821

[44] Parsek MR, Greenberg EP: Sociomicrobiology: The connections between quorum sensing and biofilms. Trends. Microbiol. 2005;**13**:27-33. DOI:10.1016/j.tim.2004.11.007

[45] Costerton JW: Anaerobic biofilm infections in cystic fibrosis. Mol. Cell. 2002;**10**: 699-700. DOI: http://dx.doi.org/10.1016/S1097-2765(02)00698-6 DOI:10.1016/S1097-2765(02)00698-6#doilink

[46] Sauer K, Camper AK, Ehrlich GD, Costerton JW, Davies DG: *Pseudomonas aeruginosa* displays multiple phenotypes during development as a biofilm. J. Bacteriol. 2002;**184**:1140-1154. DOI: 10.1128/jb.184.4.1140-1154.2002 DOI:10.1128%2Fjb.184.4.1140-1154.2002#pmc_ext

[47] Hentzer M, Eberl L, Givskov M:Transcriptome analysis of *Pseudomonas aeruginosa* biofilm development: Anaerobic respiration and iron limitation. Biofilms. 2005;**2**:37-61. DOI: http://dx.doi.org/10.1017/S1479050505001699

[48] Xu KD, Stewart PS, Xia F, Huang CT, McFeters GA: Spatial physiological heterogeneity in *Pseudomonas aeruginosa* biofilm is determined by oxygen availability. Appl. Environ. Microbiol. 1998;**64**:4035-4039. DOI: 0099-2240/98/$04.0010

[49] Davies DG, Parsek MR, Pearson JP, Iglewski BH, Costerton JW, Greenberg EP: The involvement of cell-to-cell signals in the development of a bacterial biofilm. Science. 1998;**280**:295-298. DOI: 10.1126/science.280.5361.295

[50] Hentzer M, Wu H, Andersen JB, Riedel K, Rasmussen TB, Bagge N, Kumar N, Schembri MA, Song Z, Kristoffersen P, Manefield M, Costerton JW, Molin S,Eberl L, Steinberg P, Kjelleberg S, Høiby N, Givskov M: Attenuation of *Pseudomonas aeruginosa* virulence by quorum sensing inhibitors. EMBO J. 2003;**22**:3803-3815. DOI: 10.1093/emboj/cdg366

[51] Bjarnsholt T, Jensen PØ, Burmølle M, Hentzer M, Haagensen JA, Hougen HP, Calum H, Madsen KG, Moser C, Molin S, Høiby N, Givskov M: *Pseudomonas aeruginosa* tolerance to tobramycin, hydrogen peroxide and polymorphonuclear leukocytes is quorum-sensing dependent. Microbiology. 2005;**151**:373-383. DOI: 10.1099/mic.0.27463-0

[52] Hassett DJ, Ma JF, Elkins JG, Iglewski BH: Quorum sensing in *Pseudomonas aeruginosa* controls expression of catalase and superoxide dismutase genes and mediates biofilm susceptibility to hydrogen peroxide. Mol. Microbiol. 1999;**34**:1082-1093. DOI: 10.1046/j.1365-2958.1999.01672.x

[53] Hentzer M, Teitzel GM, Balzer GJ, Heydorn A, Molin S, Givskov M, Parsek MR: Alginate overproduction affect *Pseudmonas aeruginosa* biofilm structure and function. J. Bacetriol. 2001; 183:5395-5401. DOI: 10.1128/JB.183.18.5395-5401.2001

[54] Winstanley C, O'Brien S, Brockhurst AM, *Pseudomonas aeruginosa* evolutionary adaptation and diversification in cystic fibrosis chronic lung infections. Trends. Microbiol. 2016;**24**:327-337 (in Special Issue Microbial Endurance). DOI: http://dx.doi.org/10.1016/j.tim.2016.01.008

[55] Stover CK, Pham XQ, Erwin AL, Mizoguchi SD, Warrener P, Hickey MJ, Brinkman FSL, Hufnagle WO, Kowalk DJ, Lagrou M, Garber RL, Goltry L, Tolentino E, Westbrock-Wadman S, Yuan Y, Brody LL, Coulter SN, Folger KR, Kas A, Larbig K, Lim R, Smith K, Spencer D, Wong GK-S, Wu Z, Paulsen IT, Reizer J, Saler MH, Hancock REW, Lory S, Olson MV: Complete genome sequence of *Pseudomonas aeruginosa* PAO1, an opportunistic pathogen. Nature. 2000;**406**:959-964. DOI: 10.1038/35023079

[56] Smith EE, Buckley DG, Wu Z, Saenphimmachak C, Hoffman LR, D'Argenio DA, Miller SI, Ramsey BW, Speert DP, Moskowitz SM, Burns JL, Kaul R, Olson MV: Genetic adaptation by *Pseudomonas aeruginosa* to the airways of cystic fibrosis patients. Proc. Natl. Acad. Sci. U.S.A. 2006;**103**:8487-8492. DOI: 10.1073/pnas.0602138103

[57] Boles BR, Thoendel M, Singh PK: Self-generated diversity produces "insurance effects" in biofilm communities. Proc. Natl. Acad. Sci. U.S.A. 2004;**101**:16630-16635. DOI: 10.1073/pnas.0407460101

[58] Driffield K, Miller K, Bostock JM, O'Neill AJ, Chopra I: Increased mutability of *Pseudomonas aeruginosa* in biofilms. J. Antimicrob. Chemother. 2008;**61**:1053-1056. DOI:10.1093/jac/dkn044

[59] Oliver A, Canton R, Campo P, Baquero F, Blazquez J: High frequency of hypermutable *Pseudomonas aeruginosa* in cystic fibrosis lung infection. Science. 2000;**288**:1251-1254. DOI: 10.1126/science.288.5469.1251

[60] Hogardt M, Hoboth C, Schmoldt S, Henke C, Bader L, Heesemann J: Stage-specific adaptation of hypermutable *Pseudomonas aeruginosa* isolates during chronic pulmonary infection in patients with cystic fibrosis. J. Infect. Dis. 2007;**195**:70-80. DOI: 10.1086/509821

[61] Nguyen D, and Singh PK: Evolving stealth: genetic adaptation of *Pseudomonas aeruginosa* during cystic fibrosis infections. Proc. Natl. Acad. Sci. U.S.A. 2006;**103**:8305-8306. DOI: 10.1073/pnas.0602526103 DOI:10.1073%2Fpnas.0602526103#pmc_ext

[62] Górna H, Lawnicazak Ł, Zgoła-Greśkowiak A, Kaczorek E: Differences and dynamic changes in cell surface properties of three *Pseudomonas aeruginosa* strain isolated from petroleum-pollutes soil as a response to various carbon sources and the external addition of rhamnolipids. Bioresour. Technol. 2011;**102**:3028-3033. DOI: 10.1016/j.biortech.2010.09.124

[63] Pacwa-Płociniczak M, Płaza GA, Piotrowska-Seget Z, Cameotra SS: Environmental applications of biosurfactants: Recent advances. Int. J. Mol. Sci. 2011;**12**:633-654. DOI: 10.3390/ijms12010633

[64] Fracchia L, Banat JJ, Cavallo M, Ceresa C, Banat IM: Review Potential therapeutic applications of microbial surface-active compounds. Bioengineering. 2015;**2**:144-162. DOI: 10.3934/bioeng.2015.3.144

[65] Gharaei-Fathabad E: Biosurfactants in pharmaceutical industry: A mini-review. Am. J. Drug. Discov. Dev. 2011;**1**:58-69. DOI: 10.3923/ajdd.2011.58.69 DOI:10.3923/ajdd.2011.58.69#_blank

[66] Muthusamy K, Gopalakrishnan S, Ravi TK, Sivachidambaram P: Biosurfactants: Properties, commercial production and application. Curr. Sci. 2008;**94**:736-747. DOI: 10.1016/j.chemosphere.2008.01.003

[67] Van Hamme JD, Singh A, WardOP: Surfactants in microbiology and biotechnology: Part 1. Physiological aspects. Biotechnol. Adv. 2006;**24**:604-620. DOI: doi:10.1016/j.biotechadv.2006.08.001

[68] Tahzibi A, Kamal F, Assadi MM: Improved production of rhamnolipids by a *Pseudomonas aeruginosa* mutant. Iran. Biomed. J. 2004;**8**:25-31. http://ibj.pasteur.ac.ir/browse.php?a_id=508&slc_lang=en&sid=1&ftxt=1

[69] Abalos A, Pinazo A, Infante MR, Casals M, Garcia F, Manresa A: Physicochemical and antimicrobial properties of new rhamnolipids produced by *Pseudomonas aeruginosa* AT10 from soybean oil refinery wastes. Langmuir. 2001;**17**:1367-1371. DOI: 10.1021/la0011735

[70] Abdel-Mawgoud AM, Aboulwafa MM, Hassouna NAH: Characterizations of rhamnolipid produced by *Pseudomonas aeruginosa* isolate Bs 20. Appl. Biochem. Biotechnol. 2009;**157**:329-345. DOI: 10.1007/s12010-008-8285-1

[71] Benincasa M, Abalos A, Oliveira I, Manresa A: Chemical structure, surface properties and biological activities of the biosurfactant produced by *Pseudomonas aeruginosa* LBI from soapstock. Antonie. Van. Leeuwen. 2004;**85**:1-8. DOI: 10.1023/B:ANTO.0000020148.45523.41

[72] Haba E, Abalos A, Jauregui O, Espuny MJ, Manresa A: Use of liquid chromatography-mass spectroscopy for studying the composition and properties of rhamnolipids produced by different strains of *Pseudomonas aeruginosa.* J. Surfact. Deterg. 2003;**6**:155-161. DOI: 10.1007/s11743-003-0260-7

[73] Mata-Sandoval J, Karns J, Torrens A: Effect of nutritional and environmental conditions on the production and composition of rhamnolipids by *P. aeruginosa* UG2. Microbiol. Res. 2001;**155**: 249-256. DOI: 10.1016/S0944-5013(01)80001-X

[74] Pornsunthorntawee O, Wongpanit P, Chavadej S, Abe M, Rujiravanit R: Structural and physiochemical characterization of crude biosurfactant produced by *Pseudomonas aeruginoa* SP4 isolated from petroleum-contaminated soil. Bioresour. Technol. 2008;**99**:1589-1595. DOI: 10.1016/j.biortech.2007.04.020

[75] Benincasa M, Contiero J, Manresa MA, Moraes IO: Rhamnolipid production by *Pseudomonas aeruginosa* LBI growing on soapstock as the sole carbon source. J. Food. Eng. 2002;**54**:283-288. DOI: http://dx.doi.org/10.1016/S0260-8774(01)00214-X DOI:10.1016/S0260-8774(01)00214-X#doilink

[76] Benincasa M, Accorsini FR: *Pseudomonas aeruginosa* LBI production as an integrated process using the wastes from sunflower-oil refining as substrate. Bioresour. Technol. 2008;99:3843-3849. DOI: 10.1016/j.biortech.2007.06.048

[77] Rahman KSM, Rahman TJ, McClean S, Marchant R, Banat IM: Rhamnolipid biosurfactants production by strains of *Pseudomonas aeruginosa* using low cost raw materials. Biotechnol. Prog. 2002;**18**:1277-1281. DOI: 10.1021/bp020071x

[78] Costa S.G.V.A.O., Nitschke M., Hadaad R, Eberlin MN, Contiero J: Production of *Pseudomonas aeruginosa* LBI rhamnolipids following growth on Brazilian native oils. Process. Biochem. 2006;**41**:483-488. DOI: 10.1016/j.procbio.2005.07.002

[79] Déziel E, Lépine F, Dennie D, Boismenu D, Mamer OA, Villemur R: Liquid chromatography/mass spectrometry analysis of mixtures of rhamnolipids produced by *Pseudomonas aeruginosa* strain 57RP grown on mannitol or naphthalene. Biochim. Biophys. Acta. 1999;**1440**:244-252. DOI: 10.1016/S1388-1981(99)00129-8

[80] Nitschke M, Costa SG, Contiero J: Structure and applications of a rhamnolipid surfactant produced in soybean oil waste. Appl. Biochem. Biotechnol. 2010;**160**:2066-2074. DOI: 10.1016/j.biotechadv.2010.05.013

[81] Aparna A, Srinkethan G, Smitha H: Production and characterization of biosurfactant produced by a novel *Pseudomonas* sp. 2B. Colloids. Surf. B. 2012;**95**:23-29. DOI: 10.1016/j.colsurfb.2012.01.043

[82] Nie M, Yin X, Ren C, Wang Y, Xu F, Shen Q: Novel rhamnolipid biosurfactants produced by a PAH-degrading bacterium *P. aeruginosa* strain NY3. Biotechnol. Adv. 2010;**28**:635-643. DOI: 10.1016/j.biotechadv.2010.05.013

[83] Price NPJ, Ray KJ, Vermillion K, Kuo TM: MALDI-TOF mass spectrometry of naturally occurring mixtures of monorhamnolipids and dirhamnolipids. Carbohydr. Res. 2009;**344**:204-209. DOI: 10.1016/j.carres.2008.10.013

[84] Sarachat T, Pornsunthorntawee O, Chavadej S, Rujiravanit R: Purification and concentration of a rhamnolipid biosurfactant produced by *Pseudomonas aeruginosa* SP4 using foam fractionation. Bioresour. Technol. 2010;**101**:324-30. DOI: 10.1016/j.biortech.2009.08.012

[85] Deziel E, Lepine F, Milot S, Villemur R: RhlA is required for the production of a novel biosurfactant promoting swarming motility in *Pseudomonas aeruginosa*: 3-(3-hydroxyalkanoyloxy)alkanoic acids (HAAs), the precursors of rhamnolipids. Microbiology. 2003;**149**: 2005-2013. DOI: 10.1099/mic.0.26154-0

[86] Blankenfeldt W, Asuncion M, Lam JS, Naismith JH: The structural basis of the catalytic mechanism and regulation of glucose-1-phosphate thymidylyltransferase (RmlA). EMBO J. 2000;**19**:6652-6663. DOI: 10.1093/emboj/19.24.6652 DOI:10.1093%2Femboj%2F19.24.6652#pmc_ext

[87] Cabrera-Valladares N, Richardson AP, Olvera C, Trevino LG, Deziel E, Lepine F, Soberon-Chavez G: Monorhamnolipids and 3-(3-hydroxyalkanoyloxy)alkanoic acids (HAAs) production using *Escherichia coli* as a heterologous host. Appl. Microbiol. Biotechnol. 2006;**73**:187-194. DOI: 10.1007/s00253-006-0468-5

[88] Haussler S, Becker T: The pseudomonas quinolone signal (PQS) balances life and death in *Pseudomonas aeruginosa* populations. PLoS Pathog. 2008;4(3): e1000166. DOI: http://dx.doi.org/10.1371/journal.ppat.1000166

[89] Franklin MT., Nivens DE., Weadge JT., Lynne-Howell L, Biosynthesis of *P. aeruginosa* extracellular polysacharides alginate, Pel and Psl. Front. Microbiol. 2011;**2**:1-16. DOI: 10.3389/fmicb.2011.00167

[90] Halverson LJ. Role of alginate in bacterial biofilms. In Rehm BHA editor. Alginates: Biology and Applications. Springer-Verlag, Berlin Heidelberg; 2009. pp. 135-151. DOI: 10.1007/978-3-540-92679-5_2

[91] Gulez G, Altıntas A, Fazli, M, Dechesne A, Workman CT, Tolker-Nielsen T, Smets BF: Colony morphology and transcriptome profiling of *Pseudomonas putida* KT2440 and its mutants deficient in alginate or all EPS synthesis under controlled matric potentials. Microbiol. Open. 2014;**3**:457-469. DOI: 10.1002/mbo3.180

[92] Fett WF, Wells JM, Cescutti P, Wijey C: Identification of exopolysaccharides produced by fluorescent Pseudomonads associated with commercial mushroom (*Agaricus bisporus*) production. Appl. Environ. Microbiol. 1995;**61**:513-517. DOI: 0099-2240/95/$04.0010

[93] Remminghorst U, Rehm BHA: Bacterial alginates: From biosynthesis to applications. Biotechnol. Lett. 2006;**28**:1701-1712. DOI: 10.1007/s10529-006-9156-x

[94] Hay ID, Rehman ZU, Moradali MF, Wang Y, Rehm BHA: Microbial alginate production, modification and its applications. Microb. Biotechnol. 2013;**6**:637-650. DOI: 10.1111/1751-7915.12076 DOI:10.1111%2F1751-7915.12076#pmc_ext

[95] Coulon C, Vinogradov E, Filloux A, Sadovskaya I: Chemical analysis of cellular and extracellular carbohydrates of a biofilm forming strain *Pseudomonas aeruginosa* PA14. PLoS One. 2010;**5**:e14220. DOI: 10.1371/journal.pone.001422

[96] Friedman L, Kolter R: Two genetic loci produce distinct carbohydrate-rich structural components of the *Pseudomonas aeruginosa* biofilm matrix. J. Bacteriol. 2004;**186**:4457-4465. DOI: 10.1128/JB.186.14.4457-4465.2004 DOI:10.1128%2FJB.186.14.4457-4465.2004#pmc_ext

[97] Darzins A, Frantz B, Vanags RI, Chakrabarty AM: Nucleotide sequence analysis of the phosphomannose isomerase gene (pmi) of *Pseudomonas aeruginosa* and comparison with the corresponding *Escherichia coli* gene manA. Gene. 1986; **42**:293-302. DOI: 10.1016/0378-1119(86)90233-7

[98] Deretic V, Gill JF, Chakrabarty AM: Gene algD coding for GDPmannose dehydrogenase is transcriptionally activated in mucoid *Pseudomonas aeruginosa*. J. Bacteriol. 1987;**169**:351-358. DOI: 0021-9193/87/010351-08$02.00/0

[99] Zielinski NA, Chakrabarty, AM, Berry A: Characterization and regulation of the *Pseudomonas aeruginosa* algC gene encoding phosphomannomutase. J. Biol. Chem. 1991;**266**:9754-9763. http://www.jbc.org/content/266/15/9754.full.pdf

[100] Franklin MJ, Ohman DE: Identification of algF in the alginate biosynthetic gene cluster of *Pseudomonas aeruginosa* which is required for alginate acetylation. J Bacteriol. 1993;**175**:5057-5065. DOI: 0021-9193/93/165057-09$02.00/0

[101] Franklin MJ, Chitnis CE, Gacesa P, Sonesson A, White DC, Ohman DE: *Pseudomonas aeruginosa* AlgG is a polymer level alginate C5-mannuronan epimerase. J. Bacteriol. 1994;**176**:1821-1830. DOI: 0021-9193/94/$04.00+0

[102] Goldberg JB, Hatano K, Pier GB: Synthesis of lipopolysaccharide O side chains by *Pseudomonas aeruginosa* PAO1 requires the enzyme phosphomannomutase. J. Bacteriol. 1993;**175**:1605-1611. DOI:0021-9193/93/061605-07$02.00/0

[103] Olvera C, Goldberg JB, Sanchez R, Soberon-Chavez G: The *Pseudomonas aeruginosa* algC gene product participates in rhamnolipid biosynthesis. FEMS Microbiol. Lett. 1999;**179**:85-90. DOI: http://dx.doi.org/10.1111/j.1574-6968.1999.tb08712.x

[104] Pritt B, O'Brien L, Winn W: Mucoid Pseudomonas in cystic fibrosis. Am. J. Clin. Pathol. 2007;**128**:32-34. DOI: 10.1309/KJRPC7DD5TR9NTDM

[105] Verstraeten N, Braeken K, Debkumari B, Fauvart M, Fransaer J, Vermant J, Michiels J: Living on a surface: Swarming and biofilm formation. Trends. Microbiol. 2008;**16**:496-506. DOI: 10.1016/j.tim.2008.07.004

[106] Harshey RM: Bacterial motility on a surface: many ways to a common goal. Annu. Rev. Microbiol. 2003;**57**:249-273. DOI: 10.1146/annurev.micro.57.030502.091014

[107] Caiazza NC, Shanks RMQ, O'Toole GA: Rhamnolipids modulate swarming motility patterns of *Pseudomonas aeruginosa*. J. Bacteriol. 2005;**187**:7351-7361. DOI: 10.1128/JB.187.21.7351-7361.2005 DOI:10.1128%2FJB.187.21.7351-7361.2005#pmc_ext

[108] Déziel E, Comeau Y, Villemur R: Initiation of biofilm formation by *Pseudomonas aeruginosa* 57RP correlates with emergence of hyperpiliated and highly adherent phenotypic variants deficient in swimming, swarming, and twitching motilities. J. Bacteriol. 2001;**183**:1195-1204. DOI: 10.1128/JB.183.4.1195-1204.2001

[109] Tremblay J, Richardson AP, Lépine F, Déziel E: Self-produced extracellular stimuli modulate the *Pseudomonas aeruginosa* swarming motility behaviour. Environ. Microbiol. 2007;**9**:2622-2630. DOI: 10.1111/j.1462-2920.2007.01396.x

[110] Al-Tahhan RA, Sandrin TR, Bodour AA, Maier RM: Rhamnolipidinduced removal of lipopolysaccharide from *Pseudomonas aeruginosa:* Effect on cell surface properties and interaction with hydrophobic substrates. Appl. Environ. Microbiol. 2000;**66**:3262-3268. DOI: 10.1128/AEM.66.8.3262-3268.2000

[111] Boles BR, Thoendel M, Singh PK: Rhamnolipids mediate detachment of *Pseudomonas aeruginosa* from biofilms. Mol. Microbiol. 2005;**57**:1210-1223. DOI: 10.1111/j.1365-2958.2005.04743.x

[112] Zhang YM, Miller RM: Effect of a *Pseudomonas* rhamnolipid biosurfactant on cell hydrophobicity and biodegradation of octadecane. Appl. Environ. Microbiol. 1994;**60**:2101-2106. DOI: 0099-2240/94/$04.00+0

[113] Davey ME, Caiazza NC, O'Toole GA: Rhamnolipid surfactant production affects biofilm architecture in *Pseudomonas aeruginosa* PAOI. J. Bacetriol. 2003;**185**:1027-1036. DOI: 10.1128/JB.185.3.1027-1036.2003

[114] Byrd MS, Sadovskaya I, Vinogradov E, Lu H, Sprinkle AB, Richardson SH, Ma L, Ralston B, Parsek MR, Anderson EM, Lam JS, Wozniak DJ: Genetic and biochemical analyses of the *Pseudomonas aeruginosa* Psl exopolysaccharide reveal overlapping roles for polysaccharide synthesis enzymes in Psl and LPS production. Mol. Microbiol. 2009;**73**:622-638. DOI: 10.1111/j.1365-2958.2009.06795.x DOI:10.1111%2Fj.1365-2958.2009.06795.x#pmc_ext

[115] Alhede M, Bjarnsholt T, Jensen PO, Phipps RK, Moser C, Christophersen L, Christensen LD, van Gennip M, Parsek M, Hoiby N, Rasmussen TB, Givskov M: *Pseudomonas aeruginosa* recognizes and responds aggressively to the presence of polymorphonuclear leukocytes. Microbiol. Sgm. 2009;**155**:3500-3508. DOI: 10.1099/mic.0.031443-0

[116] Høiby N: *P. aeruginosa* in cystic fibrosis patients resists host defenses, antibiotics. Microbe. 2006;**1**:571-577.

[117] Barbier M, Martínez-Ramos I, Townsend P, Albertí S: Surfactant protein A blocks recognition of *Pseudomonas aeruginosa* by CKAP4/P63 on airway epithelial cells. J. Infect. Dis. 2012;**206**:1753-1762. DOI: 10.1093/infdis/jis587

[118] Zulianello L, Canard C, Köhler T, Caille D, Lacroix JS, Meda P: Rhamnolipids are virulence factors that promote early infiltration of primary human airway epithelia by *Pseudomonas aeruginosa*. Infect. Immun. 2006;**74**:3134-3147. DOI: 10.1128/IAI.01772-05

[119] Moss J, Ehrmantraut ME, Banwart BD, Frank DW, Barieri JT: Sera from adult patients with cystic fibrosis contain antibodies to *Pseudomonas aeruginosa* type III apparatus. Infect. Immun. 2001;**69**:1185-1188. DOI: 10.1128/IAI.69.2.1185-1188.2001

[120] Winzer K, Williams P: Quorum sensing and the regulation of virulence gene expression in pathogenic bacteria. Int. J. Med. Microbiol. 2001;**291:**131-143. DOI: 10.1078/1438-4221-00110

[121] Kownatzki R, Tummler B, Doring G: Rhamnolipid of *Pseudomonas aeruginosa* in sputum of cystic fibrosis patients. Lancet. 1987;**329**:1026-1027. DOI: http://dx.doi.org/10.1016/S0140-6736(87)92286-0

[122] Read RC, Roberts P, Munro N, Rutman A, Hastie A, Shryock T, Hall R, McDonald-Gibson W, Lund V, Taylor G: Effect of *Pseudomonas aeruginosa* rhamnolipids on mucociliary transport and ciliary beating. J. Appl. Physiol. (1985). 1992;**72**:2271-2277. http://jap.physiology.org/content/72/6/2271

[123] Graham A, Steel DM, Wilson R, Cole PJ, Alton E, Geddes DM: Effects of purified *Pseudomonas rhamnolipids* on bioelectric properties of sheep tracheal epithelium. Exp. Lung. Res. 1993;**19**:77-89. DOI: http://dx.doi.org/10.3109/01902149309071082

[124] Stutts MJ, Schwab JH, Chen MG, Knowles MR, Boucher RC: Effects of *Pseudomonas aeruginosa* on bronchial epithelial ion transport. Am. Rev. Respir. Dis. 1986;**134**:17-21. DOI: 10.1164/arrd.1986.134.1.17

[125] Fung DC, Somerville M, Richardson PS, Sheehan JK: Mucusglycoconjugate complexes released from feline trachea by a bacterial toxin. Am. J. Respir. Cell. Mol. Biol. 1995;**12**:296-306. DOI: 10.1165/ajrcmb.12.3.7873196

[126] Somerville M, Taylor G, Watson D, Rendell NB, Rutman A, Todd H, Davies JR, Wilson R, Cole P, Richardson PS: Release of mucus glycoconjugates by *Pseudomonas aeruginosa* rhamnolipid feline trachea in vivo and human bronchus in vitro. Am. J. Respir. Cell. Mol. Biol. 1992;**6**:116-122. DOI: 10.1165/ajrcmb/6.1.116

[127] Cowell BA, Twining SS, Hobden JA, Kwong MS, Fleiszig MS: Mutation of *lasA* and *lasB* reduces *Pseudomonas aeruginosa* invasion of epithelial cells. Microbiology. 2003;**149**:2291-2299. DOI: 10.1099/mic.0.26280-0

[128] Lee VT, Smith RS, Tummler B, Lory S: Activities of *Pseudomonas aeruginosa* effectors secreted by the III type secretion system in vitro and during infection. Infect. Immun. 2005;**73**:1695-1705. DOI: 10.1128/IAI.73.3.1695-1705.2005

[129] Darling KE, Dewar A, Evans TJ: Role of the cystic fibrosis transmembrance conductance regulator in internalization of *Pseudomonas aeruginosa* by polarized respiratory epithelial cells. Cell. Microbiol. 2004;**6**:521-533. DOI: 10.1111/j.1462-5822.2004.00380.x

[130] Pier GB: CFTR mutation and host susceptibility to *Pseudomonas aeruginosa* lung infection. Curr. Opin. Microbiol. 2002;**5**:81-86. DOI: 10.1016/s1369-5274(02)00290-4

[131] Häussler S, Nimtz M, Domke T, Wray V, Steinmetz I: Purification and characterization of a cytotoxic exolipid of *Burkholderia pseudomallei*. Infect. Immun. 1998;**66**:1588-1593. DOI: 0019-9567/98/$04.0010

[132] Kharazmi A, Bibi Z, Nielsen H, Hoiby N, Döring G Effect of *Pseudomonas aeruginosa* rhamnolipid on human neutrophil and monocyte function. Apmis. 1989;**97**:1068-1072. DOI: 10.1111/j.1699-0463.1989.tb00519.x

[133] König B, Bergmann U, König W: Induction of inflammatory mediator release (serotonin and 12-hydroxyeicosatetraenoic acid) from human platelets by *Pseudomonas aeruginosa* glycolipid. Infect. Immun. 1992;**60**:3150-3155. DOI:10.1159/000236706

[134] Jensen PO, Bjarnsholt T, Phipps R, Rasmussen TB, Calum H, Christoffersen L, Moser C, Williams P, Pressler T, Givskov M, Hoiby: Rapid necrotic killing of polymorphonuclear leukocytes is caused by quorum-sensing-controlled production of rhamnolipid by *Pseudomonas aeruginosa*. Microbiol. Sgm. 2007;**153**:1329-1338. DOI: 10.1099/mic.0.2006/003863-0

[135] Bédard M, McClure CD, Schiller NL, Francoeur C, Cantin A, Denis M: Release of interleukin-8, interleukin-6, and colony stimulating factors by upper airway epithelial cells: implication for cystic fibrosis. Am. J. Respir. Cell. Mol. Biol. 1993;**9**:455-462. DOI: 10.1165/ajrcmb/9.4.455

[136] McClure CD, Schiller NL: Inhibition of macrophage phagocytosis by *Pseudomonas aeruginosa* rhamnolipids in vitro and in vivo. Curr. Microbiol. 1996;**33**:109-117. DOI: 10.1007/s002849900084

[137] Van Gennip M, Christensen LD, Alhede M, Phipps R, Jensen PO, Christophersen L, Pamp SJ, Moser C, Mikkelsen PJ, Koh AY, Tolker-Nielsen T, Pier GB, Hoiby N, Givskov M, Bjarnsholt T: Inactivation of the rhlA gene in *Pseudomonas aeruginosa* prevents rhamnolipid production, disabling the protection against polymorphonuclear leukocytes. Apmis. 2009;**117**:537-546. DOI: 10.1111/j.1600-0463.2009.02466.x

[138] Ernst RK, Hajjar AM, Tsai JH, Moskowitz SM, Wilson CB, Miller SI: *Pseudomonas aeruginosa* lipid A diversity and its recognition by Toll-like receptor 4. J. Endotoxin. Res. 2003;**9**:395-400. DOI:10.1179/096805103225002764

[139] Ernst RK, Moskowitz SM, Emerson JC, Kraig GM, Adams KN, Harvey MD, Ramsey B, Speert DP, Burns JL, Miller SI: Unique lipid A modifications in *Pseudomonas aeruginosa* isolated from the airways of patients with cystic fibrosis. J. Infect. Dis. 2007;**196**:1088-1092. DOI: 10.1086/521367

[140] Ernst RK, Yi EC, Guo L, Lim KB, Burns JL, Hackett M, Miller SI: Specific lipopolysaccharide found in cystic fibrosis airway *Pseudomonas aeruginosa*. Science. 1999;**286**:1561. DOI: 10.1126/science.286.5444.1561

[141] Hajjar AM, Ernst RK, Tsai JH, Wilson CB, Miller SI: Human Toll-like receptor 4 recognizes host-specific LPS modifications. Nat. Immunol. 2002;**3**:354-359. DOI: 10.1038/ni777

[142] Doring G, Pier GB: Vaccines and immunotherapy against *Pseudomonas aeruginosa*. Vaccine. 2008;**26(8):**1011-1124. DOI:10.1016/j.vaccine.2007.12.007

[143] Stuart B, Lin JH, Mogayzel PJ Jr: Early eradication of *Pseudomonas aeruginosa* in patients with cystic fibrosis. Paediatr. Respir. Rev. 2010;**11**:177-184. DOI: 10.1016/j.prrv.2010.05.003

[144] Hayes D, Feola JrDJ, Murphy BS, Kuhn RJ, Davis GA: Eradication of *Pseudomonas aeruginosa* in an adult patient with cystic fibrosis. Am. J. Health. Syst. Pharm. 2011;**68**:319-322. DOI: 10.2146/ajhp10010

[145] Chan C, Burrows LL, Deber CM: Alginate as an auxiliary bacterial membrane: binding of membrane-active peptides by polysaccharides. J. Pept. Res. 2005;**65**:343-351. DOI: 10.1111/j.1399-3011.2005.00217.x

[146] Ryan G, Singh M, Dwan K: Inhaled antibiotics for long-term therapy in cystic fibrosis. Cochrane Database Syst. Rev. 2011;**3**:CD001021. DOI: 10.1002/14651858.CD001021.pub2

[147] Ceri H, Olson ME, Stremick C, Read RR, Morck D, Buret A: The Calgary Biofilm Device: New technology for rapid determination of antibiotic susceptibilities of bacterial biofilms. J. Clin. Microbiol. 1999;**37**:1771-1776. DOI: 0095-1137/99/$04.0010

[148] Tomlin KL, Malott RJ, Ramage G, Storey DG, Sokol PA, Ceri H: Quorumsensing mutations affect attachment and stability of *Burkholderia cenocepacia* biofilms. Appl. Environ. Microbiol. 2005;**71**:5208-5218. DOI: 10.1128/AEM.71.9.5208-5218.2005

[149] Davies J A, Harrison JJ, Marques LL, Foglia GR, Stremick CA, Storey DG, Turner RJ, Olson ME, Ceri H: The GacS sensor kinase controls phenotypic reversion of small colony variants isolated from biofilms of *Pseudomonas aeruginosa* PA14. FEMS Microbiol. Ecol. 2007; **59**:32-46. DOI:10.1111/j.1574-6941.2006.00196.x

[150] Alfa MJ, Howie R: Modeling microbial survival in buildup biofilm for complex medical devices. BMC Infect. Dis. 2009;**9**:56. DOI: 10.1186/1471-2334-9-56

[151] Geske GD, Wezeman RJ, Siegel AP, Blackwell HE: Small molecule inhibitors of bacterial quorum sensing and biofilm formation. J. Am. Chem. Soc. 2005;**127**:12762-12763. DOI: 10.1021/ja0530321

[152] Rasmussen TB, Givskov M: Quorum-sensing inhibitors as anti-pathogenic drugs. Int. J. Med. Microbiol. 2006;**296**:149-161 DOI:10.1016/j.ijmm.2006.02.005

[153] Galloway WR, Hodgkinson JT, Bowden SD, Welch M, Spring DR: Quorum sensing in Gram-negative bacteria: small-molecule modulation of AHL and AI-2 quorum sensing pathways. Chem. Rev. 2011;**111**:28-67. DOI: 10.1021/cr100109t

[154] Bjarnsholt T, Tolker-Nielsen T, Hoiby N, Givskov M: Interference of *Pseudomonas aeruginosa* signalling and biofilm formation for infection control. Expert. Rev. Mol. Med. 2010;**12**:e11. DOI:10.1017/S1462399410001420

[155] Poole K: *Pseudomonas aeruginosa*: Resistance to the Max. Front. Microbiol. 2011;**2**:1-13. DOI: 10.3389/fmicb.2011.00065 DOI:10.3389%2Ffmicb.2011.00065#pmc_ext

[156] Skindersoe, ME, Alhede M, Phipps R, Yang L, Jensen PO, Rasmussen TB, Bjarnsholt T, Tolker-Nielsen T, Hoiby N, Givskov M: Effects of antibiotics on quorum sensing in *Pseudomonas aeruginosa*. Antimicrob. Agents. Chemother. 2008;**52**:3648-3656. DOI: 10.1128/AAC.01230-073.

[157] Bals, R, Hubert D, Tummler B: Antibiotic treatment of CF lung disease: From bench to bedside. J. Cyst. Fibros. 2011;**10**:146-151. DOI:10.1016/S1569-1993(11)60019-2 DOI:10.1016/S1569-1993%2811%2960019-2#_blank#Persistent link using digital object identifier

[158] Rasmussen TB, Skindersoe ME, Bjarnsholt T, Phipps RK, Christensen KB, Jensen PO, Andersen JB, Koch B, Larsen TO, Hentzer M, Eberl L, Hoiby N, Givskov M: Identity and effects of quorum-sensing inhibitors produced by *Penicillium* species. Microbiology. 2005;**151**(Pt 5):1325-1340. DOI:10.1099/mic.0.27715-0

[159] Harmsen M, Yang L, Pamp SJ, Tolker-Nielsen T: An update on *Pseudomonas aeruginosa* biofilm formation, tolerance, and dispersal. FEMS Immunol. Med. Microbiol. 2010;59(3):253-268. DOI:10.1111/j.1574-695X.2010.00690.x

[160] Hentzer M, Riedel K, Rasmussen TB, Heydorn A, Andersen JB, Parsek MR, Rice SA, Eberl L, Molin S, Hoiby N, Kjelleberg S, Givskov M: Inhibition of quorum sensing in *Pseudomonas aeruginosa* biofilm bacteria by a halogenated furanone compound. Microbiology. 2002;**148**(Pt 1):87-102.

Chapter 7

Anti-PcrV Immunization for *Pseudomonas aeruginosa* Pneumonia in Cystic Fibrosis

Yoshifumi Naito, Kiyoshi Moriyama and Teiji Sawa

Additional information is available at the end of the chapter

http://dx.doi.org/10.5772/intechopen.69767

Abstract

Propagation of multidrug-resistant *Pseudomonas aeruginosa,* which causes endemic nosocomial infections, has become a major concern in various parts of the world. In patients with cystic fibrosis, a major cause of death is respiratory tract infections with antibiotic-resistant *P. aeruginosa*. This condition has prompted medical research aimed at developing effective prophylaxis and treatments that do not rely on conventional antimicrobial agents. The pathogenesis that results in cytotoxicity and mortality in immunocompromised patients infected with *P. aeruginosa* is associated with the type III secretion system of this bacterium. Clinical isolates that are cytotoxic and drug-resistant are involved in acute exacerbation of chronic infectious diseases. The *P. aeruginosa* V-antigen PcrV, a *Yersinia* V-antigen LcrV homolog, is involved as an indispensable component in the translocational process of type III secretory (TTS) toxins. Vaccination against PcrV ensures survival of infection-challenged mice and decreases lung inflammation and injury. Furthermore, anti-PcrV IgG can inhibit translocation of TTS toxins. These observations support the hypothesis that anti-PcrV strategies have the potential as nonantibiotic immune strategies for preventing aggravation of *P. aeruginosa* infections in patients with cystic fibrosis.

Keywords: cystic fibrosis, exoenzyme, PcrV, *Pseudomonas aeruginosa,* type III secretion system, V-antigen

1. Introduction

Propagation of multidrug-resistant *Pseudomonas aeruginosa* (MDR-PA) has become a serious concern in various parts of the world [1–4]. Recent outbreaks of extensively drug-resistant

P. aeruginosa (XDR-PA) are threatening to increase XDR-PA colonization of immunocompromised and artificially ventilated patients because efficacious antimicrobial choices against XDR-PA are limited [3–5]. In patients with cystic fibrosis (CF), a major cause of death is respiratory tract infections with *P. aeruginosa*. This condition has led to medical research on the development of effective prophylaxis and treatments that do not rely on conventional antimicrobial agents [6]. Furthermore, recent reports have suggested that XDR-PA strains appear to have a greater ability to promote bacteremia and sepsis [7]. Therefore, the pathogenic mechanisms that are responsible for this infection are important for protecting patients from the lethal consequences of these infections.

The pathogenesis responsible for mortality in *P. aeruginosa* pneumonia is associated with the development of septic shock and multiple organ failure. This is because certain *P. aeruginosa* strains have the ability to cause necrosis of the lung epithelium and disseminate into the circulation [8]. Advances in genomic analysis and cellular microbiology have shown that damage to the lung epithelium is associated with expression of toxins. These toxins are directly translocated into eukaryotic cells through the type III secretion system (TTSS) of *P. aeruginosa* [9]. Unlike classic type I and type II secretion systems, the newly identified TTSS, through which bacteria directly transfer their toxins from the bacterial cytosol to the eukaryotic cell cytosol, were discovered in most pathogenic Gram-negative bacteria (**Figure 1**) [10]. Four type III secretory (TTS) toxins, called ExoS, ExoT, ExoU, and ExoY, have been identified in *P. aeruginosa* [11, 12]. ExoS is the 49-kDa form of exoenzyme S, which is a bifunctional toxin that has ADP-ribosyltransferase and GTPase-activating protein (GAP) activities [13]. ExoS disrupts endocytosis,

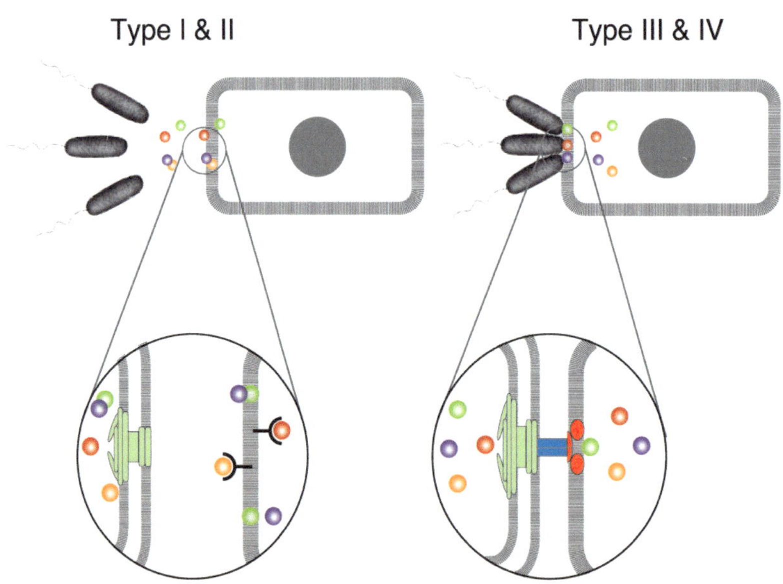

Figure 1. Toxin secretion systems in Gram-negative bacteria. In the types I and II secretion systems, bacteria secrete toxins into the extracellular space (left side of figure). As one example, secreted toxins are captured by surface receptors on the eukaryotic cell membrane and are then transferred to the cytosol. In the types III and IV secretion systems, bacteria secrete toxins directly into the cytosol of target eukaryotic cells through their secretion apparatus (right side of the figure). The mechanism whereby the secreted toxins are transferred to the eukaryotic cell cytosol is called translocation.

the actin cytoskeleton, and cellular proliferation. ExoT, which is a 53-kDa form of exoenzyme S with 75% sequence homology to ExoS, also exerts GAP activity and interferes with cell morphology and motility [13–15]. ExoY is a nucleotidyl cyclase that increases intracellular levels of cyclic adenosine and guanosine monophosphates, resulting in the formation of edema [12]. ExoU exhibits phospholipase A_2 activity activated by host cell ubiquitination after translocation. ExoU is a major pathogenic cytotoxin that causes alveolar epithelial injury and necrosis of macrophages [16–19].

In this review, we summarize the TTSS of *P. aeruginosa* and its association with CF. We also review the development of immune therapies, including passive and active immunization against the TTSS-associated virulence of *P. aeruginosa*.

2. Cytotoxic or invasive *P. aeruginosa* strains

In most acute clinical manifestations of *P. aeruginosa* infection, severe pneumonia occurs in patients under ventilatory management and in immunocompromised patients [2, 3]. Patients with severe *P. aeruginosa* pneumonia frequently develop sepsis and subsequent multiorgan failure [7].

In the mid-1990s, researchers investigating *P. aeruginosa* reported that the strains expressing ExoS (49-kDa type exoenzyme S) had low cytotoxicity to eukaryotic cells, whereas the strains that did not express ExoS had strong cytotoxicity [20, 21]. Therefore, at that time, *P. aeruginosa* strains were classified as either a cytotoxic $exoS^-$ type or an invasive $exoS^+$ type, depending on the genotypes of the 49-kDa exoenzyme S [20]. The 53-kDa exoenzyme S (ExoT) was discovered as a gene product that was distinct from ExoS [14, 15]. However, because cytotoxic $exoS^-$ type- and invasive $exoS^+$ type-strains both possessed ExoT, the mechanism for cytotoxic virulence could not be explained solely on the basis of possessing the ExoT gene. Therefore, the mechanism whereby the cytotoxic characteristics of $exoS^-exoT^+$ type-strains develop is unknown. In 1997, a new cytotoxin, ExoU, was identified [16]. *P. aeruginosa* strains that do not have *exoU* always possess *exoS*. Therefore, the genotype of cytotoxic strains is $exoS^-exoT^+exoU^+$ and the genotype of invasive strains is $exoS^+exoT^+exoU^-$ [20, 21]. While searching for major cytotoxins in *P. aeruginosa, P. aeruginosa* exoenzymes were found to translocate directly into the eukaryotic cytosol through the TTS mechanism [22]. Among the four TTS cytotoxins, ExoS, ExoT, ExoU, and ExoY, *P. aeruginosa* clinical isolates that cause severe sepsis and mortality express TTS ExoU [16, 23–25]. After discovery of ExoU, studies showed the enzymatic action of phospholipase A_2, which is activated by a eukaryotic cell factor after translocation into the eukaryotic cell cytosol [17–19].

3. Genomic analyses of *P. aeruginosa* strains

The whole genome sequencing project by the *Pseudomonas* Genome Project was completed for the *P. aeruginosa* strain PAO1 in 2000 [26]. Since this time, comparative genomics is currently on-going between the PAO1 reference strain and various clinical isolates of which the characteristics differ from PAO1 (**Figure 2**). In this research field, the major question is how much do the strains differ from each other at the gene level, especially between strains isolated from patients with acute infections and strains isolated from chronically infected patients with CF. The genetic mechanisms underlying multidrug resistance are also of major interest in these comparative genomic studies.

The clinical isolate UCBPP-PA14 is cytotoxic and is similar to the laboratory strain PA103 UCBPP-PA14 that has the TTS phenotype $ExoS^-ExoT^+ExoU^+ExoY^-$, whereas invasive PAO1 is $ExoS^+ExoT^+ExoU^-ExoY^+$ [16, 20]. Therefore, genomic analysis of UCBPP-PA14 was conducted to identify their phenotypic differences. As a result, two pathogenicity islands that do not exist in PAO1 were discovered in the UCBPP-PA14 genome [27]. Thereafter, researchers found that clinical strains containing *P. aeruginosa* pathogenicity island-2 (PAPI-2) and *exoU* display the cytotoxic phenotypes that are responsible for acute lung injury in animal models [16, 27]. Concurrently, strains harboring PAPI-2 and *exoU* were found to have deletional mutation of the *exoS* gene, which creates the *exoS*$^-$ genotype in PA103 and UCBPP-PA14 [27].

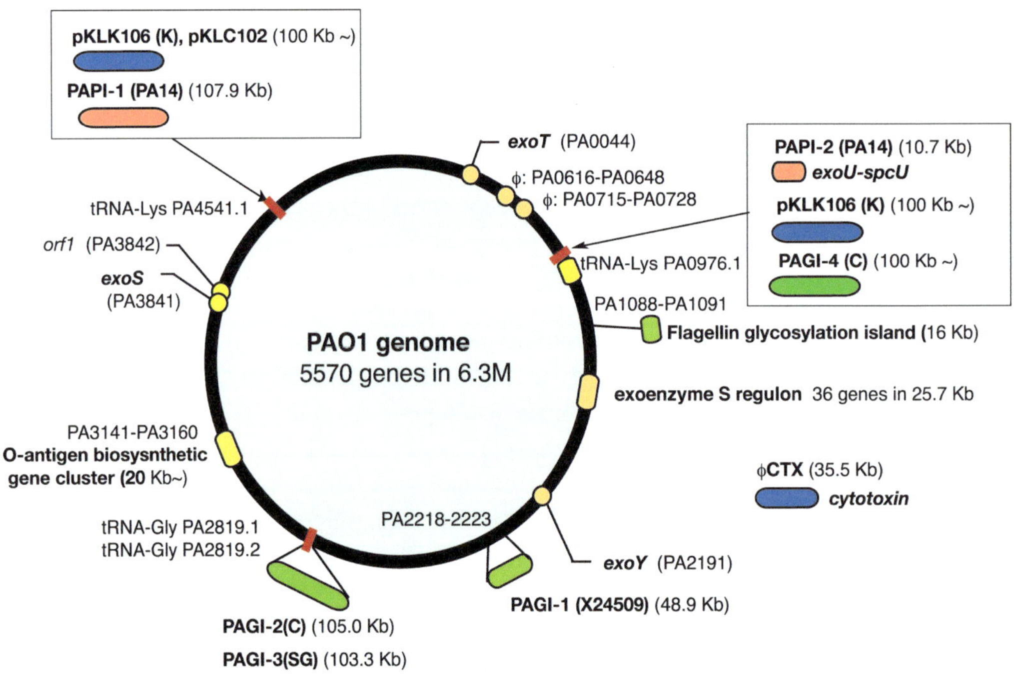

Figure 2. The PAO1 reference strain genome and its pathogenic gene configuration. The *P. aeruginosa* strain PAO1 possesses 5570 genes in its 6.3-Mb circular genome. The exoenzyme S regulon is a gene cluster (25.7 kb) for type III secretion. Type III secretory toxin genes, such as *exoS*, *exoT*, and *exoY*, are scattered throughout the genome. The *P. aeruginosa exoU* gene, which is located in an insertional pathogenic gene cluster in pathogenicity island-2 (PAPI-2), was discovered in the UCBPP-PA14 virulent clinical strain.

4. The type III secretion system of *P. aeruginosa*

4.1. Components of the type III secretion system and the exoenzyme S regulon

The TTSS is composed of the following: (1) secretion apparatus (injectisome), (2) translocators, (3) a set of secreted toxins, and (4) regulatory components [28]. In the *P. aeruginosa* genome, a pathogenic gene cluster called the exoenzyme S regulon encodes the genes for regulation, secretion, and translocation of the TTSS [9, 11] (**Figure 3**). In the exoenzyme S regulon, the *exsCBA* operon encodes the transcriptional activator protein ExsA, which regulates expression of exoenzyme S and its co-regulated proteins (**Figure 4**) [11]. Four TTS toxins, ExoS, ExoT, ExoU, and ExoY were identified in *P. aeruginosa* (**Table 1**) [11, 12, 16]. The genes for these TTS toxins are scattered in the genome [26]. In contrast, *exoU*, which is located in the insertional gene pathogenic cluster PAPI-2, is present with its chaperone protein gene *spcU* only in the genomes of cytotoxic strains, such as PA103 and UCBPP-PA14 [16, 27, 29].

4.2. The *pcrGVHpopBD* translocation operon

One operon in the exoenzyme S regulon, called *pcrGVHpopBD*, encodes five proteins associated with translocational processes for TTS toxins [11]. These proteins are PcrV, PopB, and PopD, and their chaperones are PcrG and PcrH. PcrV, which is the *P. aeruginosa* V-antigen, is a cap structure component on the tip of the injection needle formed by PscF in the secretion apparatus [30] (**Figure 5**). The genetic organization for the exoenzyme S regulon shares

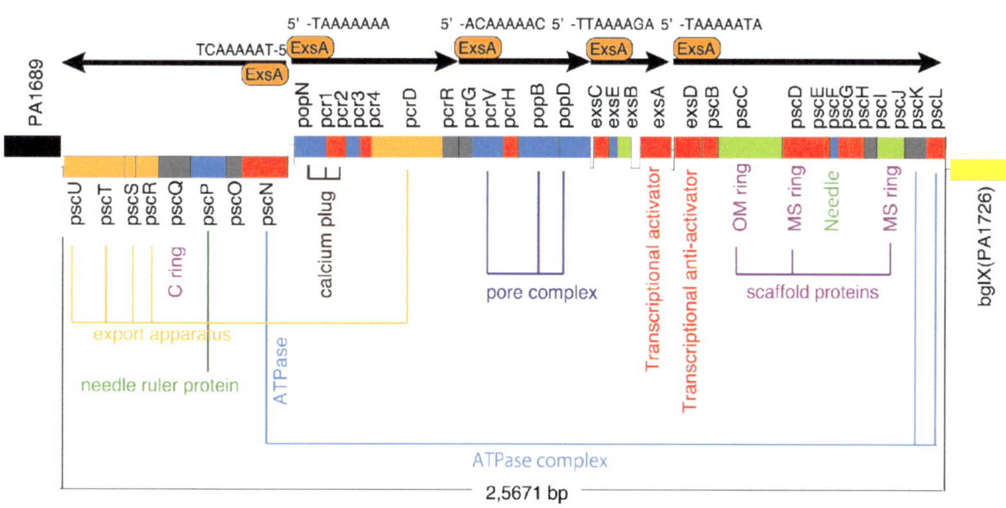

Figure 3. Genomic structure of the exoenzyme S regulon. The type III secretion regulatory region (25.5 kb), found as a gene cluster, was named the exoenzyme S regulon. The exoenzyme S regulon comprises five operons, including 36 genes for transcription (*exsA-exsD*), genes encoding the secretion apparatus (*pscB-pscU*), and others encoding translocation-related proteins (*pcrGVHpopBD*). The *exsCBA* operon encodes the transcriptional activator ExsA protein, which regulates expression of exoenzyme S and co-regulated proteins.

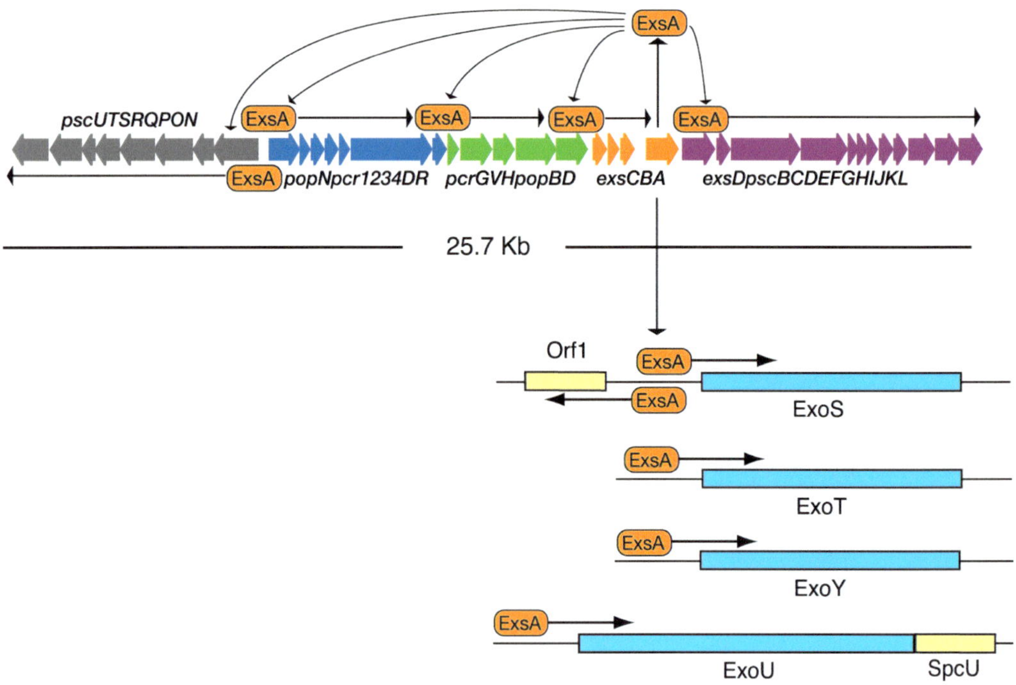

Figure 4. Type III secretion regulation in *P. aeruginosa* by the ExsA transcriptional activator. The ExsA transcriptional activator protein activates five operons in the exoenzyme S regulon via five ExsA binding motifs "TxAAAAxA". ExoT, ExoU, and ExoY were identified in *P. aeruginosa*. Genes for ExoS, ExoT, and ExoY are scattered in the genome. The *orf1* gene, which encodes a chaperone protein for ExoS, is next to *exoS*. The *exoU* gene, which is located in the insertional gene pathogenic cluster PAPI-2, is present with its chaperone protein gene *spcU* only in the genomes of cytotoxic strains, such as PA103 and UCBPP-PA14.

Toxins	Size (kDa)	Enzymatic activity	Action
ExoS	49	FAS-dependent ADP-ribosyltransferase	Antiphagocytosis, inhibition of endocytosis
ExoT	53	Small GTPase activating protein activity	Inhibition of tissue repair
ExoU	74	Phospholipase A2	Cytotoxin, lipid degradation
ExoY	42	Adenylate cyclase	Edema formation, anti-inflammatory

Table 1. Type III secretory toxins in P. aeruginosa.

the most homology with the *Yersinia* Yop virulon [31]. *Yersinia* LcrV has been reported to be a molecular target competing with TTSS virulence. Similarly, *P. aeruginosa* PcrV also is a molecular target that can compete with TTSS virulence in *P. aeruginosa* [32, 33]. This competition with TTSS virulence will be discussed later in this review.

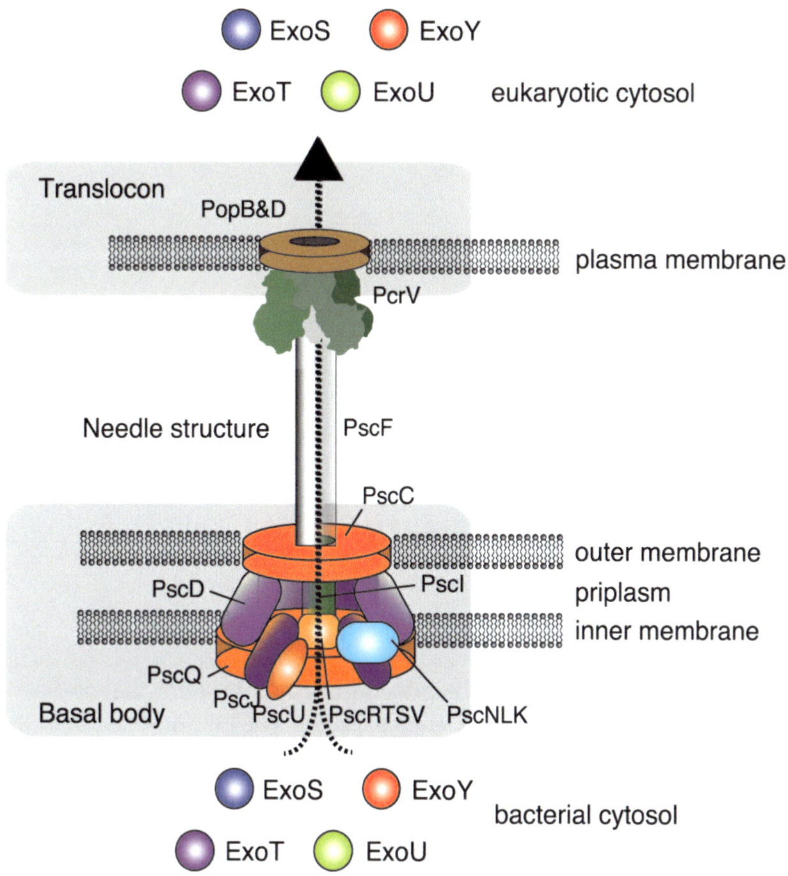

Figure 5. The type III secretory apparatus of *P. aeruginosa*. The *P. aeruginosa* type III secretory apparatus comprises many protein components as follows: a cap component, PcrV; a needle component, PscF; an outer ring component, PscC; and basal components, including PscJ, ATPase PscN, and others. Four type III secretory toxins, ExoS, ExoT, ExoU, and ExoY, are injected directly into the cytosol of target eukaryotic cells through the type III secretory apparatus. Translocated toxins are activated by specific eukaryotic cell cofactors. Following activation, ADP-ribosyltransferase activity is shown by ExoS, whereas ADP-ribosyltransferase and GTPase-activating protein activity is shown by ExoT. Activated ExoU has phospholipase A_2 activity, and ExoY exhibits adenylate cyclase activity.

4.3. *Yersinia* V-antigen LcrV and *P. aeruginosa* PcrV

Historically, *Yersinia* LcrV has been referred to as the *Yersinia* V-antigen. Approximately 50 years ago in the UK, Burrows et al. reported that *Yersinia* V-antigen was an antigen substance associated with the pathogenic toxicity [34–38] of this bacterium. They found that only *Y. pestis,* with the antigenic factor they called the V-antigen, induced immunity in a mouse model of infection [34–38]. In 1986, the gene encoding the LcrV V-antigen, *lcrV*, was cloned from the Low-calcium response (LCR) operon of the *Y. pestis* pCD1 plasmid [39]. A genetic mutation experiment then showed that LcrV is essential for translocation of the toxin [32]. Additionally, antibodies against LcrV were reported to be capable of blocking transfer of the toxin [32]. As well as *Yersinia* LcrV in the TTSS, *P. aeruginosa* PcrV is essential for transition of the TTSS toxin, and the antibody against PcrV can block transition of the TTS toxin [33]. PcrV might play a role in connecting the needle rod (composed of PscF) to the pore (formed with PopB/PopD) on the eukaryotic cell membrane. Indeed, electron microscopy has successfully visualized V-antigens as cap structures on the mushroom needle tip portion of the protein [30]. Specific blocking antibodies against the V-antigen also block translocated toxin from binding to the top part of the cap structure [32, 40].

5. *P. aeruginosa* type III secretory toxins

5.1. ExoS and ExoT

In the late 1970s, *P. aeruginosa* exoenzyme S was discovered as an adenosine diphosphate ribosyltransferase that was distinct from exotoxin A [41, 42]. However, in the mid-1990s, exoenzyme S activity was determined to be the result of two highly homologous toxins, termed ExoS (49-kDa exoenzyme S) and ExoT (53-kDa exoenzyme S), which are encoded in two separate portions of the *P. aeruginosa* genome [14, 15]. ExoS and ExoT were also found to be secreted by the TTS mechanism [15, 22].

5.1.1. ADP-ribosyltransferase activity

ExoS and ExoT are two immunologically indistinguishable proteins that co-fractionate with exoenzyme S activity [14]. ExoS and ExoT encode proteins of 457 and 453 amino acids, respectively, and share 75% amino acid identity. ExoT possesses approximately 0.2% of the ADP-ribosyltransferase activity of ExoS [14, 15]. ExoT diminishes motility of macrophages and phagocytosis, at least in part through disrupting the eukaryotic cellular actin cytoskeleton, and also blocks wound healing [43, 44]. The ExoS carboxyl terminal catalyzes transfer of the ADP-ribose moiety of nicotinamide adenine dinucleotide to a number of different proteins, including the intermediate filament protein, vimentin [45–47].

5.1.2. GTPase-activating protein activity

The amino terminal domains of ExoS and ExoT have been characterized as GAPs of Rho GTPases [48]. The Rho GAP activity of ExoS stimulates reorganization of the actin cytoskeleton by inhibiting Rac and Cdc42, and induces formation of actin stress fibers by inhibiting Rho [49]. These domains, which include catalytic arginines, share sequence homology with not only *Yersinia* YopE and *Salmonella* SptP, but also with mammalian Rho GAP proteins, such as hsp-120GAP, hsNF1, dmGAP1, and sclRA1. Biochemical studies have shown that ExoT possesses GAP activity for RhoA, Rac1, and Cdc42, and interferes with Rho signal transduction pathways, which regulate actin organization, exocytosis, cell cycle progression, and phagocytosis [50, 51].

5.2. ExoU

A specific isogenic mutant of the cytotoxic *P. aeruginosa* strain PA103, which does not have ExoS and is genetically modified to lack ExoT, is still cytotoxic *in vitro*. This mutant causes epithelial injury *in vivo*, indicating that another cytotoxin is responsible for the observed pathology [16, 17]. In 1997, ExsA-activated ExoU was discovered to be a major virulence factor causing lung injury and the *exoU* gene was cloned from the cytotoxic strain PA103 [16]. A region downstream of *exoU* encodes a small 15-kDa protein named SpcU, which functions as a chaperone for ExoU [29]. ExoU is a TTS protein of *P. aeruginosa* that is necessary for epithelial cell cytotoxicity *in vitro* and virulence in a mouse model of pneumonia [16].

5.2.1. Patatin-like phospholipase A_2 activity

ExoU contains a potato patatin-like phospholipase A (PLA) domain [17]. Patatin is a member of a multigene family of vacuolar storage glycoproteins with lipid acyl hydrolase and acyl transferase activities. Alignment of ExoU, potato patatin, and human PLA2 shows three highly conserved regions in the ExoU amino acid sequence as follows [17]: (1) a glycine-rich nucleotide binding motif, GXGXXG/A (position 111–116 in ExoU); (2) a serine-hydrolase motif, which includes a serine active site for cPLA2, GXSXG/S (position 140–144 in ExoU); and (3) an active site motif containing aspartate for cPLA2, DGG/A (position 344–347 in ExoU) (**Figure 6**).

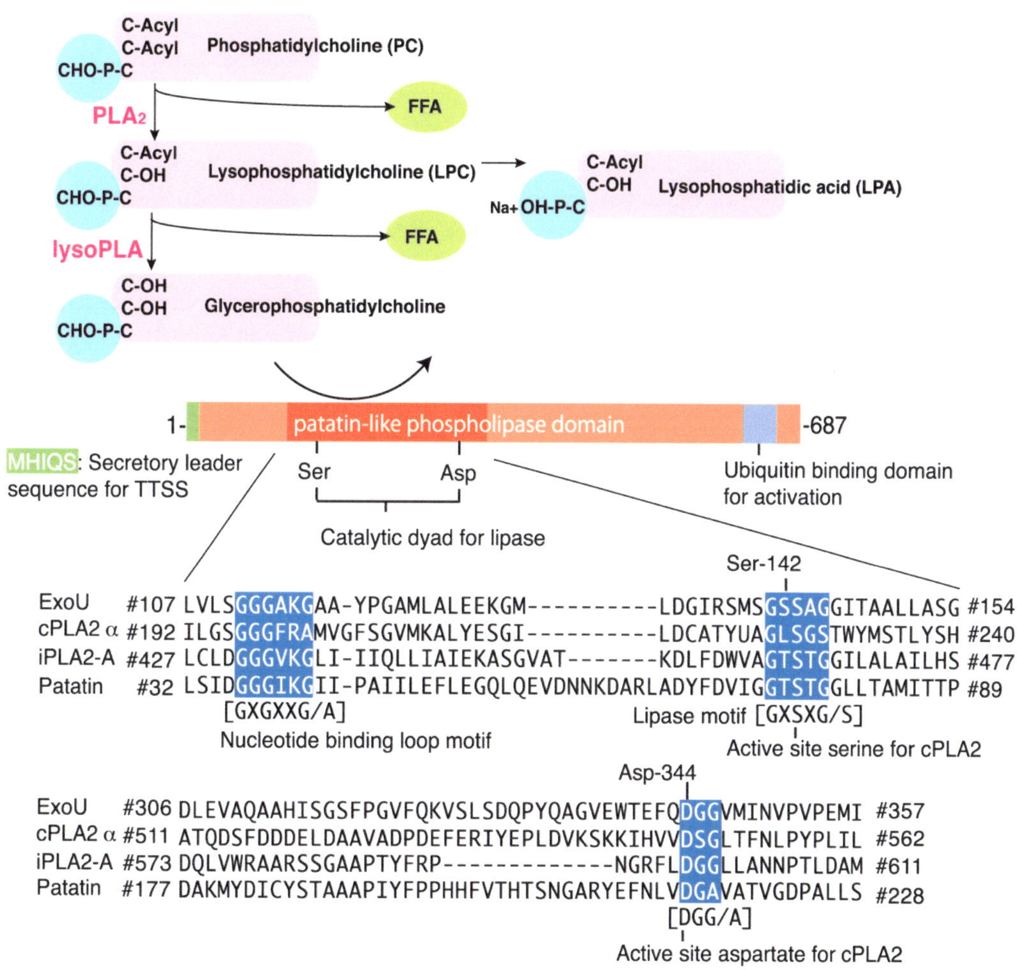

Figure 6. Enzymatic activity and consensus motifs in ExoU. *P. aeruginosa* ExoU, a major factor causing cytotoxicity and epithelial injury in the lungs, contains a patatin domain that catalyzes membrane phospholipids through its phospholipase A_2 activity. Homology in the amino acid sequence, with a catalytic dyad in the primary structure, is found among patatin, mammalian phospholipase A_2 ($cPLA_2$-α and $iPLA_2$), and ExoU. FFA: free fatty acids.

5.2.2. Phospholipase A_2 activity and acute lung injury

Site-directional mutations in the predicted catalytic site of ExoU cause a loss of lysophospholipase A activity [52]. Airspace instillation of virulent *P. aeruginosa* expressing ExoU causes acute lung injury and death in infected mice [53]. However, airspace instillation of isogenic mutants secreting catalytically inactive ExoU is non-cytotoxic and this does not cause acute lung injury or death in these mice [53]. Therefore, virulent *P. aeruginosa* causes acute lung injury, with concomitant sepsis and mortality, via cytotoxic activity derived from the patatin-like phospholipase domain of ExoU. Cells targeted by ExoU through the TTSS are not only epithelial cells, but also macrophages [54]. Through the TTSS, ExoU is activated after its translocation into the cytosol of eukaryotic cells [55–57]. Ubiquitin and ubiquitin-modified proteins are associated with the activation of ExoU [18, 19].

5.3. ExoY

ExoY has adenylate cyclase activity and is secreted by the TTS mechanism [12]. The primary ExoY sequence shares homology with sequences of the extracellular adenylate cyclases of *Bordetella pertussis* (CyaA), *Bacillus anthracis* (EF), and *Y. pestis* insecticidal toxin [12]. An unknown eukaryotic cell factor, distinct from calmodulin, enhances recombinant ExoY catalysis. Infection of eukaryotic cells with *P. aeruginosa* that produce catalytically active ExoY results in an elevation of intracellular cAMP and morphological changes in cells. ExoY increases the permeability of lung endothelial cells and alters Chinese hamster ovary cell morphology but does not result in acute cytotoxic responses. Ninety percent of clinical isolates that are tested show the presence of the *exoY* gene in DNA hybridization experiments [12]. ExoY production may play a role in protecting the bacterium from local phagocytic cells [58].

6. Cystic fibrosis and *P. aeruginosa* type III secretion

6.1. *P. aeruginosa* pneumonia and cystic fibrosis

Respiratory infections with *P. aeruginosa* are the major causes of morbidity and mortality in individuals with CF. *P. aeruginosa* isolates from newly infected patients with CF resemble those from acutely infected non-CF patients, and have a number of virulence factors including flagella, pili, pyocin, pyoverdin, and the TTSS [59, 60]. Expression of these virulence factors is considered to be essential for successful development of infection at an early stage of infection in patients with CF. However, at the chronic stage of infection, triggered by high selective pressure in CF lungs and by antibiotic treatments, *P. aeruginosa* gradually generates genotypes and phenotypes that are specially adapted to the lungs in CF. These include overproduction of alginate (mucoid phenotype), loss of lipopolysaccharide O-antigen components, loss of motility, resistance to antibiotics, virulence factor loss, and adapted metabolism [61]. These changes might be essential for *P. aeruginosa* to facilitate evasion of the host defense mechanisms and immune surveillance [62].

6.2. Epidemiological studies of isolates from patients with cystic fibrosis

In our epidemiological study that analyzed clinical isolates, there was a subset of isolates that displayed the TTS phenotype $ExoS^-ExoU^-$ with extensive drug-resistant characteristics [63]. Most of these isolates were from chronic infections in patients with CF. Therefore, clinical isolates of *P. aeruginosa* are classified into three subgroups depending on their ExoS and ExoU phenotypes. $ExoS^+ExoU^-$ strains are invasive and cause infections in burns tissues, whereas $ExoS^-ExoU^+$ strains are cytotoxic and cause acute pneumonia and sepsis. Most strains isolated from chronic infections in CF patients are $ExoS^-ExoU^-$ (**Figure 7**). *P. aeruginosa* strains that are isolated from acutely infected patients show positive phenotypes for TTS proteins (ExoS, ExoU, and PcrV) and the positive O-antigen phenotype. However, strains that are isolated from chronic infections of patients with CF are frequently the O-antigen phenotype (−), TTS protein phenotypes (−), and the mucoid phenotype (+) with increased antibiotic resistance (**Figure 8**). Recent studies have shown that TTSS production, as well as other virulence factors, such as flagella, pili, pyocin, and pyoverdine, are attenuated in many isolates from chronically infected patients with CF [64–66]. The results of several studies that investigated the relationship between CF clinical isolates and the TTSS in *P. aeruginosa* are shown in **Table 2** [61, 67–71]. Two of the six studies were longitudinal and followed the same patients with CF. Additionally, four studies performed genotype analysis on strains, and five others performed immunoblot analysis of TTS proteins. Findings from these epidemiological studies suggest that CF isolates from children are more virulent with a positive TTSS phenotype than isolates that are recovered from adults. These studies also suggest that isolates from initial infections are more virulent than isolates from subsequent infections. The ratio between $ExoS^+ExoU^-$ and $ExoS^-ExoU^+$ differed in each study. However, a more recent report from Hu et al. showed that 7 isolates among 40 in total from subsequently occurring infections were $ExoU^+$ [71]. These findings suggest the potential pathogenic involvement of ExoU-associated virulence, even in patients with CF.

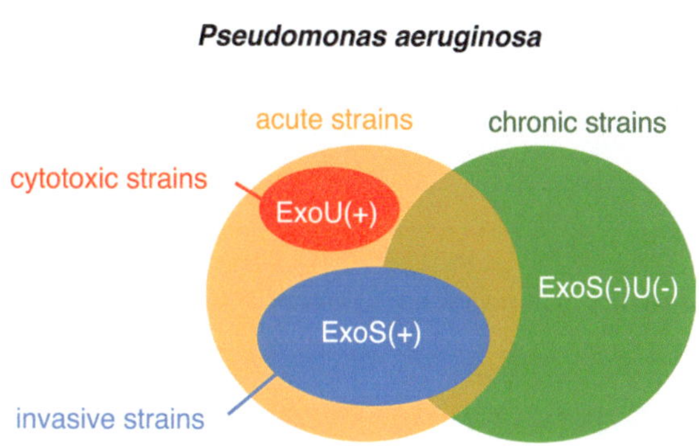

Figure 7. Type III secretory toxin phenotypes in *P. aeruginosa* clinical isolates. *P. aeruginosa* clinical isolates can be classified into three subgroups depending on their ExoS and ExoU phenotypes. ExoS(+)ExoU(−) stains are invasive and cause infections in burnt tissue, whereas ExoS(−)ExoU(+) strains are cytotoxic and cause acute pneumonia and sepsis. Most strains that are isolated from chronic infections in patients with cystic fibrosis are ExoS(−)ExoU(−)

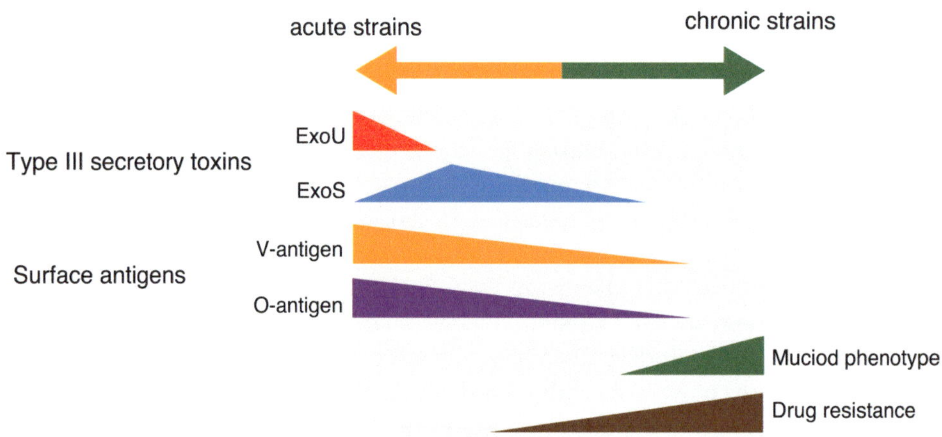

Figure 8. Phenotypic variation in *P. aeruginosa* clinical isolates. *P. aeruginosa* strains that are isolated from acutely infected patients are positive for type III secretory proteins, such as ExoS, ExoU, and PcrV, and are O-antigen positive. In contrast, strains that are isolated from chronic infections in patients with cystic fibrosis are frequently O-antigen-negative and type III secretory protein-negative, but are mucoid with increased antibiotic resistance.

6.3. Type III secretion and cystic fibrosis isolates

Most studies have reported that the proportion of *P. aeruginosa* strains secreting TTS proteins decreases over the duration of *P. aeruginosa* infection. Jain et al. showed a significant inverse correlation between the percentage of TTS proteins and the duration of *P. aeruginosa* infection [67]. They also reported an association between the proportion of TTS protein-secreting isolates and a decline in the rate of forced expiratory volume in 1 s in patients who still harbor at least some TTS-positive isolates. Other reports that investigated the genotype and phenotype of the TTSS showed that all *P. aeruginosa* strains harbor at least some TTSS genes (*exoS, exoT, exoU, exoY*), regardless of the expression of TTS proteins (ExoS, ExoT, ExoU) [66, 69–71]. This suggests that the TTSS regulon may remain intact and the expression of TTSS can be reversible. There are other variants called rough small-colony variants in *P. aeruginosa*, and these have been isolated from chronically infected patients with CF [72, 73]. These variants are hyperpiliated and hyperadherent, and differ from the mucoid phenotype in their secretion of TTS proteins. Their remarkably high resistance to several antibiotic classes enables their persistence in the lungs in CF.

6.4. Comparative genome studies on recent *P. aeruginosa* isolates

Comparative genomics on the reference PAO1 strain and isolates from patients with CF are on-going. In 2003, two comparative studies between CF isolates and PAO1 were reported. These studies demonstrated that clinical strains do not express TTSS, whereas most of them that are isolated from chronic infections possess this gene cluster [74, 75]. Additionally, these studies show that 10% of genes in CF isolates do not exist in the PAO1 genome, and half of them are newly identified genes.

Year	Author	Reference	CF clinical isolates, *n*	TTSS secretion (+), *n* (%)	Exoenzyme genotype, *n*				Exoenzyme phenotype, *n* (% positive by genotype)			
					S	*T*	*Y*	*U*	S	T	Y	U
2000	Dacheux et al.	[69]	29	8 (27.5%)	28	28	28	3	8 (28.6)	8 (28.6)	NA	0 (0)
2004	Jain et al.	[61]	235 (CI, children)	40 (18%)	NA	NA	NA	NA	35 (88)	40 (100)	NA	2 (5)
			200 (CI, adults)	8 (4%)					8 (100)	8 (100)	NA	0 (0)
			35 (NI)	17(49%)					17 (100)	17 (100)	NA	0 (0)
2005	Lee et al.	[68]	7	5 (71.4%) (initial)	7	NA	NA	0	5 (71.4)	NA	NA	0 (0)
				3 (42.8%) (subsequent)	6	NA	NA	1	2 (28.6)	NA	NA	1 (14.3)
2007	Wareham et al.	[70]	75	39 (52%)	66	75	74	12	NA	NA	NA	9 (75)
2008	Jain et al.	[67]	1299 (CI, children)	29.1%	NA	NA	NA	NA	NA	NA	NA	NA
			1217 (CI, adult)	11.5%								
			135 (NI)	45.2%								
2013	Hu et al.	[71]	52 (initial)	43 (82.7%)	44	NA	NA	8	36 (82)	NA	NA	7 (88)
			40 (subsequent)	26 (65%)	33	NA	NA	7	19 (58)	NA	NA	7 (100)

Table 2. Studies on the relationship between cystic fibrosis and type III secretion in *P. aeruginosa*.

Recent reports have indicated that the combination of carbapenem and fluoroquinolone resistance and the presence of the gene encoding the TTSS ExoU effector in *P. aeruginosa* are the strongest predictors of development of pneumonia [76–78]. Further investigations have suggested that the fluoroquinolone-resistant phenotype and the *exoU*+ genotype of *P. aeruginosa* cause poor clinical outcomes in patients with *P. aeruginosa* pneumonia [76–79]. Several genome sequence analyses of small colony variants of *P. aeruginosa* have been reported recently [80–85]. These studies showed multifactorial antibiotic-resistance mechanisms, such as overexpression of efflux mechanisms, LPS modification, and a drastic downregulation of the *Pseudomonas* quinolone signal quorum-sensing system. These reports suggest that, over the last 15 years, wide-spread global carbapenem and fluoroquinolone use has rapidly enhanced propagation of virulent and drug-resistant *P. aeruginosa* strains.

7. Anti-PcrV strategies in *P. aeruginosa* infections

Recent outbreaks of XDR-PA are threatening to increase colonization by MDR-PA in immunocompromised patients because efficacious antimicrobial choices are extremely limited. Therefore, this situation requires development of new prophylactic or therapeutic strategies that do not rely on conventional antimicrobial agents [86, 87].

7.1. Active and passive immunization against *P. aeruginosa* PcrV

The first experimental trial on immunotherapy against the TTSS of *P. aeruginosa* was performed using *E. coli*-derived recombinant PcrV protein to actively immunize mice [33]. In this experiment, the immunized mice survived lethal challenge infections with *P. aeruginosa* pneumonia. Together with the active immunization trial, passive immunization was carried out in mice with a purified protein A binding γ-globulin fraction, which was separated from the sera of rabbits that were actively immunized with recombinant PcrV [30]. In this series, the immunized mice survived pulmonary administration of a lethal dose of *P. aeruginosa*. A correlation between the survival rate of the mice and the dose of the polyclonal anti-PcrV antibody was found. The effects of this polyclonal anti-PcrV antibody were later tested in various animal models of burns and chronic bacterial pneumonia [88, 89].

The mechanism responsible for the positive effect of the polyclonal anti-PcrV antibodies, in terms of whether the effect depends on the Fc-portion of the antibody, was investigated. The anti-PcrV polyclonal antibody $F(ab)'_2$ was tested in a rabbit model, and the same effect as whole IgG was confirmed [90]. This finding strongly suggests that the prophylactic and therapeutic effects of anti-PcrV polyclonal antibodies are derived by blocking the action involved in the pathogenicity of the antigen. Monoclonal antibody screening on normal mouse hybridomas was then performed and the clone mAb166 was discovered as the strongest TTSS blocker [40]. The clone mAb166 displayed equivalent therapeutic and prophylactic effects to those of the anti-PcrV polyclonal antibody [40, 91, 92]. The mAb166 Fab fragment also conferred the same therapeutic effect as the original whole IgG in *P. aeruginosa* pneumonia [85]. In particular, mAb166 exerted a strong therapeutic effect following airway administration of *P. aeruginosa* in a pneumonia model in rats [93]. By using this mAb166 antibody as a template with the bacteriophage gene shuffling recombination technology, the US venture company KaloBios Inc. started a project to create a humanized anti-PcrV antibody. Consequently, KB001-A was developed as a humanized monoclonal antibody [94]. This antibody underwent phase I and phase II clinical trials in the USA and France [95, 96].

7.2. Immunization against PcrV in immunocompromised models

Active immunization with PcrV was examined in immunocompromised mice that were pre-treated with cyclophosphamide [97]. Cyclophosphamide treatment induced immunosuppression in the mice, decreased immunity against *P. aeruginosa*, and decreased the lethal dose of *P. aeruginosa*. In this study, five truncated PcrV fragments and full-length-PcrV were tested as vaccine candidates in a mouse model of *P. aeruginosa* pneumonia. Acute systemic infection was introduced by intraperitoneal injection of a lethal dose of *P. aeruginosa* in this mouse model [97]. This study showed that active immunization with either full-length $PcrV_{1–294}$ or $PcrV_{139–294}$, both of which contain the $_{PcrV144–257}$ blocking epitope region of monoclonal anti-PcrV IgG mAb166, successfully protected the immunocompromised mice from lethal *P. aeruginosa* infection. This finding suggested that the anti-PcrV strategy might be effective in neutropenic conditions in which human patients frequently develop *P. aeruginosa* infections.

The intravenous immunoglobulin (IVIG) was recently shown to confer significant protection against lethal infection with virulent *P. aeruginosa* [98, 99]. The effect of administrating 2.5 mg of IVIG was comparable with that of administrating 10 μg of specific anti-PcrV polyclonal IgG. The mechanism of protection is likely to involve the synergic action of anti-PcrV titers and some surface antigen to block the TTSS-associated virulence of *P. aeruginosa* [98]. There is considerable variation in anti-PcrV titers in adult subjects without any obvious history of infection with *P. aeruginosa* [100]. IVIG extracted from high anti-PcrV titer human sera confers protective effects in a mouse model of lethal *P. aeruginosa* pneumonia [101]. These results suggest that, not only monoclonal strategies against PcrV, but serum-derived immunoglobulin therapy with specific titers against PcrV also has great potential as effective immunotherapeutic tool against lethal *P. aeruginosa* infections.

8. Conclusions

In this review, we summarize the current status of research on the pathogenesis and treatment of *P. aeruginosa* infections from the viewpoint of acute and chronic infections. First, there are two phenotypes of *P. aeruginosa* strains: one causes acute types of infection, whereas the other causes chronic types of infection. Genomic level differences exist between these two phenotypes. In the course of evolution, acquisition of virulence gene cassettes, especially PAPI-2, created subtypes with increasing toxicity. Second, exposure to antibiotics enhances their drug resistance together with a loss of cytotoxicity and antigenicity that can be targeted by host immunity. Third, some mutant cytotoxic and drug-resistant *P. aeruginosa* strains may be involved in acute exacerbation of chronic infectious diseases. The lifespan of patients with CF has improved via various medical advances. Rather than focusing on eradication of infectious pathogens, prophylaxis against lethal pathogenic factors to avoid acute exacerbation during the chronic infection state should probably be given more priority at present. Currently, the monoclonal antibody strategies that are used against bacterial infections have not yet reached the level of practical application that is found in cancer therapy. The on-going challenge for anti-PcrV immunotherapy is realizing its potential to improve the clinical outcome of *P. aeruginosa* infections occurring in patients with CF.

Acknowledgements

This work was supported by the Japan Society for the Promotion of Science, Grants-in-Aid for Scientific Research (KAKENHI Nos. 24390403, 26670791, and 15H05008), and The Ministry of Education, Culture, Sports, Science and Technology, Japan to Teiji Sawa.

Abbreviations

CF	cystic fibrosis
GAP	GTPase-activating protein
IVIG	intravenous immunoglobulin
MDR-PA	multidrug-resistant *Pseudomonas aeruginosa*
PAPI-2	*P. aeruginosa* pathogenicity island-2
PLA	Phospholipase A
TTS	Type III secretory
TTSS	Type III secretion system
XDR-PA	extensively drug-resistant *P. aeruginosa*

Author details

Yoshifumi Naito[1], Kiyoshi Moriyama[2] and Teiji Sawa[1]*

*Address all correspondence to: anesth@koto.kpu-m.ac.jp

1 Department of Anesthesiology, Kyoto Prefectural University of Medicine, Kyoto, Japan

2 Department of Anesthesiology, School of Medicine, Kyorin University, Mitaka, Japan

References

[1] Viale P, Giannella M, Tedeschi S, et al. Treatment of MDR-Gram negative infections in the 21st century: A never ending threat for clinicians. Current Opinion in Pharmacology. 2015;**24**:30-37. DOI: 10.1016/j.coph.2015.07.001

[2] Ramirez-Estrada S, Borgatta B, Rello J. *Pseudomonas aeruginosa* ventilator-associated pneumonia management. Infection and Drug Resistance. 2016;**9**:7-18. DOI: 10.2147/IDR.S50669

[3] Grgurich PE, Hudcova J, Lei Y, et al. Management and prevention of ventilator-associated pneumonia caused by multidrug-resistant pathogens. Expert Review of Respiratory Medicine. 2012;**6**:533-555. DOI: 10.1586/ers.12.45

[4] Quartin AA, Scerpella EG, Puttagunta S, et al. A comparison of microbiology and demographics among patients with healthcare-associated, hospital-acquired, and ventilator-associated pneumonia: A retrospective analysis of 1184 patients from a large, international study. BMC Infectious Diseases. 2013;**13**:561. DOI: 10.1186/1471-2334-13-561

[5] Parker CM, Kutsogiannis J, Muscedere J, Cook D, et al. Ventilator-associated pneumonia caused by multidrug-resistant organisms or *Pseudomonas aeruginosa*: Prevalence, incidence, risk factors, and outcomes. Journal of Critical Care. 2008;**23**:18-26. DOI: 10.1016/j.jcrc.2008.02.001

[6] Winstanley C, O'Brien S, Brockhurst MA. *Pseudomonas aeruginosa* evolutionary adaptation and diversification in cystic fibrosis chronic lung infections. Trends Microbiology. 2016;**24**:327-337. DOI: 10.1016/j.tim.2016.01.008.

[7] Pena C, Gomez-Zorrilla S, Suarez C, et al. Extensively drug-resistant *Pseudomonas aeruginosa*: Risk of bloodstream infection in hospitalized patients. European Journal of Clinical Microbiology & Infectious Diseases. 2012;**31**:2791-2797. DOI: 10.1007/s10096-012-1629-3

[8] Sawa T, Shimizu M, Moriyama K, et al. Association between *Pseudomonas aeruginosa* type III secretion, antibiotic resistance, and clinical outcome: A review. Critical Care. 2014;**18**:668. DOI: 10.1186/s13054-014-0668-9

[9] Sawa T. The molecular mechanism of acute lung injury caused by *Pseudomonas aeruginosa*: From bacterial pathogenesis to host response. Journal of Intensive Care. 2014;**2**:10. DOI: 10.1186/2052-0492-2-10

[10] Notti RQ, Stebbins CE. The structure and function of type III secretion systems. Microbiology Spectrum. 2016;**4**:1-30. DOI: 10.1128/microbiolspec.VMBF-0004-2015

[11] Frank DW. The exoenzyme S regulon of *Pseudomonas* aeruginosa. Molecular Microbiology. 1997;**26**:621-629

[12] Yahr TL, Vallis AJ, Hancock MK, et al. ExoY, an adenylate cyclase secreted by the *Pseudomonas aeruginosa* type III system. Proceedings of the National Academy of Sciences of the United States of America. 1998;**95**:13899-13904

[13] Barbieri JT. *Pseudomonas aeruginosa* exoenzyme S, a bifunctional type-III secreted cytotoxin. International Journal of Medical Microbiology. 2000;**290**:381-387

[14] Goranson J, Frank DW. Genetic analysis of exoenzyme S expression by *Pseudomonas aeruginosa*. FEMS Microbiology Letters. 1996;**135**:149-155

[15] Yahr TL, Barbieri JT, Frank DW. Genetic relationship between the 53- and 49-kilodalton forms of exoenzyme S from *Pseudomonas aeruginosa*. Journal of Bacteriology. 1996;**178**:1412-1419

[16] Finck-Barbancon V, Goranson J, Zhu L. ExoU expression by *Pseudomonas aeruginosa* correlates with acute cytotoxicity and epithelial injury. Molecular Microbiology. 1997;**25**:547-557

[17] Sato H, Frank DW, Hillard CJ, et al. The mechanism of action of the *Pseudomonas aeruginosa*-encoded type III cytotoxin, ExoU. EMBO Journal. 2003;**22**:2959-2969

[18] Stirling FR, Cuzick A, Kelly SM, et al. Eukaryotic localization, activation and ubiquitinylation of a bacterial type III secreted toxin. Cell Microbiology. 2006;**8**:1294-1309. DOI: 10.1016/j.bpj.2011.01.056

[19] Anderson DM, Schmalzer KM, Sato H, et al. Ubiquitin and ubiquitin-modified proteins activate the *Pseudomonas aeruginosa* T3SS cytotoxin, ExoU. Molecular Microbiology. 2011;**82**:1454-1467. DOI: 10.1111/j.1365-2958.2011.07904.x

[20] Fleiszig SM, Wiener-Kronish JP, Miyazaki H, et al. *Pseudomonas aeruginosa*-mediated cytotoxicity and invasion correlate with distinct genotypes at the loci encoding exoenzyme S. Infection and Immunity. 1997;**65**:579-586

[21] Sawa T, Ohara M, Kurahashi K, et al. In vitro cellular toxicity predicts *Pseudomonas aeruginosa* virulence in lung infections. Infection and Immunity. 1998;**66**:3242-3249

[22] Yahr TL, Goranson J, Frank DW. Exoenzyme S of *Pseudomonas aeruginosa* is secreted by a type III pathway. Molecular Microbiology. 1996;**22**:991-1003

[23] Kurahashi K, Kajikawa O, Sawa T, Ohara M, Gropper MA, Frank DW, Martin TR, Wiener-Kronish JP. Pathogenesis of septic shock in *Pseudomonas aeruginosa* pneumonia. The Journal of Clinical Investigation. 1999;**104**:743-750

[24] Hauser AR, Cobb E, Bodi M, et al. Type III protein secretion is associated with poor clinical outcomes in patients with ventilator-associated pneumonia caused by *Pseudomonas aeruginosa*. Critical Care Medicine. 2002;**30**:521-528

[25] Howell HA, Logan LK, Hauser AR. Type III secretion of ExoU is critical during early *Pseudomonas aeruginosa* pneumonia. mBio. 2013;**4**:e00032-00013. DOI: 10.1128/mBio.00032-13

[26] Stover CK, Pham XQ, Erwin AL, et al. Complete genome sequence of *Pseudomonas aeruginosa* PAO1, an opportunistic pathogen. Nature. 2000;**406**:959-964

[27] He J, Baldini RL, Deziel E, et al. The broad host range pathogen *Pseudomonas aeruginosa* strain PA14 carries two pathogenicity islands harboring plant and animal virulence genes. Proceedings of the National Academy of Sciences of the United States of America. 2004;**101**:2530-2535

[28] Galan JE, Collmer A. Type III secretion machines: Bacterial devices for protein delivery into host cells. Science. 1999;**284**:1322-1328

[29] Finck-Barbancon V, Yahr TL, Frank DW. Identification and characterization of SpcU, a chaperone required for efficient secretion of the ExoU cytotoxin. Journal of Bacteriology. 1998;**180**:6224-6231

[30] Mueller CA, Broz P, Muller SA, et al. The V-antigen of *Yersinia* forms a distinct structure at the tip of injectisome needles. Science. 2005;**310**:674-676

[31] Cornelis GR, Wolf-Watz H. The *Yersinia* Yop virulon: A bacterial system for subverting eukaryotic cells. Molecular Microbiology. 1997;**23**:861-867

[32] Pettersson J, Holmstrom A, Hill J, et al. The V-antigen of *Yersinia* is surface exposed before target cell contact and involved in virulence protein translocation. Molecular Microbiology. 1999;**32**:961-976

[33] Sawa T, Yahr TL, Ohara M, et al. Active and passive immunization with the *Pseudomonas* V antigen protects against type III intoxication and lung injury. Nature Medicine. 1999;**5**:392-398

[34] Burrows TW. An antigen determining virulence in *Pasteurella pestis*. Nature (London). 1956;**177**:426-427

[35] Burrows TW. Biochemical properties of virulent and avirulent strains of bacteria: Salmonella typhosa and *Pasteurella pestis*. Annals of the New York Academy of Sciences. 1960;**88**:1125-1135

[36] Burrows TW, Bacon GA. The basis of virulence in *Pasteurella pestis*: Attempts to induce mutation from avirulence to virulence. British Journal of Experimental Pathology. 1954;**35**:129-133

[37] Burrows TW, Bacon GA. The basis of virulence in *Pasteurella pestis*: An antigen determining virulence. British Journal of Experimental Pathology. 1956;**37**:481-493

[38] Burrows TW, Bacon GA. The effects of loss of virulence determinants on the virulence and immunogenicity of strains of *Pasteurella pestis*. British Journal of Experimental Pathology 1958;**39**:278-291

[39] Perry RD, Harmon PA, Bowmer WS, et al. A low-Ca^{2+} response operon encodes the V antigen of *Yersinia pestis*. Infection and Immunity. 1986;**54**:428-434

[40] Frank DW, Vallis A, Wiener-Kronish JP, et al. Generation and characterization of a protective monoclonal antibody to *Pseudomonas aeruginosa* PcrV. Journal of Infectious Diseases. 2002;**186**:64-73

[41] Iglewski BH, Sadoff J, Bjorn MJ, et al. *Pseudomonas aeruginosa* exoenzyme S: An adenosine diphosphate ribosyltransferase distinct from toxin A. Proceedings of the National Academy of Sciences of the United States of America. 1978;**75**:3211-3215

[42] Bjorn MJ, Pavlovskis OR, Thompson MR, et al. Production of exoenzyme S during *Pseudomonas aeruginosa* infections of burned mice. Infection and Immunity. 1979;**24**:837-842

[43] Garrity-Ryan L, Kazmierczak B, Kowal R, et al. The arginine finger domain of ExoT contributes to actin cytoskeleton disruption and inhibition of internalization of *Pseudomonas aeruginosa* by epithelial cells and macrophages. Infection and Immunity 2000;**68**:7100-7113

[44] Geiser TK, Kazmierczak BI, Garrity-Ryan LK, et al. *Pseudomonas aeruginosa* ExoT inhibits in vitro lung epithelial wound repair. Cell Microbiology. 2001;**3**:223-236

[45] Coburn J, Dillon ST, Iglewski BH, et al. Exoenzyme S of *Pseudomonas aeruginosa* ADP-ribosylates the intermediate filament protein vimentin. Infection and Immunity. 1989;**57**:996-998

[46] Coburn J, Kane AV, Feig L, et al. *Pseudomonas aeruginosa* exoenzyme S requires a eukaryotic protein for ADP-ribosyltransferase activity. Journal of Biological Chemistry. 1991;**266**:6438-6446

[47] Kulich SM, Frank DW, Barbieri JT. Purification and characterization of exoenzyme S from *Pseudomonas aeruginosa* 388. Infection and Immunity. 1993;**61**:307-313

[48] Goehring UM, Schmidt G, Pederson KJ, et al. The N-terminal domain of *Pseudomonas aeruginosa* exoenzyme S is a GTPase-activating protein for Rho GTPases. Journal of Biological Chemistry. 1999;**274**:36369-36372

[49] Krall R, Sun J, Pederson KJ, et al. In vivo rho GTPase-activating protein activity of *Pseudomonas aeruginosa* cytotoxin ExoS. Infection and Immunity. 2002;**70**:360-367

[50] Sundin C, Henriksson ML, Hallberg B, et al. Exoenzyme T of *Pseudomonas aeruginosa* elicits cytotoxicity without interfering with Ras signal transduction. Cell Microbiology. 2001;**3**:237-246

[51] Kazmierczak BI, Engel JN. *Pseudomonas aeruginosa* ExoT acts in vivo as a GTPase-activating protein for RhoA, Rac1, and Cdc42. Infection and Immunity. 2002;**70**:2198-2205

[52] Tamura M, Ajayi T, Allmond LR, et al. Lysophospholipase A activity of *Pseudomonas aeruginosa* type III secretory toxin ExoU. Biochemical and Biophysical Research Communications. 2004;**316**:323-331

[53] Pankhaniya RR, Tamura M, Allmond LR, et al. *Pseudomonas aeruginosa* causes acute lung injury via the catalytic activity of the patatin-like phospholipase domain of ExoU. Critical Care Medicine. 2004;**32**:2293-2299

[54] Diaz MH, Hauser AR. *Pseudomonas aeruginosa* cytotoxin ExoU is injected into phagocytic cells during acute pneumonia. Infection and Immunity. 2010;**78**:1447-1456. DOI: 10.1128/IAI.01134-09

[55] Schmalzer KM, Benson MA, Frank DW. Activation of ExoU phospholipase activity requires specific C-terminal regions. Journal of Bacteriology. 2010;**192**:1801-1812. DOI: 10.1128/JB.00904-09

[56] Tyson GH, Hauser AR. Phosphatidylinositol 4,5-bisphosphate is a novel coactivator of the *Pseudomonas aeruginosa* cytotoxin ExoU. Infection and Immunity. 2013;**81**:2873-2881. DOI: 10.1128/IAI.00414-13

[57] Benson MA, Komas SM, Schmalzer KM, et al. Induced conformational changes in the activation of the *Pseudomonas aeruginosa* type III toxin, ExoU. Biophysical Journal. 2011;**100**:1335-1343

[58] Hritonenko V, Mun JJ, Tam C, et al. Adenylate cyclase activity of *Pseudomonas aeruginosa* ExoY can mediate bleb-niche formation in epithelial cells and contributes to virulence. Microbial Pathogenesis. 2011;**51**:305-312. DOI: 10.1016/j.micpath.2011.08.001

[59] Fegan M, Francis P, Hayward AC, Davis GH, Fuerst JA. Phenotypic conversion of *Pseudomonas aeruginosa* in cystic fibrosis. Journal of Clinical Microbiology. 1990;**28**:1143-1146

[60] Burns JL, Gibson RL, McNamara S, Yim D, Emerson J, Rosenfeld M, Hiatt P, McCoy K, Castile R, Smith AL, et al. Longitudinal assessment of *Pseudomonas aeruginosa* in young children with cystic fibrosis. Journal of Infectious Diseases. 2001;**183**:444-452

[61] Jain M, Ramirez D, Seshadri R, Cullina JF, Powers CA, Schulert GS, Bar-Meir M, Sullivan CL, McColley SA, Hauser AR. Type III secretion phenotypes of *Pseudomonas aeruginosa* strains change during infection of individuals with cystic fibrosis. Journal of Clinical Microbiology. 2004;**42**:5229-5237

[62] Smith EE, Buckley DG, Wu Z, et al. Genetic adaptation by *Pseudomonas aeruginosa* to the airways of cystic fibrosis patients. Proceedings of the National Academy of Sciences of the United States of America. 2006;**103**:8487-8492

[63] Roy-Burman A, Savel RH, Racine S, et al. Type III protein secretion is associated with death in lower respiratory and systemic *Pseudomonas aeruginosa* infections. Journal of Infectious Diseases. 2001;**183**:1767-1774

[64] Luzar MA, Thomassen MJ, Montie TC. Flagella and motility alterations in *Pseudomonas aeruginosa* strains from patients with cystic fibrosis: Relationship to patient clinical condition. Infection and Immunity. 1985;**50**:577-582

[65] Romling U, Fiedler B, Bosshammer J, et al. Epidemiology of chronic *Pseudomonas aeruginosa* infections in cystic fibrosis. Journal of Infectious Diseases. 1994;**170**:1616-1621

[66] De Vos D, De Chial M, Cochez C, et al. Study of pyoverdine type and production by *Pseudomonas aeruginosa* isolated from cystic fibrosis patients: Prevalence of type II pyoverdine isolates and accumulation of pyoverdine-negative mutations. Archives of Microbiology. 2001;**175**:384-388

[67] Jain M, Bar-Meir M, McColley S, et al. Evolution of *Pseudomonas aeruginosa* type III secretion in cystic fibrosis: A paradigm of chronic infection. Translational Research. 2008;**152**:257-264. DOI: 10.1016/j.trsl.2008.10.003

[68] Lee VT, Smith RS, Tummler B, et al. Activities of *Pseudomonas aeruginosa* effectors secreted by the Type III secretion system in vitro and during infection. Infection and Immunity. 2005;**73**:1695-1705. DOI: 10.1128/IAI.73.3.1695-1705.2005

[69] Dacheux D, Toussaint B, Richard M, et al. *Pseudomonas aeruginosa* cystic fibrosis isolates induce rapid, type III secretion-dependent, but ExoU-independent, oncosis of macrophages and polymorphonuclear neutrophils. Infection and Immunity. 2000;**68**:2916-2924

[70] Wareham DW, Curtis MA. A genotypic and phenotypic comparison of type III secretion profiles of *Pseudomonas aeruginosa* cystic fibrosis and bacteremia isolates. International Journal of Medical Microbiology. 2007;**297**:227-234. DOI: 10.1016/j.ijmm.2007.02.004

[71] Hu H, Harmer C, Anuj S, et al. Type 3 secretion system effector genotype and secretion phenotype of longitudinally collected *Pseudomonas aeruginosa* isolates from young children diagnosed with cystic fibrosis following newborn screening. Clinical Microbiology and Infection. 2013;**19**:266-272. DOI: 10.1111/j.1469-0691.2012.03770.x

[72] von Gotz F, Haussler S, Jordan D, et al. Expression analysis of a highly adherent and cytotoxic small colony variant of *Pseudomonas aeruginosa* isolated from a lung of a patient with cystic fibrosis. Journal of Bacteriology. 2004;**186**:3837-3847. DOI: 10.1128/JB.186.12.3837-3847.2004

[73] Moyano AJ, Lujan AM, Argarana CE, et al. MutS deficiency and activity of the error-prone DNA polymerase IV are crucial for determining mucA as the main target for mucoid conversion in *Pseudomonas aeruginosa*. Molecular Microbiology. 2007;**64**:547-559. DOI: 10.1111/j.1365-2958.2007.05675.x

[74] Spencer DH, Kas A, Smith EE, et al. Whole-genome sequence variation among multiple isolates of *Pseudomonas aeruginosa*. Journal of Bacteriology. 2003;**185**:1316-1325

[75] Ernst RK, D'Argenio DA, Ichikawa JK, et al. Genome mosaicism is conserved but not unique in *Pseudomonas aeruginosa* isolates from the airways of young children with cystic fibrosis. Environmental Microbiology. 2003;**5**:1341-1349

[76] Wong-Beringer A, Wiener-Kronish J, Lynch S, et al. Comparison of type III secretion system virulence among fluoroquinolone-susceptible and -resistant clinical isolates of *Pseudomonas aeruginosa*. Clinical Microbiology and Infection. 2008;**14**:330-336. DOI: 10.1111/j.1469-0691.2007.01939.x

[77] Agnello M, Wong-Beringer A. Differentiation in quinolone resistance by virulence genotype in *Pseudomonas aeruginosa*. PLoS One. 2012;**7**:e42973. DOI: 10.1371/journal.pone.0042973

[78] Sullivan E, Bensman J, Lou M, et al. Risk of developing pneumonia is enhanced by the combined traits of fluoroquinolone resistance and type III secretion virulence in respiratory isolates of *Pseudomonas aeruginosa*. Critical Care Medicine. 2014;**42**:48-56. DOI: 10.1097/CCM.0b013e318298a86f

[79] El-Solh AA, Hattemer A, Hauser AR, et al. Clinical outcomes of type III *Pseudomonas aeruginosa* bacteremia. Critical Care Medicine. 2012;**40**:1157-1163. DOI: 10.1097/CCM.0b013e3182377906

[80] Wei Q, Tarighi S, Dotsch A, et al. Phenotypic and genome-wide analysis of an antibiotic-resistant small colony variant (SCV) of *Pseudomonas aeruginosa*. PLoS One. 2011;**6**:e29276. DOI: 10.1371/journal.pone.0029276

[81] Eckweiler D, Bunk B, Sproer C, et al. Complete genome sequence of highly adherent *Pseudomonas aeruginosa* small-colony variant SCV20265. Genome Announcements. 2014;**2**:e01232-13. DOI: 10.1128/genomeA.01232-13

[82] Sabra W, Haddad AM, Zeng AP. Comparative physiological study of the wild type and the small colony variant of *Pseudomonas aeruginosa* 20265 under controlled growth conditions. Journal of Microbiology and Biotechnology. 2014;**30**:1027-1036. DOI: 10.1007/s11274-013-1521-z

[83] Tielen P, Wibberg D, Blom J, et al. Genome sequence of the small-colony variant *Pseudomonas aeruginosa* MH27, isolated from a chronic urethral catheter infection. Genome Announcements. 2014;**2**:e01174-13. DOI: 10.1128/genomeA.01174-13

[84] Wang D, Dorosky RJ, Han CS, et al. Adaptation genomics of a small-colony variant in a *Pseudomonas chlororaphis* 30-84 biofilm. Applied and Environmental Microbiology. 2015;**81**:890-899. DOI: 10.1128/AEM.02617-14

[85] Idris SN, Desa MN, Aziz MN, et al. Antimicrobial susceptibility pattern and distribution of exoU and exoS in clinical isolates of *Pseudomonas aeruginosa* at a Malaysian hospital. The Southeast Asian Journal of Tropical Medicine and Public Health. 2012;**43**:116-123

[86] Sawa T, Wiener-Kronish JP. A therapeutic strategy against the shared virulence mechanism utilized by both *Yersinia pestis* and *Pseudomonas aeruginosa*. Anesthesiology Clinical of North America. 2004;**22**:591-606

[87] Sawa T, Ito E, Nguyen VH, Haight M. Anti-PcrV antibody strategies against virulent *Pseudomonas aeruginosa*. Human Vaccines & Immunotherapeutics. 2014;**10**:2843-2852. DOI: 10.4161/21645515.2014.971641

[88] Neely AN, Holder IA, Wiener-Kronish JP, et al. Passive anti-PcrV treatment protects burned mice against *Pseudomonas aeruginosa* challenge. Burns. 2005;**31**:153-158. DOI: 10.1016/j.burns.2004.09.002

[89] Imamura Y, Yanagihara K, Fukuda Y, et al. Effect of anti-PcrV antibody in a murine chronic airway *Pseudomonas aeruginosa* infection model. European Respiratory Journal. 2007;**29**:965-968. DOI: 10.1183/09031936.00147406

[90] Shime N, Sawa T, Fujimoto J, et al. Therapeutic administration of anti-PcrV F(ab')(2) in sepsis associated with *Pseudomonas aeruginosa*. Journal of Immunology. 2001;**167**:5880-5886

[91] Wang Q, Li H, Zhou J, Zhong M, et al. PcrV antibody protects multi-drug resistant *Pseudomonas aeruginosa* induced acute lung injury. Respiratory Physiology & Neurobiology. 2014;**193**:21-28. DOI: 10.1016/j.resp.2014.01.001

[92] Song Y, Baer M, Srinivasan R, et al. PcrV antibody-antibiotic combination improves survival in *Pseudomonas aeruginosa*-infected mice. European Journal of Clinical Microbiology & Infectious Diseases. 2012;**31**:1837-1845. DOI: 10.1007/s10096-011-1509-2

[93] Faure K, Fujimoto J, Shimabukuro DW, et al. Effects of monoclonal anti-PcrV antibody on *Pseudomonas aeruginosa*-induced acute lung injury in a rat model. Journal of Immune Based Therapies and Vaccines. 2003;**1**:2

[94] Baer M, Sawa T, Flynn P, et al. An engineered human antibody fab fragment specific for *Pseudomonas aeruginosa* PcrV antigen has potent antibacterial activity. Infection and Immunity. 2009;**77**:1083-1090. DOI: 10.1128/IAI.00815-08

[95] Francois B, Luyt CE, Dugard A, et al. Safety and pharmacokinetics of an anti-PcrV PEGylated monoclonal antibody fragment in mechanically ventilated patients colonized with *Pseudomonas aeruginosa*: A randomized, double-blind, placebo-controlled trial. Critical Care Medicine. 2012;**40**:2320-2326. DOI: 10.1097/CCM.0b013e31825334f6

[96] Milla CE, Chmiel JF, Accurso FJ, et al. Anti-PcrV antibody in cystic fibrosis: A novel approach targeting *Pseudomonas aeruginosa* airway infection. Pediatric Pulmonology. 2013;**49**:650-658. DOI: 10.1002/ppul.22890

[97] Moriyama K, Wiener-Kronish JP, et al. Protective effects of affinity-purified antibody and truncated vaccines against *Pseudomonas aeruginosa* V-antigen in neutropenic mice. Microbiology and Immunology. 2009;**53**:587-594. DOI: 10.1111/j.1348-0421.2009.00165.x

[98] Katoh H, Yasumoto H, Shimizu M, et al. IV Immunoglobulin for acute lung injury and bacteremia in *Pseudomonas aeruginosa* pneumonia. Critical Care Medicine. 2016;**44**:e12-e24. DOI: 10.1097/CCM.0000000000001271

[99] Shimizu M, Katoh H, Hamaoka S, et al. Protective effects of intravenous immunoglobulin and antimicrobial agents on acute pneumonia in leukopenic mice. Journal of Infection and Chemotherapy. 2016;**22**:240-247. DOI: 10.1016/j.jiac.2016.01.006

[100] Yasumoto H, Katoh H, Kinoshita M, et al. Epidemiological analysis of serum anti-*Pseudomonas aeruginosa* PcrV titers in adults. Microbiology and Immunology. 2016;**60**:114-120. DOI: 10.1111/1348-0421.12353

[101] Kinoshita M, Kato H, Yasumoto H, et al. The prophylactic effects of human IgG derived from sera containing high anti-PcrV titers against pneumonia-causing *Pseudomonas aeruginosa*. Human Vaccines & Immunotherapeutics. 2016;**12**:2833-2846. DOI: 10.1080/21645515.2016.1209280